Clinical Oncology
The Foundations of Current Patient Management
(and Selected Therapeutic Developments)

Clinical Oncology

The Foundations of Current Patient Management
(and Selected Therapeutic Developments)

EDITED BY

Jesús Vicente, M.D.

Head, Oncology Department
Fundación Jimenez Diaz, Madrid, Spain

Hernán Cortes-Funes, M.D., Ph.D.

Head, Cancer Chemotherapy Section
Hospital 1º de Octubre, Madrid, Spain

Pablo Viladiu, M.D.

Head, Oncology Department
Hospital Santa Catalina, Gerona, Spain

Franco M. Muggia, M.D.

Director, Division of Oncology
New York University Medical Center

MASSON Publishing USA, Inc.

New York • Paris • Barcelona • Milan • Mexico City • Rio de Janeiro

FOREWORD

THE ORIGIN of the book is reflected throughout its pages. Having emanated from the deliberations of the Torremolinos meeting, by design of its organizers it portrays both the *leading edges* of clinical oncology with its new concepts in clinical trails and the *application* of these concepts in the sophisticated and yet conservative environment of Spanish medicine. This amalgamation of views should be recognized by the reader as he or she peruses the chapters in greater and lesser detail. I shall illustrate the point further with specific examples.

The treatment of malignant lymphomas constitutes one of the most successful developments in clinical oncology of the last two decades. The direction of future studies from the vantage point of the National Cancer Institute, U.S.A., where many of the advances originated, is described. On the other hand, Dr. Vicente's encyclopedic and well-referenced view of historical developments constitutes a unique account of his personal experience as these landmarks of progress were unfolding. His own data vastly confirm the logical sequence of studies performed by the innovating clinics of the world. His careful documentation constitutes, therefore, a valuable account of clinical investigation from a captive and prepared field worker.

In breast cancer, an analogous theme can be discerned. The truly daring, but well-conceived, executed sequence of studies of the Instituto Nazionale Tumori, Milano have revolutionized our concepts of biology and treatment in this coming decade. The results of these studies have been interpreted differently by various authors, and its effects on the conservative trends of the surgeon and the radiotherapist can be discerned. Although I do not subscribe to the views expressed in these respective chapters, they illustrate in an extensively referenced way the basis for resisting the introduction of new concepts of adjuvant chemotherapy, and they amply document areas of controversy. Since similar themes and arguments are raised in the United States and in other countries, this annotated controversy is particularly noteworthy.

Finally, the coverage of the treatment of lung cancer presents the up-to-now futile attempts of clinical oncology to deal with an overwhelming disease by use of combined modalities. Only surgery appears to hold consistent curative promise in cell types other than in the chemosensitive small cell carcinoma. The well-studied Spanish series add yet another discouraging chapter in treatment with radiotherapy, chemotherapy, or both. The presentation is very useful, however, not only in pointing out limitations of treatment, but also in the proper application of diagnostic techniques and selection of patients for surgery. The global reporting of their experience, without the selection often presented in surgical series in the United States, is a particularly valuable aspect. These chapters bring out the contributions that well-integrated chest services with all diagnostic and therapeutic disciplines can make in the treatment of patients afflicted with an illness associated with a discouraging outlook.

In summary, this book on clinical oncology is a blend of the innovation of clinical trials emanating principally, but not exclusively, out of therapeutic research influenced by the National Cancer Institute (U.S.), and the documentation of application of old and new concepts in the experience of various institutions throughout Spain. The readers should be cognizant of these trends and the inherent controversies represented as they delve through its chapters.

FRANCO M. MUGGIA, M.D.

CANCER MANAGEMENT

Luther W. Brady and Vincent T. DeVita, Jr., Series Editors

PREFACE

RECENTLY, the Sociedad Española de Quimioterapia Oncologica (SEQUIO, Spanish Cancer Chemotherapy Society) held an International Seminar on Medical Oncology. Beyond in-depth workshops on the latest advances in the therapy of patients with malignant lymphomas, and breast and lung cancers, the meeting gave special emphasis to concepts guiding the application of cancer chemotherapy and to the methodology of cancer clinical trials. The selection of topics and speakers was a most felicitous one. The result was a productive exchange on an international scale on very important aspects of cancer treatment. Thus, from a meeting originally organized by SEQUIO to update physicians and specialists in oncology on the important recent developments in chemotherapy, valuable contributions emanated, which should be of general interest to clinical and laboratory researchers of the cancer problem. This valuable exchange led the participants and organizers to gather all individual contributions into one volume.

With this as a background for the seminar, the reader should not expect an encyclopedic treatise on cancer treatment or of the selected areas covered. On the other hand, the assembling of representatives from major treatment research entities of two continents gives particular breadth to the items covered. These contributions, intermixed with reviews from prominent Spanish specialists, provide insight into research trends and the ingredients in their successful application. A unique contribution of this seminar, in fact, was the coverage of clinical trial methodology and resources. This coverage, coupled with specific examples of the landmark studies which established the role of chemotherapy in treatment of specific cancers, provides a most illuminating overview of such methodology and of the ingredients of success.

Undoubtedly, as with many other books dealing with science, some items will require updating even as they are being printed. Of greater permanence in this volume, however, is the demonstration of productivity in treatment research leading to advances in clinical science for the benefit of patients afflicted with cancer. Thus, we hope the reader will recognize—as those of us who attended the seminar have—the foundations of the future. Such foundations span across international boundaries. Individual countries also need to recognize the climate which ignites clinical research and collaboration.

SENIOR CONTRIBUTORS

J. ALBERT SOLIS, M.D. *Servicio de Radioterapia, Fundacion Jimenez Diaz, Madrid, Spain.*

P. ALBERTO, M.D. *Centre d'Onco-Hematologic des Policliniques et de l'Hôpital Cantonal, Geneve, Switzerland.*

K. D. BAGSHAWE, M.D. *Department of Clinical Oncology, Charing Cross Hospital, London, U.K.*

A. BRUGAROLAS, M.D. *Servicio de Quimioterapia e Inmunoterapia, Hospital General de Asturias, Oviedo, Spain.*

P. P. CARBONE, M.D. *Department of Human Oncology, Wisconsin Clinical Cancer Center, Madison, Wisconsin*

J. C. CATALAN FERNANDEZ, M.D. *Centro Regional de Oncología, Palma de Mallorca, Baleares, Spain.*

E. H. COOPER, M.D. *Unit for Cancer Research, University of Leeds, Leeds, U.K.*

H. CORTES-FUNES, M.D. *Sección de Quimioterapia Oncológica, Hospital 1º de Octubre, Madrid, Spain.*

M. DE LENA, M.D. *Instituto Nazionale per lo Studio e la cura dei Tumori, Milan, Italy.*

L. GIMENO ALFOS, M.D. *Departamento de Radioterapia, Hospital "Enrique Sotomayor," Bilbao, Spain.*

D. GONZALEZ GONZALEZ, M.D. *Department of Radiotherapy, Wilhelmina Gasthuis, Amsterdam, The Netherlands*

E. M. GREENSPAN, M.D. *Mount Sinai School of Medicine, New York, New York.*

C. HERRANZ, M.D. *Seccion Oncologia Médica, Hospital "La Fe," Valencia, Spain.*

J. J. LOPEZ LOPEZ, M.D. *Servicio de Oncologia, Hospital San Pablo, Barcelona, Spain.*

A. MORENO NOGUEIRA, M.D. *Servicio de Oncologia Médica, Hospital "Virgen del Rocio," Seville, Spain.*

F. M. MUGGIA, M.D. *Director, Division of Oncology, New York University Medical Center, New York, New York.*

J. H. MULDER, M.D. *Department of Internal Medicine, Radiotherapeutic Institute, Rotterdam, The Netherlands.*

H. OLIVA ALDAMIZ, M.D. *Departamento de Anatomia Patológica, Fundación Jimenez Diaz, Madrid, Spain.*

J. OTERO LUNA, M.D. *Servicio de Radioterapia, Clinica Puerta de Hierro, Madrid, Spain.*

F. PARIS ROMEUU, M.D. *Servicio de Cirugía Torácica, Hospital "La Fe," Valencia, Spain.*

S. PAVLOSKY, M.D. *Instituto de Investigaciones Hematológicas, Buenos Aires, Argentina.*

M. RIBAS MUNDO, M.D. *Departamento de Medicina Interna, Universidad Autónoma, Barcelona, Spain.*

M. C. RIVAS, M.D. *Departamento de Anatomía Patológica, Fundación Jimenez Diaz, Madrid, Spain.*

S. A. ROSENBERG, M.D. *Division of Medical Oncology, Stanford University School of Medicine, Stanford, California.*

M. ROZENCWEIG, M.D. *Division of Cancer Treatment, National Cancer Institute, Bethesda, Maryland.*

R. SACOZZI, M.D. *Instituto Nazionale per lo Studio e la, Cura dei Tumori, Milano, Italy.*

M. STAQUET, M.D. *EORTC Data Center, Institute Jules Bordet, Brussels, Belgium.*

J. VICENTE, M.D. *Servicio de Oncología, Fundacion Jimenez Diaz, Madrid, Spain.*

P. VILADIU, M.D. *Servicio de Oncología, Hospital Santa Catalina, Gerona, Spain.*

CONTENTS

PART 3:   Breast Cancer

PART 4:   Malignant Lymphomas

A. Hodgkin's Disease

B. Non-Hodgkin's Lymphomas

Foreword: Challenges and perspectives

J. Vicente, M.D.

Only a little more than three decades have elapsed since cancer chemotherapy was officially born, at the end of the Second World War, with the introduction of polyfunctional alkylating agents.[18] At about the same time, hormonal manipulations had led to some success in cancer.[8,14] Past was the prehistory of arsenicals and Coley toxins, which filled almost a century of little more than good wishes, and an exponential growth phase ensued,[5] which, fortunately enough, still continues.

Almost two decades were necessary, however, to go from simple serial testing on pure empirical grounds to a sort of experimental and clinical trials which have firmly based the present achievements. By 1964, Karnofsky[13] listed only four neoplastic diseases in which chemotherapy could be considered as a specific form of therapy, and these included female fetal choriocarcinoma, acute leukemia, especially lymphoblastic leukemia in children, metastatic Wilms' tumor, and retinoblastoma, but only as an adjuvant to radiotherapy in the latter. By that time, chemotherapy already was the treatment of choice for these tumors and yielded substantial prolongation of life, but the word "cure" was only used with caution for trophoblastic disease. Patients with some other tumors could benefit, without increase in life span, from chemotherapy as an alternative form of treatment or in a marginal manner, and most were not. Only a decade later, the panorama had completely changed[4,28]: more than 20 tumors respond in some proportion to chemotherapy and, when they do, there is a substantial prolongation of host survival; moreover, not less than 11 tumors, to which a 12th may now be added,[27] may permit a normal life span in some patients, that is to say, they may have been literally

Department of Oncology, Fundación Jiménez Diaz, Madrid, Spain.

cured by chemotherapy. These include the four neoplasms listed by Karnofsky in 1964 (acute lymphoblastic leukemia of children, Wilms' tumor, retinoblastoma, and fetal trofoblastic disease) plus other tumors frequent in childhood, namely, embryonal rhabdomyosarcoma and Ewing's sarcoma, in addition to testicular carcinomas, some skin cancers, and four lymphomas: Hodgkin's disease, Burkitt's tumor, nodular follicular mixed lymphomas, and Rappaport's histiocytic lymphoma. There is no doubt that cancer chemotherapy has now reached a status we could not dream of merely 15 years ago.

These results have been achieved not only through the development of new drugs, but also by means of a deeper understanding of the pharmacobiology of anticancer agents, which has substituted data for pure enthusiastic empiricism. Unfortunately, the available data are most incomplete, and this fact precludes further advancement; this is the main challenge of present day's chemotherapy. We know that we have potent weapons against cancer: the above results support it, but we have to learn to use them better in order to control a greater proportion of presently curable tumors, make curable most presently responsive neoplasms, and identify the factors which may render the remainder more responsive.

In fact, there are many gaps in our knowledge of the available antineoplastic agents. We group them as antimetabolites, alkylating agents, antimitotics, antibiotics, enzymes, hormones, and miscellaneous, and this is a highly heterogeneous classification, bringing together classes of drugs by their mechanism of action in some cases, and by their origin or source in other cases. This generally indicates that if we know much about the biochemistry of the final action of many drugs, we know very little about that of other substances which are in clinical use today and that this is something which we have to learn as soon as possible.

In order to achieve a response, the drugs that we use against tumors should act with some selective toxicity, that is, they should kill, preferentially at least, cancer cells, but not normal cells. On pure semantic grounds, however, and according to their mechanisms of action, all the available drugs are only cytostatic, not carcinostatic, which means that they do not, in fact, recognize cancer cells for their toxic action, and there is evidence of this in their low therapeutic index and secondary or collateral effects.[1] Nevertheless, that some selective toxicity exists in the usable drugs is clearly demonstrated by the actual cure of some proportion of 12 classes of malignant tumors in man.

This was also shown experimentally, early in the 1960s by the work of Skipper and co-workers, which culminated in the already classical paper on the criteria and kinetics associated with curability of experimental leukemia[22] and related ones, which defined for the first time one of the most useful concepts for cancer chemotherapy: anticancer drugs kill cancer cells in a logarithmic or exponential fashion, following a pseudo-first-order kinetics, and a given dose of a particular drug will kill a reasonably constant fraction of the susceptible cells, not a fixed number of them, regardless of the amount present. They also established the need of killing the last cell, which will need the same dose as the first millions of cells according to this kinetics, in order to cure the disease, and postulated that the viable tumor cell burden would be able to limit the possibility of cure, as it has been indeed the case. It has been demonstrated more recently by the same authors, that this is due to the selection of drug-resistant cells.[23]

How our cytostatic drugs preferentially kill cancer cells is still very incompletely understood. Drugs progress to clinical use through diverse phases of laboratory investigations, including toxicity and pharmacological studies on animals, followed by human pharmacological and toxicity studies (Phase I) and screening tumor trials (Phase II).[6] The final effect of a drug on its target depends from a series of factors,[1] starting with the pharmaceutical availability profile.

The pharmacokinetic phase, however, which comprises absorption, distribution, metabolic activation or inactivation and excretion is essential because it determinates the drug availability in the target tissues. Alkylating agents, for instance, which are highly chemically reactive compounds, are prone to easy inactivation by nucleophilic centers in many substances before they reach their target molecules, and others need specific activation before they can act on them. Therefore, differences in activity among the various compounds of this class are likely to be due to pharmacokinetic differences.[12] All the problems concerning extracellular disposition of drugs are highly complex and need a deep investigation for each substance for its better usage, but cellular processes are by no means less intricate, starting at transport through tissue boundaries and cellular membranes.[2] One of today's most interesting chemotherapeutic techniques, namely, high-dose Methotrexate followed by Citrovorum Factor rescue, is based on the magnitude of the active transport process through cell membrane,[11] experimentally reported 20 years before[7] but still incompletely known. Transport mechanisms may also be exploitable for the design of selective agents based on the lipid solubility of the moiety. For example, some folate antagonists like pyrimethamine or the more active dichloro derivatives, can enter cerebrospinal fluid, brain, and even Methotrexate-resistant cells, in which they persist with clearance time of several days[16]. It may also be feasible to incorporate drugs into selective carrier molecules or into liposomes to act through more or less selective endocytosis.[1] Thus, generally speaking, a complete pharmacokinetic profile is necessary for the optimal use of a drug, and, unfortunately, we lack much information on this regard. Recent developments, however, permitting the measurement of minute amounts of drugs in tissues and body fluids, would facilitate the use of pharmacokinetic models and computer simulation of compartmental drug distribution to aid a better choice of drug dosage and schedules of administration.[16]

The pharmacodynamic phase covers the drug-receptor interaction in the target tissue cells, which, through a sequence of biochemical and physico-chemical events, leads to the final effect. This ultimate phase is, by no means, simpler than previous ones, and there are many obstacles here for the drug to overcome.[2] The appearance of a resistant population by increased production of target molecules, changes in enzyme specificity, or alternate pathways which bypass drug-inhibited reactions are the most prone to take place; according to Hutchison,[10] they need not be considered pessimistically, since when one or more pathways are changed it may be possible to take advantage of the resistance phenomenon by the convenient use of the associated collateral sensitivity. On similar grounds is based the presently widespread use of combination chemotherapy, namely, multiple inhibition of a single enzyme, sequential blockade, concurrent, complementary, and concerted inhibition, in addition to some pharmacokinetic phenomena still not completely elucidated.[15]

Many aspects of today's known selectivity and most pharmacodynamic mechanisms are actually concerned with cell cycle kinetics. The work of Bruce, et al.[3] and of Van Putten and Lelieveld[25] have enabled us some understanding of these pharmacodynamic mechanisms and the classification of drugs into two well-defined classes: those highly cell cycle-phase specific, nearly always antimetabolites and antimitotic substances, and those cell cycle-stage nonspecific, for the remainder. The former are able to kill the cells only in one fraction of the cell cycle, DNA-synthesis (S) phase for most antimetabolites and mitosis (M) phase for antimitotic drugs, and sensitivity depends on the fraction of cells passing through these phases during drug action; the latter kill cells in all or most fractions of the cycle, and sensitivity depends on the fraction of cells in the proliferative state. Individual drugs may be then studied and entered in one or other class,[9] and these properties form the basis for scheduling. This is also a very complex problem, however, taking into account all the preceding facts, only solvable in part thanks to experimental animal models.

Generally speaking, cell cycle-phase specific agents need to be given in a more or less continuous fashion, in order to permit the whole population of dividing cells to go through the corresponding S or M phase, that is, they have to be administered at a constant rate for a time at least twice the duration of the whole cell cycle of the particular tumor, whereas cell cycle-stage nonspecific drugs are best administered at high single doses. These facts stem from the experiments of Skipper on L1210 leukemic mice.[21] One example of cell cycle-phase specific agent, arabinosylcytosine, will achieve cures if administered continuously q. 3 hr/day every 5 days, four times, because this schedule of almost continuous administration is the only one that is able to kill leukemic cells faster than they are being replaced. On the other hand, maximum tolerated *daily* doses of a cell cycle-stage nonspecific agent, cyclophosphamide, do not kill leukemic cells as fast as they are being replaced, so that it should be administered as separated high single doses in order to achieve cures. If we were able to synchronize more cells or all the cells[24] to the cycle phase in which the drug acts (cell doubling time of leukemia L1210 is about 0.5 days), we will need less prolonged drug action, since killing per dose should be faster and host toxicity lower. This should be particularly useful for tumors that, like this leukemia, have short doubling times and high growth fractions, and which resemble other tumors also used for screening drugs and for these, such scheduling works. This also may explain why we can control at present some human tumors and not others: all of them share, in fact, these characteristics of rapid doubling and high growth fraction, which may render them amenable to cure. This is also the basis of adjuvant therapy: although most human tumors are not controllable by chemotherapy because they are in a plateau phase of growth when diagnosed, they can be treated in an exponential phase of growth when only a few cells are left after surgery,[20] and these are more amenable to chemotherapy as we use it today.[19] Clinical testing of these concepts is in progress and will be reported in other chapters of this book.

Nevertheless, presently, controllable human tumors represent only less than 10% of all cancer patient population,[28] so that we need to turn our eyes to the remainder 90%. All of them share a low growth fraction and long doubling time; thus, many established facts for rapidly growing tumors may not apply to them. In addition to adjuvant therapy for locally advanced tumors, we must seek some other possibility of recruiting cells from resting state to proliferate[24] and thus rendering them sensitive to present-day chemotherapy. Alternatively we ought to use animal experimental models with slow-growing[26] and/or properly transplanted human tumors[17] for the screening of drugs and scheduling studies, aided by direct studies in man. Finally, we must prepare the most carefully designed clinical trials in addition to the pharmacological, biochemical, and kinetic investigations so that we can improve on the present situation, all of which is eagerly needed. These intriguing questions will be covered in the next chapters.

References

1. Ariëns, E. J.: Drug design and cancer. In *Pharmacological Basis of Cancer Chemotherapy*. Williams and Wilkins, Baltimore, 1975, pp. 127–152.

2. Ball, C. R.: Intracellular factors influencing the response of tumors to chemotherapeutic agents. In *Scientific Basis of Cancer Chemotherapy*, G. Mathe, Ed., Springer-Verlag, Heidelberg, 1969, pp. 26–40.

3. Bruce, W. R., Meeker, B. E., and Valeriote, F. A.: Comparison of the sensitivity of normal hematopoietic and transplanted lymphoma colony-forming cells to chemotherapeutic agents administered in vivo. *J Natl Cancer Inst, 37*: 233–245, 1966.

4. De Vita, V. T., Jr., Young, R. C., and Canellos, G. P.: Combination versus single agent chemotherapy: A review of the basis for selection of drug treatment of cancer. *Cancer 35*: 98–110, 1975.

5. Frei, E., III: Prospectus for cancer chemotherapy. *Cancer 30*: 1656–1661, 1972.

6. Gehan, E. A.: The determination of the number of patients required in a preliminary and a follow-up trial of a new chemotherapeutic agent. *J Chron Dis 13*: 346–353, 1961.

7. Goldin, A., Venditti, J. M., Humphreys, S. R., Dennis, D., Mantel, N., and Greenhouse, S. W.: Factors influencing the specificity of action of an antileukemic agent (amethopterin). Multiple treatment schedules plus delayed administration of Citrovorum Factor. *Cancer Res. 15*: 57–69, 1955.

8. Huggins, C., and Hodges, C. V.: Studies on prostatic cancer. I. Effect of castration, estrogen and of androgen injection on serum phosphatases in metastatic carcinoma of the prostate. *Cancer Res 1: 293–297*, 1941.

9. Humphrey, R. M., and Barranco, S. C.: Cellular Pharmacology. In *Pharmacological Basis of Cancer Chemotherapy*. Williams and Wilkins, Baltimore, 1975, pp. 85–103.

10. Hutchison, D. J.: Cross resistance and collateral sensitivity studies in cancer chemotherapy. *Adv Cancer Res 7*: 235–350, 1963.

11. Jaffe, N., Frei, E., III, Traggis, D., and Bishop, Y.: Adjuvant Methotrexate and Citrovorum Factor treatment of osteogenic sarcoma. *N Engl J Med 291*: 994–997, 1974.

12. Karnofsky, D. A., et al.: Comparative clinical and biological effects of alkylating agents. *Ann NY Acad Sci 68: 657–1266*, 1958.

13. Karnofsky, D. A.: Chemotherapy of cancer and its present position in the management of neoplastic diseases. In *Chemotherapy of Cancer*, P. A. Plattner, Ed., Elsevier, Amsterdam, 1964, pp. 3–17.

14. Loeser, A. A.: Mammary carcinoma. Response to implantation of male hormone and progesterone. *Lancet 2: 698–700, 1941*.

15. Mihich, E., and Grindey, G. B.: Multiple basis of combination chemotherapy. *Cancer 40: 534–543*, 1977.

16. Nichol, C. A.: Pharmacokinetics. Selectivity of action related to physicochemical properties and kinetic patterns of anticancer drugs. *Cancer 40: 519–528*, 1977.

17. Povlsen, C. O., and Jacobsen, G. K.: Chemotherapy of a human malignant melanoma transplanted in the nude mouse. *Cancer Res 35: 2790–2796, 1975*.

18. Rhoads, C. P.: Nitrogen Mustards in the treatment of neoplastic disease. Official statement. *JAMA 131: 656–658, 1946*.

19. Schabel, F. M.: Surgical adjuvant chemotherapy of metastatic murine tumors. *Cancer 40: 558–568*, 1977.

20. Simpson-Herren, L., Sanford, A. H., and Holmquist, J. P.: Effects of surgery on cell kinetics of residual tumor. *Cancer Treat Rep 60: 1749–1760, 1976*.

21. Skipper, H. E.: The cell cycle and chemotherapy of cancer. In *The Cell Cycle and Cancer*, R. Baserga, Ed. M. Dekker, New York, 1971, pp. 358–387.

22. Skipper, H. E., Schabel, F. M., and Wilcox, W. S.: Experimental evaluation of potential anticancer agents. XIII. On the criteria and kinetics associated with "curability" of experimental leukemia. *Cancer Chemother Rep 35: 1–111, 1964*.

23. Skipper, H. E., Schabel, F. M., and Lloyd H. H.: Experimental therapeutics and kinetics: Selection and overgrowth of specifically and permanently drug-resistant tumor cells. *Sem. Hematol 15: 207–219*, 1978.

24. Van Putten, L. M.: Are cell kinetics data relevant for the design of tumor chemotherapy schedules? *Cell Tissue Kinet 7: 493–504, 1974*.

25. Van Putten, L. M., and Lelieveld, P.: Factors determining cell killing by chemotherapeutic agents *in vivo*. II. Melphalan, Chlorambucil and Nitrogen Mustard. *Eur J Cancer 7: 11–16, 1971*.

26. Venditti, J. M.: Relevance of transplantable animal-tumor systems to the selection of new agents for clinical trial. In *Pharmacological Basis of Cancer Chemotherapy*. Williams and Wilkins, Baltimore, 1975, pp. 245–270.

27. Young, R. C., Anderson, T., and Bender, R. A.: Nodular mixed lymphoma (NML): Another potentially curable non-Hodgkin's lymphoma. *Proc Am Assoc Cancer Res and ASCO 18: 356, 1977*.

28. Zubrod, C. G.: Chemical control of Cancer. *Proc US Natl Acad Sci 69: 1042–1047, 1972*.

Basic cancer chemotherapy: Obstacles and future pharmacologic aspects and selective toxicity

2

Abraham Goldin, Ph.D.

Selective toxicity has been defined as that property of a drug that enables it to injure one kind of cell while leaving other kinds unaffected even when these cells are close neighbors.[1,2] The cells which are to be injured are referred to as the uneconomic cells and the cells which are to be spared are referred to as the economic cells. In antitumor chemotherapy, the uneconomic cells that are to be injured are the tumor cells and the cells which are to be spared are the vital cells of the host.[1,2] Any consideration of selective toxicity, in order to have meaning in antitumor chemotherapy, should take into account the host–tumor–drug relationship.[9,13,24] In general terms, antitumor selective toxicity may be increased: a) by increasing the antitumor effect relative to limiting toxicity for the host; b) by diminishing the toxicity for the host with retention of antitumor effectiveness; c) by a diminution in the appearance of resistant tumor cells and more effective treatment of drug resistors once they have appeared; and d) by an increase in the host response against tumor growth. There are a variety of ways in which antitumor selective toxicity may be increased, taking into account the host–tumor–drug relationship, and a number of these will be discussed in this paper.

First, it is important to review the various ways in which antitumor selective toxicity may be measured. In the determination of the antitumor activity of drugs, the effect of the drug on the tumor can be measured without taking into account

the effect on the host. This methodology provides no basis for determination of the selective toxicity of antitumor agents since the limitation of host toxicity would not enter as a factor in the assay. This methodology would be similar to that which is employed in *in vitro* tissue culture systems and is subject to the same limitations in terms of measuring selective toxic action. However, the introduction of host parameters can be entered into this type of assay system where, for example, toxicity for the host is measured in terms of drug lethality or as body weight loss. In one type of system frequently used, comparison is made of the ratio of T/C where T is the average weight or size of treated tumors and C is the control average. This type of procedure permits comparison of the relative degree of effectiveness of compounds; i.e., comparisons may be made of T/C at a maximum tolerated dose, with those compounds producing greater inhibition of tumor growth being considered as having more extensive selective toxic action against tumor.

Although routine screening procedures have in the past commonly employed tumor size or tumor weight as the basis for estimating antitumor effect, assay systems involving the influence of therapy on the survival time of tumorous animals may more closely approximate the clinical situation and have been utilized in more recent times to a considerably greater extent. For this purpose, assay systems have been developed in which antitumor agents and alternative chemotherapies may be compared on the basis of the survival-time response of the tumorous host.[9,13,17,24,41] In one system that was developed employing leukemia L1210, a specificity index was used to determine the relative effec-

Division of Cancer Treatment, National Cancer Institute, Bethesda, Maryland.
Reprinted from Cancer Clinical Trials 2: 119–127, 1978.

tiveness of drugs and comparative therapies.[24] In this system, a temporal separation was made of deaths resulting from drug-dose mortality and deaths attributable to progressive growth of tumor. This then permitted determination, in the comparison of two drugs or therapies, of the relationship between antitumor effect and dosage, the relationship of lethal toxicity to the host and dosage, and the comparative antitumor effect of the drugs or therapies in relation to the limiting lethal toxic effect on the host.[24] Thus, the antitumor activity of two drugs could be determined at equal cost in drug-dose mortality for the host. It was determined by employing this type of procedure that at equal calculated probit of toxic mortality for the host (equal toxicity), amethopterin was more effective than aminopterin in increasing the survival time of mice succumbing to leukemia L1210, indicating that the former had a higher specificity index against tumor as a result of selective toxic action.[18] In another study which employed this methodology, it was observed that at equivalent probit of drug-dose mortality, intermittent treatment with aminopterin was more effective than daily treatment in increasing the survival time of leukemic animals.[16] It was also determined that on delay of administration of citrovorum factor for 12–24 hours following aminopterin, as opposed to concomitant administration, there was an increase in therapeutic antileukemic efficacy.[14,15] This resulted from differential protection for the host by the citrovorum factor with retention of antifolic toxicity against the leukemic cells, thereby permitting utilization of higher dosage of the folic acid antagonist. It was also demonstrated, by using this procedure, that the combination of intermittent therapy with aminopterin plus delayed administration of citrovorum factor provided further increases in therapeutic efficacy.[19] Thus, the initial demonstration, in dose–response studies, that the selective toxicity of antitumor agents is subject to alteration by appropriate application of drug therapy was accomplished using this methodology.

It was also demonstrated, using the specificity index system, that at equal mortality response there was a sharp loss in therapeutic efficacy of aminopterin when it was administered as a single dose against advanced leukemic L1210 disease as compared with treatment of early disease.[16]

Theoretically, if an antitumor agent were non-toxic for the host, the dosage of the drug could be increased indefinitely until the point where total eradication of the tumor cell population would occur. However, this has not been too readily achievable since with all of the known antitumor agents, the toxicity for the host is limiting. With an active drug, such as amethopterin, as the dosage is increased in the treatment of responsive tumors such as leukemia L1210, the survival time is increased progressively until such point where the toxicity of the amethopterin for the host becomes dominant, and the survival time then diminishes.[41] This severe limitation to therapeutic success, namely, the lethal toxicity of the drug for the host, has provided an additional basis for the comparison of the selective therapeutic action of antitumor agents and treatment modalities. In this system, no effort is made to separate toxic and tumor deaths. Dose–survival time response curves are established for the drugs or treatment modalities being investigated, and comparison is generally made of the maximum increases in survival time elicited at optimal dosage. In addition, it is possible to compare the therapeutic indexes (margin of safety) with which the drugs or treatment modalities may be employed, as reflected in the width of the dose–response curves. The therapeutic index has been defined for this system as the dose yielding the optimal increase in survival time divided by the dose giving a 40% increase in survival time.[41] In a typical experiment a comparison was made of the relative effectiveness of methotrexate, 6-thioguanine, 6-mercaptopurine and azaserine in increasing the survival time of mice with leukemia L1210, and it was clear that at the optimal dose methotrexate was approximately twice as effective as 6-thioguanine and 6-mercaptopurine, which in turn were somewhat more effective than azaserine.[24] It is of interest to note that although 6-mercaptopurine and 6-thioguanine are two closely related analogs, the dosage range over which they were effective was considerably different (80–180 mg/kg for 6-mercaptopurine; 3–16 mg/kg for 6-thioguanine).

Employing the dose–survival time response system, in general there was good agreement with the results obtained with the therapeutic specificity index methodology discussed above. In this system it was again observed that amethopterin was more effective than aminopterin in increasing the survival time of leukemic animals.[20] With this system, dichloromethotrexate and bromochloromethotrexate were found to be considerably more effective than methotrexate in increasing the survival time of animals with advanced leukemia L1210, when treatment was initiated several days prior to death at a time when the disease was systemic and could be recovered from the various organs and blood of the animals.[10] This system is suitable for measuring comparative selective toxicity as reflected not only in relative increases in survival time but also as reflected in the ability to elicit more extensive cure-rate levels.[8] The system has been employed successfully in studies of metabolite–antimetabolite relationships; combination chemotherapy with pairs of drugs and in polychemotherapy with multiple drug combinations; and in combined modalities with surgery, radiation, and immunotherapy. It has been employed in studies of schedule dependency of drug action, the origin and treatment of tumor cell resistance and tumor cell sequestration and metastasis. The above studies have been conducted both from the point of view of extension of survival time of tumorous animals and the elicitation of significant cure rate. Associated pharmacologic and biochemical parameters and cytokinetic investigations have been incorporated in studies utilizing this methodology.[7–9,12,13,22–24,29,43]

It is important to consider ways in which antitumor selective toxicity may be improved. One approach is the classic one, namely, to conduct a screening program in the search for new antitumor agents that will have increased antitumor activity. Such screening can be conducted on a random basis or on the basis of some rational approach. In this regard, the current "new screen" at the National Cancer Institute, employing human tumors growing in athymic mice, and the selection of compounds with known biological activity for testing, based on surveillance of the literature, may be considered as a prospective experimental approach designed to determine whether screening with human tumors will improve the selection of new and more potent antitumor agents for the clinic. The discovery of antitumor activity for N-(phosphonacetyl)-L-aspartic acid (PALA), a transition-state inhibitor of aspartate transcarbamylase, was based on the rationale of the new prospective screen.[30] Based on biochemical rationale it bypassed the P388 leukemia pre-screen, where it was only marginally active, and despite lack of activity against leukemia L1210 it demonstrated definitive

activity against Lewis lung carcinoma and other tumors.

Within a class of known antitumor agents, considerable effort may be expended to increase selective action by a search for more effective congeners. It is of interest to cite the antitumor antibiotic adriamycin as a notable example. Interest in adriamycin stemmed from a demonstration that it was more effective than daunomycin, albeit only moderately so, in increasing the survival time of animals carrying leukemia L1210.[38] It was also demonstrated to be more effective than daunomycin in the leukemia P388 system and in a variety of other tumor systems.[11,38]

With respect to the host–tumor–drug relationship, there are both pharmacologic and biochemical factors that may influence the extent of selectivity of action or degree of resistance to chemotherapeutic agents. Pharmacologic factors that may influence the extent of selective toxicity or resistance to antitumor agents are summarized in Table 1.[12] The concentration of the drug that is reached at the site of the tumor and the duration of its maintenance there (concentration and time; $C \times T$) are most important pharmacologic factors. Important elements contributing to $C \times T$ include the drug dosage that can be employed without the elicitation of limiting host toxicity and the route and schedule of the administration of drug. Selection of an appropriate route or schedule may result in an extensive increase in the effectiveness of a drug. In most instances, when therapy is initiated clinically there is a relatively large body burden of tumor cells, and this may influence the concentration of drug that can be achieved in the tumor cells. In general, the greater the number of tumor cells or the greater the number of resistant cells, the less effective the drug will be. The location in the host of the tumor cells may determine the $C \times T$ that can be achieved, particularly for advanced tumor where there is infiltration in the neighboring tissues, or metastasis and sequestration in various organs. The host may have an effect on the pharmacokinetics of a drug, resulting in increased metabolic inactivation or excretion, and where this occurs it must be overcome in order to obtain and maintain a level of drug adequate to elicit selective action. Where a drug is immunogenic it may be inactivated by being bound to antibody and ways must be sought to avoid this inactivation. $C \times T$ may be altered by a variety of factors pertaining to the host–tumor–drug interrelationship, and these are worthy of extensive investigation.

It is of interest to note an example in which the choice of appropriate scheduling of therapy was influenced by the body burden of tumor cells. For methotrexate, as cited above for aminopterin, intermittent therapy initiated early in the course of the disease was highly effective in the treatment of leukemia L1210. However, for very advanced stages there was a loss in therapeutic effectiveness for the intermittent schedule.[22] Nevertheless, it was possible to overcome this apparent loss in selectivity by utilization of a second drug, 1,3-bis(2-chloroethyl)-1-nitrosourea (BCNU). This drug is highly cytotoxic for leukemia L1210, and when it was administered as a single dose to animals with advanced leukemia it reduced the tumor cell population to such an extent that subsequent administration with methotrexate on an intermittent schedule again became highly effective.[44] Thus, administration of BCNU by sharply diminishing the tumor cell population essentially converted advanced disease to early disease, making the intermittent schedule again more selective. A similar observation has been made in the clinic where an intermittent schedule with methotrexate was demonstrated to be more effective than daily treatment for remission maintenance of acute lymphocytic leukemia of children following reduction of a large body burden of tumor by remission induction therapy.[39]

In another example, it was observed that single treatment with BCNU of animals with advanced leukemia L1210 reduced the body burden of leukemic cells sufficiently so that when this was followed by treatment with cytosine arabinoside daily, starting the next day, there was a marked increase in the percentage of survivors.[8]

Surgical adjuvant approaches constitute a highly important means for increasing pharmacologic sensitivity of the tumor cells that remain. A study conducted by Mayo et al.,[34] involving advanced Lewis lung tumor, demonstrated that surgery alone was incapable of eliciting increased survival time or cure of the animals, because of the presence of a metastatic population localized primarily in the lungs. The disease was also relatively resistant to treatment with cyclophosphamide or methyl CCNU. Combination treatment with cyclophosphamide plus methyl CCNU did yield a marked increase in survival time but failed to result in any

survivors. Nevertheless, when surgery was followed by treatment with cyclophosphamide and methyl CCNU, a survival rate of 50% of the animals was achieved.

It has been demonstrated that the presence of a small number of resistant cells in a tumor population may result rapidly in therapeutic resistance.[43] Therefore, it is necessary to diminish or delay the origin of resistant cells in order to maintain or increase selective action.

Where tumor cell sequestration occurs, it is important to employ drugs that will be capable of penetrating to the sequestered site where they may exert a therapeutic effect. For example, on extensive treatment of leukemia L1210 with methotrexate, the leukemic cells may cross the blood–brain barrier and since methotrexate is incapable of reaching the intracranial site, treatment subsequently fails. However, drugs such as BCNU are capable of crossing the blood–brain barrier and it is possible to employ this type of drug to eradicate tumor cells that have become sequestered in the brain.[27,42]

In addition to the search for new analogs of known antitumor agents, attempts may be made to alter the physical or chemical characteristics of drugs in order to improve their pharmacologic behavior and therapeutic selectivity. Increased solubilization of an insoluble drug may increase $C \times T$ at the tumor site. If a drug can be made more lipophilic it may improve its ability to cross the blood–brain barrier. A drug may be incorporated in liposomes in order to improve its delivery to the target site.[25] The formation of carrier-complexes has been attempted to increase selective delivery of a drug to the target site, such as with the formation of complexes of anthracyclines and DNA.[5]

The competitive relationship of an antimetabolite with a metabolite may determine the extent of selective action. For example, it was demonstrated in one study that as the relative concentration of citrovorum factor was increased, it was necessary to increase the aminopterin dosage in order to maintain the therapeutic effectiveness of the folic acid antagonist.[21] The timing of administration of a metabolite in relation to an antimetabolite may be critical. As indicated above, on treatment with aminopterin plus delayed administration of citrovorum factor there was an increase in the therapeutic response,[14] whereas when citrovorum factor

TABLE 1

Pharmacologic Factors Influencing the Extent of Selective Toxicity and Resistance to Antitumor Agents[a]

I. Concentration and Time ($C \times T$) of Drug at Tumor Cell Site
   A. Drug dosage
   B. Drug route
   C. Drug scheduling
   D. Body burden of tumor cells
      1. Total number of sensitive cells
      2. Relative number of resistant cells
   E. Location of tumor cells: infiltration, metastasis, and sequestration
   F. Host pharmacokinetics: increased metabolic inactivation, excretion rate
   G. Immunologic factors that may alter drug availability
II. Change in Characteristics of Drug
   A. Improved solubility
   B. Change in lipophilic characteristics
   C. Liposomes, carrier complex formation, etc.
III. Competition with Metabolite
   A. Relative concentration of metabolite
   B. Extent of precursor formation to active metabolite
   C. Relation to metabolic pools
IV. Influence of Other Drugs
   A. Other antitumor agents
   B. Antibiotics, etc.
V. Alteration of Cell Membrane (or intracellular membranes)
   A. Biochemical
   B. Pharmacologic
VI. Kinetic Considerations
   A. Tumor growth, drug response (log kill), and recovery rates
   B. Length of S and other phases of cell cycle
   C. Size of nondividing pool (G_0)
VII. Relative Uptake and Toxicity for Tumor and Vital Tissues of Host

[a] See Goldin and Johnson.[12]

and aminopterin were administered simultaneously, there was a net loss of therapeutic effectiveness.[15]

Additional pharmacologic factors that may influence the extent of tumor cell selectivity are listed in Table 1. Therapeutic effectiveness may be influenced by the utilization of other antitumor agents and antibiotics as well as by other drugs. Physical, biochemical or pharmacologic alteration of the cell membrane or intracellular membranes may influence drug effectiveness. Kinetic considerations are of great importance involving factors such as rate of tumor growth, the percentage log

cell kill, and rates of recovery of the tumor cell population and of vital host tissues. Any alteration in the phases of the cell cycle may influence drug effectiveness. The size of the nondividing pool (G_0) as well as of the proliferating pool may influence drug effectiveness. Any means for stimulating G_0 cells to enter the proliferating pool may increase the sensitivity to therapy. In addition, the extent of tumor cell selectivity or resistance may be determined by the relative uptake and toxicity of the antitumor agents for tumor cells and vital tissues of the host.

An interesting study involves the influence of other drugs on the uptake of methotrexate by L1210 cells *in vitro*. It was observed that hydrocortisone, cephalothin, methyl prednisolone, and L-asparaginase inhibited methotrexate uptake, while vinblastine and vincristine increased the uptake of the drug.[45] This was reflected in *in vivo* studies where with vinblastine or vincristine plus methotrexate an improved therapeutic response was observed, in contrast to a reduction of therapeutic effect for the drugs that reduced methotrexate uptake.[45]

Biochemical factors pertaining to the extent of antitumor drug selectivity and resistance are listed in Table 2.[12,33] It is important to increase or to avoid the limitation of any decrease in the intracellular concentration of drugs. The latter could result from

TABLE 2

Biochemical Mechanisms Pertaining to Selective Toxicity and Resistance[a]

I. Extent of Intracellular Concentration of Drug
   A. Reduction of transport
   B. Decrease of activating enzymes
   C. Induction or activation of drug-catabolizing enzymes
II. Minimize Direct Effect on Target Enzymes
   A. Increase in concentration of inhibited enzyme or a coenzyme
   B. Alteration of target enzyme resulting in decreased sensitivity to drug
III. Cell can Skirt Action of Drug
   A. Development of or increased utilization of alternate pathways
   B. Decreased requirement for product of inhibited reaction
IV. Cell Survives by Repair
   A. Induction or activation of repair mechanisms

[a] See Goldin and Johnson[12] and Lane.[33]

reduction in transport or a decrease in an essential activating enzyme. The induction or activation of enzymes that catabolize the drug could lead to rapid inactivation and thereby interfere with its ability to reach the tumor cell target. A decrease in essential activating enzyme has been observed, for example, with 6-mercaptopurine[3] or 6-thioguanine.[6]

An increase in the concentration of inhibited enzyme or coenzyme could tend to minimize the direct effect of a drug on target enzymes. A notable example of this is the increase in the enzyme dihydrofolate reductase that has been observed to occur on progressive treatment of leukemia with methotrexate.[36] It is also possible for alteration of the target enzyme to occur, resulting in diminished sensitivity to drug therapy.[26] Additional kinds of biochemical mechanisms of resistance involve the capability of the tumor cells to skirt the action of the drug, as the result of an increase in the utilization of alternate pathways or a decreased requirement for the product of the metabolic reaction that is inhibited. Also, the tumor cells may develop improved repair mechanisms following exposure to the drug which would increase their survival value. It is clear that there is a reciprocal relationship between the development of biochemical resistance to a drug and the extent of therapeutic activity. Any means for preventing or overcoming biochemical resistance will result in an increase in the selectivity of drug action.

Biochemical mechanisms of tumor cell resistance, involving antimetabolites primarily, have been reviewed by Lane.[33] For 6-mercaptopurine or 6-thioguanine, a decrease in hypoxanthine-guanine phosphoribosyl transferase or an increase in alkaline phosphohydrolase may occur. For 6-thioguanine there could also be a decrease in ribonucleotide reductase or an increase in guanine deaminase. For 5-fluorouracil a variety of alterations could account for resistance, including a decrease in uridine phosphorylase, a decrease in uridine kinase, a decrease in pyrimidine phosphoribosyl transferase, an increase or a decrease in thymidine kinase, or an increase in degradation of nucleosides and deoxyribonucleosides. With cytosine arabinoside there could be a decrease in deoxycytidine kinase or an increase in pyrimidine nucleoside deaminase. With methotrexate there could be an increase in dihydrofolate reductase or a decrease in transport into the tumor cells. With

daunomycin and actinomycin D, a decrease in transport may occur as well as a decrease in the intracellular retention, or a decrease in drug–DNA interaction. With alkylating agents there may be an increase in repair of DNA or a decrease in transport.

For purposes of improvement of antitumor activity, it is clear that more extensive *in vivo* investigations are required on the relationship of pharmacologic and biochemical mechanisms of drug selectivity and resistance to in *vivo* therapeutic response. It is of interest to cite a study of Kessel and Hall[32] in which they compared the uptake of methotrexate and the survival time of animals carrying a variety of murine leukemias. It was observed that in general, the higher the uptake of the drug, the greater was the therapeutic response. In another study, with a series of murine tumors, a good correspondence was also observed between the extent of phosphorylation of cytosine arabinoside and the survival time of the animals.[32]

Following the origin of biochemical or pharmacologic resistance, it is still possible to employ a second drug with a differing mechanism of action which does not show cross-resistance to the initial drug. Skipper et al. have prepared a comprehensive summary on the cross-resistance characteristics of antitumor agents to serve as a guide in the selection of drugs to be used once tumor cell resistance has occurred to the initial drug.[40]

In one investigation an adriamycin-resistant subline of leukemia P-388 was established and its cross-resistance characteristics investigated (Table 3).[12,31] It was found to be cross-resistant to "non-covalent" DNA binders, mitotic spindle poisons, several protein synthesis inhibitors and ICRF 159. On the other hand, it retained sensitivity to "co-valent" DNA binders, antimetabolites, alkylating agents, the protein synthesis inhibitors anguidine and bruceantin and additional drugs including neocarzinostatin, camptothecin and indicine-N-oxide. This information may serve as a guide in the choice of drugs following the origin of tumor cell resistance to adriamycin.

The phenomenon of collateral sensitivity,[28] in which the origin of resistance to one drug leads to increased sensitivity to another, is of potential importance. Collateral sensitivity may have a biochemical or immunologic basis and is worthy of extensive investigation since it may lead to the improvement of therapy. In one study, a number

TABLE 3

Cross-Resistance of P388 Leukemia (Adriamycin-Resistant) to Antitumor Agents[a]

Cross-Resistant	Sensitive
"Noncovalent" DNA Binders	"Covalent" DNA Binders
Anthracyclines	Mitomycin C
Actinomycins	Anthramycin
Mithramycin	
Ellipticine	Antimetabolites
Other intercalators	Methotrexate
	5-Fluorouracil
Mitotic Spindle Poisons	Arabinosyl cytosine
Vinca alkaloids	Glutamine antagonists
Maytansine	
Podophyllotoxins	Alkylating Agents
	Cyclophosphamide
Protein Synthesis Inhibitors	Nitrosoureas
Emetine	cis-Platinum
Pactamycin	Piperazinedione
Homoharringtonine	Other mustards
T2 toxin	
Streptovitacin A	Protein Synthesis Inhibitors
	Anguidine
Miscellaneous	Bruceantin
ICRF 159	
Terephthalanilides	Miscellaneous
	Neocarzinostatin
	Camptothecin
	Indicine N-oxide

[a] See Goldin and Johnson[12] and Johnson et al.[31]

of L1210 sublines resistant to various drugs were shown to have collateral sensitivity to BCNU. For these resistant sublines, the collateral sensitivity appeared to be based on alteration of the antigenicity of the resistant leukemic sublines since the collateral sensitivity to BCNU was diminished when the animals were immunosuppressed with cyclophosphamide prior to inoculation of the leukemic cells.[4,37] The collateral sensitivity of a methotrexate-resistant subline of leukemia L1210 possessing high levels of dihydrofolate reductase to tetrahydrohomofolate derivatives provides an example where a biochemical alteration may account for the increased sensitivity.[35]

In summary, in reference to the obstacles and future approaches pertaining to the pharmacologic and biochemical aspects of selective toxicity, means are at hand for the manipulation of the host–tumor–drug relationship in favor of improvement

of therapeutic response. The effectiveness of individual drugs and drug combinations may be improved by the alteration of schedules and routes of drug administration, and these may be supplemented by combined modality approaches including surgery, radiation and immunotherapy plus chemotherapy. These procedures may lead to the manipulation of the tumor cell population with regard to increased cytotoxic and cytostatic activity, prevention and more effective treatment of resistant variants, and prevention and treatment of tumor cell dissemination including infiltration and metastasis. Means are also at hand for the treatment of sequestered tumor cells. The host may be manipulated with respect to its immunologic response and metabolic factors that may lead to resistance against tumor growth. Taking into account all of these factors, over a relatively short period of years there has been considerable progress in the treatment of both experimental animal and human tumors. Although much progress has been made, much remains to be done. Undoubtedly, before too long, success in therapy will be sufficiently extensive so that the focus will have to be on tumor cell reinduction either as the result of the carcinogenic action of antitumor agents or as the result of viral reinduction.

References

1. Albert, A.: Selective toxicity. In *Pharmacological Basis of Cancer Chemotherapy*. The Williams and Wilkins Co. Baltimore, 1975, pp. 153–164.

2. Albert, A.: *Selective Toxicity (5th ed.)*, Chapman and Hall, London, 1973, p. 597.

3. Brockman, R. W.: A mechanism of resistance to 6-mercaptopurine: Metabolism of hypoxanthine and 6-mercaptopurine by sensitive and resistant neoplasms. *Cancer Res 20: 643–653, 1960.*

4. Bonmassar, E., Bonmassar, A., Vadlamudi, S., and Goldin, A.: Immunological alteration of leukemic cells in vivo after treatment with an antitumor drug. *Proc Natl Acad Sci USA 66: 1089–1095, 1970.*

5. De Duve, C., De Baray, T., Poole, B., Trouet, A., Tulkens, P., and Van Hoof, F.: Lysomotropic agents. *Biochem Pharmacol 23: 2495–2531, 1974.*

6. Ellis, D. B., and Le Page, G. A.: Biochemical studies of resistance to 6-thioguanine. *Cancer Res 23: 436–443, 1963.*

7. Goldin, A.: The employment of methods of inhibition analysis in the normal and tumor-bearing mammalian organism. In *Advances in Cancer Research*, J. Greenstein and A. Haddow, Eds. Academic Press, New York, 1956, Vol. 4, pp. 113–48.

8. Goldin, A.: Factors pertaining to complete drug-in-

duced remission of tumor in animals and man. *Cancer Res 29: 2285–2291, 1969.*

9. Goldin, A.: Preclinical methodology for the selection of anticancer agents. In *Methods in Cancer Research,* H. Busch, Ed. Academic Press, New York, 1968, Vol. 4, pp. 193–254.

10. Goldin, A., Humphreys, S. R., Venditti, J. M., and Mantel, N.: Prolongation of the lifespan of mice with advanced leukemia (L1210) by treatment with halogenated derivatives of amethopterin. *J Natl Cancer Inst 22: 811–823, 1959.*

11. Goldin, A., and Johnson, R. K.: Experimental tumor activity of adriamycin (NSC 123127). *Cancer Chemother Rep* (Pt. III) 6: 137–145, 1975.

12. Goldin, A., and Johnson, R. K.: Resistance to antitumor agents. In *Recent Advances in Cancer Treatment,* H. J. Tagnon and M. J. Staquet, Eds. Raven Press, New York, 1977, pp. 155–169.

13. Goldin, A., Johnson, R. K., and Venditti, J. M.: Preclinical characterization of candidate antitumor drugs. *Cancer Chemother Rep (Pt 2)* 5 (1): 21–81, 1975.

14. Goldin, A., Mantel, N., Greenhouse, S. W., Venditti, J. M., and Humphreys, S. R.: Effect of delayed administration of citrovorum factor on the antileukemic effectiveness of aminopterin in mice. *Cancer Res 14: 43–48, 1954.*

15. Goldin, A., Mantel, N., Greenhouse, S. W., Venditti, J. M., and Humphreys, S. R.: Estimation of the antileukemic potency of the antimetabolite aminopterin, administered alone and in combination with citrovorum factor or folic acid. *Cancer Res 13: 843–850, 1953.*

16. Goldin, A., Mantel, N., Greenhouse, S. W., Venditti, J. M., and Humphreys, S. R.: Factors influencing the specificity of action of an antileukemic agent (aminopterin) time of treatment and dosage schedule. *Cancer Res 14: 311–314, 1954.*

17. Goldin, A., and Venditti, J. M.: A manual on quantitative drug evaluation in experimental tumor systems. Part II. Quantitative assessment of various classes of agents employing advanced leukemia L1210 in mice. *Cancer Chemother Rep 17: 145–178, 1962.*

18. Goldin, A., Venditti, J. M., Humphreys, S. R., Dennis, D., Mantel, N., and Greenhouse, S. W.: A quantitative comparison of the antileukemic effectiveness of two folic acid antagonists in mice. *J Natl Cancer Inst 15: 1657–64, 1955.*

19. Goldin, A., Venditti, J. M., Humphreys, S. R., Dennis, D., Mantel, N., and Greenhouse, S. W.: Factors influencing the specificity of action of an antileukemic agent (aminopterin). Multiple treatment schedules plus delayed administration of citrovorum factor. *Cancer Res 15: 57–61, 1955.*

20. Goldin, A., Venditti, J. M., Humphreys, S. R., and Mantel, N.: Comparison of the relative effectiveness of folic acid congeners against advanced leukemia in mice. *J Natl Cancer Inst 19: 1133–1135, 1957.*

21. Goldin, A., Venditti, J. M., Humphreys, S. R., and Mantel, N.: Influence of the concentration of leukemic inoculum on the effectiveness of treatment. *Science 123: 840, 1956.*

22. Goldin, A., Venditti, J. M., Humphreys, S. R., and Mantel, N.: Modification of treatment schedules in the management of advanced mouse leukemia with amethopterin. *J Natl Cancer Inst 17: 203–212, 1956.*

23. Goldin, A. Venditti, J. M., and Mantel, N.: Combination chemotherapy: Basic considerations. In *Handbook of Experimental Pharmacology, New Series,* A. C. Sartorelli and D. G. Johns, Eds. Springer-Verlag, Berlin, Heidelberg, New York, 1974, pp. 411–448.

24. Goldin, A., Venditti, J. M., and Mantel, N.: Preclinical screening and evaluation of agents for the chemotherapy of cancer: A review. *Cancer Res 21: 1334–1351, 1961.*

25. Gregoriadis, G., and Neerunjun, E. D.: Treatment of tumor bearing mice with liposome-entrapped actinomycin D prolongs their survival. Research communications. *Chem Pathol Pharmacol 10: 351–362, 1975.*

26. Heidelberger, C., Kaldor, G., Mukherjee, K. L., and Danneberg, P. B.: Studies on fluorinated pyrimidines XI. In vitro studies on tumor resistance. *Cancer Res 20: 903–909, 1960.*

27. Humphreys, S. R., Thomas, L. B., Chirigos, M. A., Goldin, A., Crawford, E. J., and Friedkin, M.: Use of dihydrofolate reductase as a biochemical index of therapy. *Nature (Lond) 195: 453–455, 1962.*

28. Hutchison, D. J.: Cross-resistance and collateral sensitivity studies in cancer chemotherapy. *Adv Cancer Res 7: 235–350, 1963.*

29. Johnson, R. K., and Goldin, A.: The clinical impact of screening and other experimental tumor studies. *Cancer Treat Rev 2: 1–31, 1975.*

30. Johnson, R. K., Inouye, T., Goldin, A., and Stark, G. R.: Antitumor activity of N-(phosphonacetyl)-L-aspartic acid, a transition-state inhibitor of aspartate-transcarbamylase. *Cancer Res 36: 2720–2725, 1976.*

31. Johnson, R. K., Ovejera, A. A., and Goldin, A.: Activity of anthracyclines against an adriamycin (NSC-123127)-resistant subline of P388 leukemia with special emphasis on cinarubin A(NSC-18334). *Cancer Treat Rep 60: 99–102, 1976.*

32. Kessel, D., and Hall, T. C.: Biochemical predictive tests. In *Cancer Medicine,* J. F. Holland and E. Frei, III, Eds. Lea and Febiger, Philadelphia, 1973, pp. 699–706.

33. Lane, M.: General mechanisms of clinical resistance to cancer chemotherapy. *Biochem Pharmacol (Suppl. 2) 23: 83–88, 1974.*

34. Mayo, J. G., Laster, W. R., Jr., Andrews, C. M., and Schabel, F. M., Jr.: Success and failure in the treatment of solid tumors. III. "Cure" of metastatic Lewis lung carcinoma with methyl-CCNU (NSC-95441) and surgery-chemotherapy. *Cancer Chemother Rep 56: 183–195, 1972.*

35. Mead, J. A. R., Goldin, A. Kisliuk, R. L. Friedkin, M., Plante, L., Crawford, E. J., and Kwok, G.: Pharmacologic aspects of homofolate derivatives in relation to amethopterin-resistant murine leukemia. *Cancer Res 26: 2374–2379, 1965.*

36. Misra, D. K., Humphreys, S. R., Friedkin, M., Goldin, A., and Crawford, E. J.: Increased dihydrofolate reductase activity as a possible basis of drug resistance in leukemia. *Nature (Lond) 189: 39–42, 1961.*

37. Nicolin, A., Vadlamudi, S., and Goldin, A.: Antigenicity of L1210 leukemic sublines induced by drugs. *Cancer Res 32: 653–657, 1972.*

38. Sandberg, J. S., Howsden, F. L., DiMarco, A., and Goldin, A.: Comparison of the antileukemic effect in mice of adriamycin (NSC-123127) with daunomycin (NSC-82151). *Cancer Chemother Rep (Pt 1) 54 (1): 1–7, 1970.*

39. Selawry, O. S., Hananian, J., Wolman, I. J., et al.: Cooperative study, acute leukemia group B: New treatment schedule with improved survival in childhood leukemia. *JAMA 194: 75–81, 1965.*

40. Skipper, H. E., Hutchison, D. J., Schabel, F. M. Jr., Schmidt, L. H., Goldin, A., Brockman, R. W., Venditti, J. M., and Wodinsky, I.: A quick reference chart on cross-resistance between anticancer agents. *Cancer Chemother Rep 56: 493–498, 1972.*

41. Skipper, H. E., and Schmidt, L. H.: A manual on quantitative drug evaluation in experimental tumor systems. Part I. Background, description of criteria, and presentation of quantitative therapeutic data on various classes of drugs obtained in diverse experimental tumor systems. *Cancer Chemother Rep 17: 1–143, 1962.*

42. Thomas, L. B., Chirigos, M. A., Humphreys, S. R., et al.: Development of meningeal leukemia (L1210) during treatment of subcutaneously inoculated mice with methotrexate. *Cancer 17: 352–360, 1964.*

43. Venditti, J. M., and Goldin, A.: Drug synergism in antineoplastic chemotherapy. In *Advances in Chemotherapy*, A. Goldin and F. Hawking, Eds. Academic Press, New York, 1964, Vol. 1, pp. 397–497.

44. Venditti, J. M., Kline, I., Tyrer, D. D., and Goldin, A. 1,3-bis (2-chloroethyl)-1-nitrosourea (NSC-409962) and methotrexate (NSC-740) as combination therapy for advanced mouse leukemia L1210. *Cancer Chemother Rep 48: 35–39, 1965.*

45. Zager, R. F., Frisby, S. A., and Oliverio, V. T.: The effects of antibiotics and cancer chemotherapeutic agents on the cellular transport and antitumor activity of methotrexate in L1210 murine leukemia. *Cancer Res 33: 1670–1676, 1973.*

3

Cell synchrony and cancer treatment

A note of caution

E. H. Cooper

PROGRESS IN CELL SYNCHRONIZATION is briefly reviewed. The major obstacles to the application of chemical synchronizing methods to man are discussed. In the main, these are the heterogeneity of human tumor cell populations with respect to their distribution in the phases of the cell cycle, cell cycle times and growth fraction.

Although the study of cell kinetics and tumor biology and that of the mode of action of many anticancer drugs have advanced considerably during the past 10 years, one should beware of accepting the idea that our knowledge is sufficient to be able to talk about cell synchronization as a reality in the treatment of human cancer. It would be very advantageous if, out of the random disorder that is present in all human tumors, some form of order could be imposed which would confer immense therapeutic advantage. There are, today, some people who believe they can do it and indeed publish remarkable recipes for such procedures. However, I believe that these claims should be examined with critical skepticism; are they really able to synchronize cells, or are these just further examples of empiricism bolstered with mis-applied scientific jargon? There is no convincing scientific proof that cell synchrony has been attained consistently in human tumors or that such synchrony is the reason why a particular regime has a good therapeutic effect; see Steel[5] for review.

Unfortunately, there is still much confusion in the minds of some chemotherapists on translating what can be achieved in the test tube or the experimental animal to man. There are immense problems that must first be solved if a regime involving synchrony is to be tailored to the individual patient's needs other than being yet another recipe in polychemotherapy that enters into the normal trial-and-error method that has been the basis of the advance in chemotherapy so far.

It is well known to biologists that there are many ways in which cells can be synchronized in the laboratory. Indeed, these manipulations are one of the more powerful techniques that have been de-

Unit for Cancer Research, University of Leeds, Leeds, England.

Reprinted from Cancer Clinical Trials 2; 175–178, 1979.

vised in recent years that have helped immensely in the understanding of the mechanisms of action of radiation and a wide range of anticancer drugs. Cell survival as a function of cell cycle phase has often been worked out in terms of one dose of the treatment. This is particularly true in relation to drugs because of the enormous amount of work involved in investigating multiple doses of drugs. The degree of the success of experiments and their interpretation depends on the effectiveness of the synchrony that is produced, and the interpretation is also dependent on whether a noxious agent is being used to synchronize the cells or whether they are synchronized by some mechanical technique. The combination of mitotic selection coupled with thymidine suicide can produce a population of cells in G_1 (that is, in the first period after mitosis prior to the synthesis of DNA); other populations in G_2 (that is, the period that follows DNA synthesis prior to mitosis) can also be produced, hence the ability of the cells in these compartments to survive a particular insult can be studied with accuracy.

From studies of the irradiation, certain general rules have emerged.[4] The cells are most sensitive in mitosis. They are resistant in G_1, and this is a time-dependent phenomenon; that is, the longer they are in G_1, the lower their resistance becomes. In the S phase, their resistance increases towards the end of S while the sensitivity in G_2 and in mitosis is about equal.

One of the techniques most frequently used in the laboratory is the study of the growth of colonies of cells *in vitro*, so that the clonogenic behavior of individual surviving cells can be identified and related to the time in the cell cycle at which they were damaged. The most widely used techniques of synchronization of cells are essentially concerned with proliferating cells, such as the mitotic selection technique, but it is well known that in both experimental tumors and in human tumors that a great many of the cells are not proliferating.

To study out of cycle cells (G_o), two techniques are commonly used. The first is to use cells that have ceased to proliferate in tissue culture for one of two reasons, possibly because the cells have grown to form close contact one with another and in this state untransformed cells exhibit a process known as contact inhibition—that is, the inhibition of division as a result of physical contact of one cell with another. The second approach is to deprive the cells of certain vital nutrients so that they stop

growing because of exhaustion in the media. Synchronous growth can be initiated by either subculturing the cells so that the contact inhibition is broken or to provide the missing nutrients. However, these two phenomena are quite different from the point of their biochemistry and biology.

It is well established that cells in contact can communicate and exchange low molecular weight compounds. Hence, disrupting these communications can have many effects other than inducing growth.[2] On the other hand, the addition of a missing metabolite may recommence division within communicating cell network. Hence, even at the level of the test tube there are many factors that can influence the interpretation of the experiments. Nevertheless, from a variety of systems of this character, it has been proven that the chemotherapeutic agents can be broadly divided into those that have a maximum effect related to a particular phase of the cell cycle and those whose action appears to be independent of the cell cycle. Examples of these different types of drugs are listed in Table 1. It is frequently the frontier between one phase of the cell cycle and another that is a critical interface for the action of certain drugs.

It is possible in experimental tumors grown in

TABLE 1

Phase Blocking and Greatest Lethal Sensitivity of some Cancer Chemotherapy Agents[a]

Agent	Phase of Blocking Action	Phase of Greatest Lethal Sensitivity
Vincristine	M	S
Chlorambucil		M_1G_1
Thiotepa	All phases	M_1G_1, G_2
BCNU		S
CCNU		G_1/S, S/G_2
Hydroxyurea	G_1/S	S
Cytosine arabinoside	G_1/S	S
Methotrexate	G_1/S	S, G_1/S
5-Fluorouracil		All phases
Adriamycin	G_1, G_2	M, G_1/S
Bleomycin		M, G_2
Daunomycin	G_2	S
Mitomycin C		G_1

[a] Modified from Steel.[5]

vivo to produce synchrony by the injection of drugs such as hydroxyurea which cause cells to be held up at the G_1/S interface as well as killing cells in S; subsequently, as the cells release from the block there is a partial synchrony, but such synchronous waves soon disappear mainly because of the variation of cell cycle times within the tumor cell population.[3,6] After cells which have been held up by synchronizing process are released, they often overshoot their normal behavior. This phenomenon is not only a property of tumor cells but is also seen in the host's normal tissues such as the bone marrow and the gut and may make them more vulnerable to certain forms of anticancer drugs.

When we come to apply this knowledge to clinical therapy, we move from the tissue culture situation where it is possible to analyze in detail many of the chemical and biophysical properties associated with synchrony to the middle ground of transplanted tumors many of which have a relatively narrow phenotypic expression to reach the problems of human tumors that are characterized by a very wide phenotypic expression, marked variation in growth fraction and often unpredictable behavior. The proof of synchrony itself is very difficult to obtain in human tumors. Essentially, it requires the demonstration that a substantial part of the population accumulated in a particular phase of the cell cycle, usually the G_1/S interface. There is an intrinsic problem of how representative one or two biopsies from a tumor are of the population as a whole. Frequently there is a wide distribution of DNA contents of cells in G_1 due to chromosome anomalies, and in most human tumors except a few embryonal and hematological malignancies that for a while grow nearly exponentially. Many of the cells are out of cycle and are not directly affected by the synchronization process. Furthermore, it is probable that in many of the common cancers, such as those of the breast, lung and bowel, it is only a fraction of the whole population that has the clonogenic activity to maintain the tumor growth.

It is these considerations which would seem to bedevil the application of the new techniques such as impulse cytofluorimetry to study shifts in the phase of the population, even though the technique has considerable attraction in model systems. But the real dilemma is how to devise studies that can show there has been a manipulation of clonogenic cells to induce them into synchrony, thereby rendering them more susceptible to treatment.

The theory of the chemotherapy of tumors is not limited to the consideration of cell kinetics alone, although the concept of cycle-dependent and cycle-independent drugs is helpful when devising polychemotherapy schedules. The pharmacokinetics of the agent, that is, distribution in tissues, half life and metabolism, are of equal importance as are the various sequellae that follow the disruption of a tumor's organization with respect to its vascularization, inflammatory response, and secondary endocrine changes which can profoundly influence the nature of the target for subsequent attacks by chemotherapy.

When we examine critically those tumors where chemotherapy appears to be really effective in the presence of widespread disease, we are concerned mainly with Hodgkin's disease, leukemias in children and certain embryonal and mesenchymal tumors in children. As has been described by Bagshawe,[1] such tumors often have very high intrinsic cell death, so that a relatively small proportion of the tumor contributes towards the tumor growth even when the tumor is growing relatively quickly. On the other hand, tumors that have a low intrinsic cell death rate are extremely difficult to treat with chemotherapy, and it is these that form the bulk of the adenocarcinomas seen in normal hospital practice.

In retrospect, then, there has been real progress in the science of the manipulation of cells under carefully controlled conditions. There are immense biological obstacles to the application of such manipulation to the wild type tumor population encountered in clinical practice. The main obstacles to progress in tumors being identified can be summarized briefly as follows:

The tumors grow slowly, and they have a broad distribution into mitotic times so that they are often a highly random population. Ischemia enhances the production of resistant cells. The stem cell population is frequently a minor portion of the tumor rather than its major portion. Host resistance mechanisms to various chemotherapeutic agents are not well understood and need much greater attention. There is definitive evidence that it is possible to synchronize cells in the test tube. It is also possible to achieve a transient partial synchrony in the laboratory animal *in vivo*, where one can take unprecedented risks in order to achieve the objective. There is a probability that synchrony may produce a slight decrease in the randomness of disorder in human tumors. This may be at the expense of increasing the susceptibility of normal tissues to damage by a particular agent.

Finally, to prove scientifically that synchronization has in fact occurred is not only a problem of scientific design, but it is also one of the means for repeated invasive investigations to satisfy scientific curiosity which in the minds of many doctors are still unacceptable as ethical procedures.

References

1. Bagshawe, K. D.: Tumor growth and anti-mitotic action. *Br J Cancer 68: 698–713, 1968.*

2. Pitts, J. D.: Junctional communication and cellular growth control. In *Intercellular Junctions and Synapses*, J. Feldman, N. B. Giluka, and J. D. Pitts, Eds. Chapman Hall, London, 1978, pp. 63–79.

3. Rajewsky, M. F.: Synchronization in vitro: Kinetics of a malignant cell system following temporary inhibition of DNA synthesis with hydroxyurea. *Exp Cell Res 60: 269–270, 1970.*

4. Sinclair, W. K.: Cyclic x-ray responses in mammalian cells in vitro. *Rad Res 33: 620–643, 1968.*

5. Steel, G. G.: *The Growth of Tumours.* Clarendon Press, Oxford, 1977, pp. 268–306.

6. Tubiana, M., Frindel, E., and Vassort, F.: Critical survey of experimental data on in vivo synchronization by hydroxyurea. *Rec Results Cancer Res 52: 187–205, 1975.*

4

Basic cancer chemotherapy: experimental models — strategy

J. H.Mulder, M.D.

In my view, the results of cancer chemotherapy for advanced disease are disappointing. In Table 1, the approximate response rate and survival prolongation in patients treated for the most common tumors such as lung, mammary, and gastrointestinal tract cancer are given. Although a significant increase in the disease-free interval can be obtained with adjuvant chemotherapy in some tumor types, the number of long-term survivors with no evidence of disease is still very low. Therefore, it seems to me appropriate to discuss the following subjects:

First, I will give reasons for the low response rate in patients with advanced disease to cancer chemotherapy, with the ultimate intention to analyze some unknown factors related to adjuvant chemotherapy. Second, I will suggest what the experimentalist should do to improve our treatment results in adjuvant chemotherapy.

If a patient with advanced metastatic disease shows minor tumor response or no response at all on cytostatic treatment, we should reckon with the following mechanisms of tumor resistance (Table 2). The neoplastic cell may be insensitive to the drugs administrated. The permeability of the cell membrane for the drug may be limited either by a transport deficiency or by a competitive effect of endogenous products against cellular drug uptake. Another well-known cause of drug resistance is the lack of drug activating enzymes. A typical example of secondary or acquired resistance of tumor cells is the development of deactivating enzymes. The second type of resistance is based on cell kinetics. During tumor growth, the fraction of tumor cells actually involved in DNA synthesis decreases. The low growth fraction of an advanced solid tumor

results in a relatively ineffectiveness of cell cycle phase-specific drugs. This can result in a tumor resistance to treatment. Recognition of drug resistance and high volume resistance have stimulated chemotherapists to start treatment early in the course of the disease, immediately after the primary treatment of the tumor. This has resulted in the practice of adjuvant chemotherapy, a subject I will discuss in the second half of my paper. Drug penetration in metastasis to the brain can be limited and therefore result in a treatment failure. Resistance as a consequence of tumor deposits in sanctuaries is a typical example of relative resistance.

How do we establish whether drug resistance or high volume resistance is an important factor in advanced tumor disease? When no shrinkage can be observed in a large tumor mass after the administration of presumably active cytostatic drugs, we should give serious consideration to a drug-induced tumor cell kill which we simply cannot observe clinically. We must investigate whether there is a discrepancy in tumor response in high tumor volumes and in micrometastases. The clinically most relevant experimental model to test this hypothesis is the one in which measurements can be performed on the primary tumor and concomitantly on metastases in the same animal.

In Table 3, data for CCNU- and 5FU-treated mice with subcutaneously inoculated Lewis lung tumor cells are given. Note that the primary tumor shows no volume reduction. However, the number of lung metastases is significantly reduced in comparison with control mice. If you want to cure the animals, the obvious procedure is to remove the primary tumor by surgical excision and to repeat the treatment postoperatively (the adjuvant model). However, referring to Table 3, the point I want to make in general is the following. In our so-called clinical screening studies, new investigational drugs are screened for their efficacy in far advanced cancer patients. When a low tumor response rate is established, the drug is dropped from further

From the Radiobiological Institute TNO, Rijswijk; and Department of Internal Medicine, Radiotherapeutic Institute, Rotterdam , The Netherlands.
Reprinted from Cancer Clinical Trials 1: 129–134, 1978.

TABLE 1

Efficacy of Current Cancer Chemotherapy in Advanced Tumor Disease

Cancer Incidence by Site		Response Rate and Effect on Survival
Leukemia and lymphomas	8%	60–90% with prolongation[a]
Breast (females)	26%	60% minor prolongation
Lung (males)	21%	30–40% no prolongation
Colon and rectum	15%	35% no prolongation
Uterus and cervix	13%	30% no prolongation
Prostate	16%	20% no prolongation
Urinary	7%	20% no prolongation

[a] Often in combination with surgery and/or radiotherapy.

investigations. This crude method of drug screening may be quite unrealistic. A new agent may be effective in micrometastases but, because of the negative results in screening studies, not evaluated further. Once a drug has been accepted for large-scale clinical investigations, the exact response rate in advanced disease will be established. Various drugs which show promising results in particular tumors will be combined, and in due course one ends up with the "best" drug combination for each type of malignancy. When adjuvant studies are considered, the most effective combination tested in advanced disease is chosen in the adjuvant format. For example, in the U.S. in nine out of 13 adjuvant studies on colon–rectal tumors, 5-Fluorouracil in combination with MeCCNU is given.[2] Is this the right policy? Let us briefly analyze Bonnadonna's CMF and Fisher's L-PAM studies as typical examples of this policy (Table 4).

TABLE 2

Causes of Treatment Failure with Cancer Chemotherapy

Resistance based on:
    Biochemical mechanisms (drug resistance)
    Cell kinetics (high volume resistance)
Relative resistance due to the host, e.g.:
    Tumor sanctuaries
    Low Kornofsky index
    Compromised bone marrow reserve
    Side effects of treatment not acceptable
Pseudoresistance due to treatment, e.g.:
    Drug dosages not optimal
    Drug antagonism
    Time interval between courses too long
    Total length of treatment too short
    Protocol violations

The 60% response rate with CMF in late breast cancer was considered promising enough to evaluate the effect of CMF in early disease. L-PAM given in advanced disease resulted in a relatively low response rate of 20%. In contrast to CMF therapy, the L-PAM drug is extremely convenient to handle and hardly any acute side effects are known. The results of both treatment schedules when given postoperatively in selected mammary cancer patients are well known.[1,3] Based on the significantly different antitumor effects in advanced disease, I do not understand why the results (expressed in relapse rate) in both adjuvant studies are so similar. It is frustrating to find that CMF therapy did not lead to far better results than the treatment with L-PAM. Consequently, the policy of extrapolation from late to early treatment should be reevaluated.

I have discussed reasons why treatment may fail in late disease. Is it a matter of resistance, or do we fail to observe the cell kill? As discussed, both possibilities may have an opposite consequence for the planning of adjuvant chemotherapy.

The adjuvant model mentioned earlier has been extensively used by the group of investigators at the Southern Research Institute, Alabama.[10,11] Their animal adjuvant studies gave a big boost to clinical research. "Small is sensitive and therefore curable" was the message. The lower the number of tumor cells, the fewer biochemically resistant cell lines, the higher the growth fraction, the better the drug penetration into the tumor and, as a consequence of all of these factors, the more effective our anticancer agents when applied in early disease. Resistance was circumvented and the fractional cell-kill hypothesis promised us long-term disease-free survivors.

TABLE 3

Effect of Treatment on Primary Tumor and on Spontaneous Lung Metastases in Lewis Lung Carcinoma

Treatment	Growth Delay (days) Mean ± S.E.	Number of Lung Metastases per Mouse Mean ± S.E.
Control	0 ± 0.5	16 ± 4
CCNU 20 mg/kg i.p.	0 ± 0.5	1 ± 0.5
5FU 100 mg/kg i.p.	1.0 ± 0.3	3 ± 1

Note: One million Lewis lung carcinoma cells were injected s.c. into groups of five C57BL/Ka mice on day 0. Treatment was given on day 11 when the tumor volume was approximately 800 mm^3. In the primary tumor no significant response on treatment was observed. Lung metastases were counted on day 30.

The translation of these experimental findings to clinical thinking has been fruitful; that is to say, the concept of micrometastases treatment is fully acknowledged by every medical oncologist. Data from mice were applied in men. In the second half of this paper, I will explore clinical problems related to adjuvant chemotherapy which should be translated back to experimental research (Table 5).

Accepting the experimental results obtained in the Adjuvant Model and, after appreciation of the theory of micrometastases, the next logical step is: How do we select effective drug schedules for our clinical trials in adjuvant chemotherapy?

The choice of drugs has always been based on tumor-specific late-disease studies. This policy, as discussed earlier, may be inappropriate. Cell cycle phase-specific drugs like AraC and MTX are generally ineffective in advanced disease but may have an effect in microtumors. As mentioned earlier, who will suggest a Cytosine Arabinoside adjuvant study for Duke's C colon carcinoma instead of adjuvant 5FU–MeCCNU combination therapy? In comparison, we should be aware that, in clinical adjuvant studies, immune stimulating agents such as BCG and *Corynebacterium parvum* are used indiscriminately for all types of tumors. As far as I know, no randomized clinical trial in advanced disease has ever shown a clear-cut effect of these agents in any neoplastic disease. The optimal choice of drugs as well as the optimal drug dosages and the effect of scheduling should be further investigated, not in men but in mice. Our group has investigated the possible effect of drug scheduling.[5,6] I would like to call attention to two features of our sequential treatment studies. First of all, we always compared the effect of the most optimal antitumor schedule investigated with the effect on critical normal tissue, the bone marrow stem cells. Only when a differential effect on tumor and on stem cells can be established is the drug schedule worthwhile for clinical investigations. The second feature of our work involved the testing of drug scheduling on different tumor cell lines. If the same drug sequence is optimal in various experimental tumor cell lines, extrapolation to clinical practice seems more justifiable then when only one mouse tumor is tested. In my view, more experimental work in this line should be done.

The next variable in adjuvant chemotherapy is the time interval between treatment courses. The

TABLE 4

Chemotherapy of Breast Cancer

Tumor Response Rate in Advanced Disease	Response in Early Disease (% with relapse)			
	Subpopulation[a]		Total Population[b]	
	control	L-PAM	control	L-PAM
L-PAM: 20%	26%	6%	31%	23%
	control	CMF	control	CMF
CMF: 60%	30%	5%	37%	20%

[a] Percent with relapse at 24 months after mastectomy in premenopausal women with 1–3 nodes.
[b] relapse rate at 24 months after mastectomy.

TABLE 5

Adjuvant Chemotherapy: Treatment Variables

1. Choice of drugs
2. Type of drugs
3. Dosages and sequences
4. Time interval
5. Total length of treatment

treatment is normally repeated as soon as the bone marrow has recovered. We are all aware of the risk of drug-induced bone marrow hypoplasia. However, the longer the treatment delay, the more tumor regrowth. Lloyd's formula is shown in Figure 1 and, as can be seen, the smaller the tumor volume doubling time and the longer the time interval between the treatment courses, the more tumor cells will recover.[11] Generally, clinicians choose the dosages of their drugs according to their accepted treatment protocol; intuitively the major violation of adjuvant study protocols is the lengthening of the time interval between treatment courses. I have to admit I am personally more interested in cell kill than in regrowth which is, according to Lloyd's formula, a misconception of what really happens during treatment.

How long is long enough or what should be the total length of adjuvant treatment? The desired total tumor cell kill to obtain cures depends on cell kill per treatment course, tumor regrowth per course and the number of tumor cells left behind after primary treatment. Referring to the last point, the total number of tumor cells immediately after the primary treatment may be between approximately 10^8 and 10^1, a difference of at least seven decades. The most accurate way to establish the number of cells left behind postoperatively is to integrate various prognostic factors, such as number of lymph nodes involved, in order to define subpopulation in our patients material. According to the fractional cell-kill hypothesis, an expected high total number of tumor cells requires more intensive and more prolonged adjuvant treatment than a low number of cells. The fractional cell-kill hypothesis, however, was based on the results of L1210 experiments and was subsequently extrapolated to solid tumors. I am personally inclined to think that the percentage of cell kill per treatment course and the regrowth rate are hypothetical figures as soon as we are talking about solid tumors, especially when we speculate on subclinical solid tumors.

Very recently, Norton at the Mt. Sinai Hospital in New York has presented an alternative hypothesis to the fractional cell-kill theory.[7] The growth curve of a solid tumor (Fig. 2, curve A) can be described according to a Gompertzian formula. Simply stated, this means exponential growth with exponentially increasing tumor volume doubling time. The most likely explanation for the Gompertzian growth is the ever-decreasing growth fraction as a result of nutritional imbalances inside

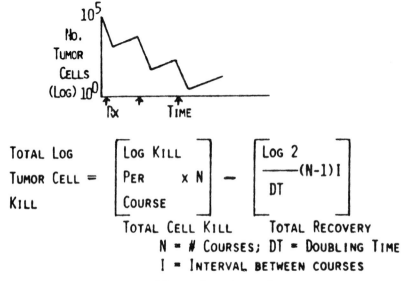

FIGURE 1.   Adjuvant chemotherapy: kinetics.

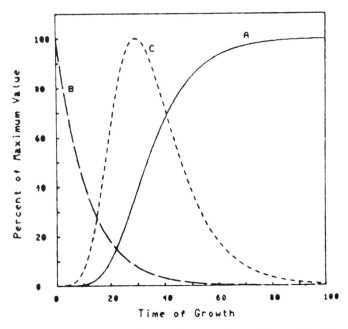

FIGURE 2.   Curve *A* represents Gompertzian growth, curve *B* growth fraction and curve *C* growth rate. The maximum growth rate occurs when the tumor volume is approximately 37% of its maximum size.

the tumor (curve *B*). The growth rate pattern in course of time, however, is very different: the maximum growth rate is at the halfway point of the subclinical growth phase (curve *C*). If the overall effect of treatment correlates, as suggested by Norton, with growth rate and not with actual tumor cell number, then in order to obtain curves, we should end our treatment program with very intensive treatment courses. I wonder whether, in the present adjuvant studies, the opposite policy is not the trend.

The first experimental model I discussed was the adjuvant animal model and I have tried to indicate some areas for experimental research. They are summarized in Table 6. My second and last experimental model most relevant to adjuvant chemotherapy is an *in vitro* model. A surgical specimen from a woman operated on for breast cancer should be used to obtain all the information needed for selecting the most promising drug treatment. Measurements of various hormone receptors have given us a lead as to how to select candidates for hormonal manipulation. A method to determine the sensitivity of cancer cells to drugs is the administration of cytostatic drugs to nude mice inoculated with human tumor material. Practically and economically, this procedure is too slow and too

TABLE 6

Adjuvant Chemotherapy: Areas For Experimental Research

1. Should the choice of drugs be based on advanced disease results?
2. Is the disease-oriented approach the right one?
3. Should we prefer sequential treatment and/or cyclic combination chemotherapy?
4. Is a less toxic treatment possible, e.g., cell cycle phase-specific drugs?
5. Can Norton's hypothesis be proven?
6. Is it possible to select drugs *in vitro*?

laborious for clinical application. The same arguments can be raised against tumor cell inoculation techniques with immune deprived mice carrying micropore diffusion chambers. I am fully aware of all of the disadvantages of an *in vitro* sensitivity test. For instance, metabolic activation of cyclophosphamide by liver enzymes is impossible *in vitro*: a false negative *in vitro* prediction should then be expected. Concentration and exposure time of the test drug in an *in vitro* system may be highly artificial, and therefore the value for prediction of tumor sensitivity may be nil. The more we know about drug kinetics, the better we are able to simulate *in vivo* situations *in vitro*. Human tumor stem cell colonies, growing as spheroids in agar, can presently be cultivated immediately after tumor operation, and the application of this model in predicting tumor response to drugs used in adjuvant chemotherapy should be urgently investigated. The conditions of the culture medium as well as the relevant criterium to assess drug-induced cell lethality are bottlenecks of the model, but as soon as the possible clinical applications are recognized by all investigators involved in this field of research, I am convinced that something workable will result.[4,8,9,12,13]

In conclusion, two experimental models seem to me most relevant to basic cancer chemotherapy: first, the adjuvant model as described, for example, for Lewis lung carcinona and, second, the *in vitro* microcolony model for drug sensitivity testing. The results of investigations in both models should help us to select the most effective antitumor and the least toxic drug treatment for adjuvant chemotherapy in the near future.

References

1. Bonnadonna, G., Rossi, A., Valagussa, P., Banfi, A., and Veronesi, U.: Adjuvant chemotherapy with CMF in breast cancer with positive axillary nodes. *Adjuvant Therapy of Cancer*, S. E. Salman and S. E. Jones, Eds. Elsevier (North Holland Biomedical Press Amsterdam, 1977, pp. 83–94.

2. *Compilation of Clinical Protocol Summaries* (2nd ed.) U.S. Dept. of Health, Education, and Welfare. National Cancer Institute, November 1977.

3. Fisher, B., and Redmond, C.: Studies of the National Surgical Adjuvant Breast Project (NSABP). In *Adjuvant Therapy of Cancer*, S. E. Salman and S. E. Jones, Eds. Elsevier (North Holland Biomedical Press, Amsterdam, 1977, pp. 67–81.

4. Hamburger, A. W., and Salmon, S. E.: Primary bioassay of human tumor stem cells. *Science 197: 461, 1977.*

5. Mulder, J. H., Edelstein, M. B., Lelieveld, P., and van Putten, L. M.: Synergism and schedule dependent cytotoxicity of Cyclophosphamide and CCNU in experimental chemotherapy. *Eur J Cancer* (in press).

6. Mulder, J. H., Smink, T., and van Putten, L. M.: Schedule dependent effectiveness of CCNU and 5-Fluorouracil in experimental chemotherapy. *Eur J Cancer 13: 1123, 1977.*

7. Norton, L., and Simon, R.: Tumor size, sensitivity to therapy, and design of treatment schedules. *Cancer Treat Rep 61: 1307, 1977.*

8. Park, C. H., Savin, M. A., Hoogstraten, B., Amare, M., and Hathaway, P.: Improved growth of in vitro colonies in human acute leukemia with the feeding culture method. *Cancer Res 37: 4595, 1977.*

9. Roper, P. R., and Drewinko, B.: Comparison of in vitro methods to determine drug-induced cell lethality. *Cancer Res 36: 2182, 1976.*

10. Schabel, F. M., Jr.: Concepts for systemic treatment of micrometastases. *Cancer 35: 15, 1975.*

11. Skipper, H. E., and Schabel, F. M., Jr.: Quantitative and cytokinetic studies in experimental tumor systems. In *Cancer Medicine*, J. F. Holland and E. Frei, III, Eds. In press.

12. Volm, M., Hummet, H., and Mattern, J.: Ubereinstimmung von Zytostatika effecten in vivo und im kurzzeittest (in vitro) bei der leukämie L1210. *Blut 35: 65, 1977.*

13. Yuhas, J. M., Li, A. P., Martinez, A. O., and Ladman, A. J.: A simplified method for production and growth of multicellular tumor spheroids. *Cancer Res 37: 3639, 1977.*

5

Adjuvant chemotherapy

K. D. Bagshawe

The term adjuvant chemotherapy has come to be applied to the use of cytotoxic agents where the primary site and histological type of cancer has been identified, where the primary tumor and in some cases the local lymph nodes also have been completely excised or ablated by radiotherapy, where full and appropriate investigations have failed to reveal residual or metastatic lesion, but where historical or statistical evidence indicates a high probability that metastatic spread has occurred.

The concept of adjuvant chemotherapy is not new and goes back at least to the 1960s.[6,10] Some early experimental tumor studies were dramatic but the early clinical studies, however, did not produce spectacular results. The heightened interest of the past 3 years stems, of course, from two well-known randomized trials in carcinoma of the breast.[1,5] Ironically, these two randomized trials appear to have precipitated a great many nonrandomized trials. I think this came about because many were, in general, too readily convinced of the likely efficacy of this approach and because we are all conditioned by the frustration of treating advanced cancer with inadequate means. Alas, the inadequacy of one therapeutic approach merely emphasizes the need for new approaches, but there is no assurance that another method will be superior. In cancer work it is regrettably true that practices suddenly change and that "bandwagons" often start to roll on the basis of inadequate evidence. Few of these nonrandomized trials provide information of the quality required, and it is surely time to look critically at the underlying thesis of adjuvant therapy to see what we can expect from it with present-day agents and to see how far we are falling short.

The rationale for the approach, reduced to its simplest terms, is the proposition that small tumor masses can be eradicated more easily than large ones. However, most workers would extend the objectives and potential benefits to include prolonged survival and more particularly prolonged disease-free survival where eradication is not achieved. It is also appropriate to look at the price to be paid in terms of both its actual and potential disadvantages.

A crucial consideration is the level of probability that a patient has micrometastatic disease. What is an acceptable price in terms of risk and morbidity when the probability of recurrent disease is 90% is different from a risk of 50% and different again from that at 10%. Moreover, we need to define whether we are talking of recurrence within 1 year or recurrence within 10 years. The implications are clearly profoundly different and these differences are themselves strongly related to patient age.

The probability of micrometastatic disease is of course known to correlate with various factors at the time of primary surgery. The greater the size of the primary mass, the greater appears the risk.[16] Similar considerations apply to local node involvement. Histological type is another prognostic factor, as may be the extent of mononuclear cell infiltration.

Clearly, the clinical material submitted to adjuvant chemotherapy is highly heterogenous, and trials which take too little account of the known variables may be worthless. Indeed, one of the "spin-offs" from properly conducted trials is their ability to define hitherto unsuspected components in this heterogeneity.

The financial costs of chemotherapy can be formidable and in some situations even prohibitive when set against marginal benefits. But I think we can accept the view[4] that if the treatment proves effective, costs will eventually fall to acceptable levels. It is a current problem but it has to be seen in the perspective of a long time span and against the cost advantages of successful treatment.

Toxicity is another matter. Once we move from

From the Department of Medical Oncology, Charing Cross Hospital, London, England.
Reprinted from Cancer Clinical Trials 1: 135–138, 1978.

the therapy of detectable disease to the therapy of undetectable disease, we accept that toxicity is being inflicted on all the members of a group for the potential benefit of a subset of the group. It is appropriate for the physician to ask whether he or she would submit to the toxicity likely to be incurred for the benefits which can be realistically, not optimistically, expected. The toxicity spectrum includes myocardial damage from adriamycin and includes death. Death from drug toxicity is always unexpected.

Second cancers occurring many years later are acceptable if metastatic disease were present at the time chemotherapy was given but are a high penalty if it were not. De Vita[4] has asserted that it is not a question whether second tumors occur so much as how many occur; and this will take decades to answer fully.

Perhaps the most common and least discussed penalty is the period of medication itself. If prolonged disease-free survival is to be scored as one of the benefits of adjuvant chemotherapy, we need some measure of the penalty of medication. To the physician, detectable disease may be an index of therapeutic failure, but for the patient an asymptomatic secondary in the lung or liver may be preferable to a bald head and a sore mouth. Although the quality of life in periods of medication, in periods of detectable but asymptomatic disease and in periods of symptomatic disease are not easy to assess, failure to attempt this is liable to lead, if not to delusions of grandeur, at least to its oncological equivalent, delusions of success. If we measure disease-free survival as an index of success, shouldn't we also measure medication-free survival?

To look briefly at the field of adjuvant therapy trials inevitably does them, and the problems they attempt to solve, less than justice. But it is appropriate to do so here and I hope that my somewhat cavalier summary is not wildly at variance with the most recent evidence.

In breast cancer there is evidence that both single-agent[7] and multiagent therapy[2] are producing a modest extension of disease-free survival and a modest increase in percentage surviving in premenopausal subjects, especially in those with one to three nodes positive and to a lesser extent in postmenopausal subjects with four or more nodes positive, compared with conventionally treated controls. The possibility that the drugs work in

premenopausal women through ovarian ablation has not been fully excluded but seems to be unlikely to be the case.[14] In Hodgkin's disease at stage I–III, recent evidence[11,13] confirms earlier reports of the value of therapy in the adjuvant role. In Wilm's tumor and rhabdomyosarcoma, adequately controlled trials have established the value of adjuvant therapy.[17] When one turns to other tumors, the situation is less satisfactory either because the results of adjuvant therapy so far have been disappointing or because of the way the trials have been conducted. It seems very likely[12] that adjuvant therapy is capable of altering prognosis in osteosarcoma of the limbs but the use of historical controls leaves some doubt in the situation. Even so, the question whether untreated controls in this disease can be accepted is now debatable. In colorectal cancer some perceive advantages in the results so far reported,[4] whereas others[3,8] remain uncommitted. In lung cancer,[9] the importance of histological type has emerged in recent years and, at least for the small cell type, chemotherapy is emerging as the primary therapy. Elsewhere, and notably for melanoma, evidence of benefit from adjuvant chemotherapy has yet to emerge.

It seems clear that adjuvant chemotherapy is falling far short of the highest hopes which some set for it but it is not failing altogether. Obviously the limitation is the relative ineffectiveness of present agents against the most common cancers. Treatment that lives up to expectations does not seem to demand rationale; it is only when expectations are not met that we look more closely at the mechanisms. Therefore, it is legitimate and timely to ask what might be expected of present agents in the adjuvant context.

Schabel[16] has drawn on murine tumor models to show that the biggest single factor in risk of micrometastatic disease is the presurgical bulk of tumor. His emphasis has also been on experience from those models which indicate that small cell populations are more susceptible than large populations. Evidence from marker-bearing human tumors such as choriocarcinoma is consistent with the view that small populations are more amenable than large ones, but the rate of response does not appear to be fundamentally different.

Schabel also suggests that small tumors may respond to agents which are ineffective against large populations of the same type. This evidence is in apparent conflict with the view that only agents of known cytoreductive potential should be used, although this conflict draws our attention to the question of what we mean by an effective agent. Logically, it should perhaps be one that reduces the rate of growth of the tumor cell population rather than one which produces a net reduction in tumor volume which is the usual criteria. Nevertheless, the trials that have been instituted have relied on drugs that have been demonstrated to be capable of inducing at least partial remissions in the corresponding clinically detectable disease.

Salmon[15] pointed to the importance of the stem cells in the tumor population as being critically important both in terms of cell numbers and in terms of mean doubling time. He suggests that something of the order of $< 10^4$ cells, remaining after surgery, is a possibility for eradication by adjuvant therapy. This would seem to be the order of magnitude for breast cancer cells that could be eliminated, although my estimate would be of the order of 10^3 cells, and even this may be too high a figure for, say, colorectal cancer and many others.

If we accept such a figure, we need to known what proportion of postsurgical patients have fewer than 10^4 cells and what proportion have more. The former patients are potentially curable. Given that up to 4 log cytoreduction might be obtained with a series of courses of therapy, the effects on the disease-free survival curves and on the survival curves would be crudely predictable. A small percentage would be expected to be cured. The remainder would be expected to have somewhat longer disease-free survival but not necessarily prolonged survival. Unfortunately, the number of patients who have micrometastatic cell numbers within the range susceptible to present agents is likely to be small.

The results obtained so far are, I think, consistent with what might be expected from these considerations. The potential to achieve eradication depends on making full use of the drugs and reduction in dosage or extension of the interval between courses in the interests of sparing toxicity are likely to result in fewer eradications of residual disease. On the other hand, it can be argued that since the maximum impact of cytotoxic agents occurs in the early months of treatment of tumors such as choriocarcinoma and malignant teratoma, where precise observations can be made, if eradication is going to be achieved it seems likely that it will be done then. I suggest that prolonged adjuvant therapy beyond 6 months would be hard to justify on present evidence and the worst of both worlds would seem to be suboptimal dosage given for a prolonged period.

Improved results can be reasonably anticipated from the use of better drug combinations but ultimately, as with treatment of overt disease, we are dependent on more effective agents. We should not precipitate our own disillusionment by having unrealistic expectations about what might be achieved with present-day agents in a cytotoxic role.

References

1. Bonadonna, G., Brusamolino, E., Valagussa, P., et al.: Combination chemotherapy as an adjuvant treatment in operable breast cancer. *N Engl J Med 294: 406–410, 1976.*

2. Bonadonna, G., Rossi, A., Valagussa, P., Banfi, A., and Veronesi, U.: Adjuvant chemotherapy with CMF in breast cancer with positive axillary nodes. In *Adjuvant Therapy of Cancer*, S. E. Salmon and S. E. Jones, Eds. North Holland Publishing Co., Amsterdam, 1977, pp. 83–94.

3. Carter, S. K.: Correlation of chemotherapy activity in advanced disease with adjuvant results. In *Adjuvant Therapy of Cancer*, S. E. Salmon and S. E. Jones, Eds. North Holland Publishing Co., Amsterdam, 1977, pp. 586–596.

4. De Vita, V. T.: Adjuvant therapy—An overview. In *Adjuvant Therapy of Cancer*, S. E. Salmon, and S. E. Jones, Eds. North Holland Publishing Co., Amsterdam, 1977 pp. 613–641.

5. Fisher, B., Carbone, P., Economon, S. G., et al.: L-Phenylalanine mustard (L-PAM) in the management of primary breast cancer. A report of early findings. *N Engl J Med 292: 117–122, 1975.*

6. Fisher, B., Ravdin, R. G., Ausman, R. K., et al.: Surgical adjuvant chemotherapy in cancer of the breast. Result of a decade of co-operative investigation. *Ann Surg 168: 337–356, 1968.*

7. Fisher B., and Rodmond, C.: Studies of the National Surgical Adjuvant Breast Project (NSABP). In *Adjuvant Therapy of Cancer*, S. E. Salmon and S. E. Jones, Eds. North Holland Publishing Co., Amsterdam, 1977, pp. 67–81.

8. Higgins, G. A., Humphrey, E., Juler, G. L., Le Veen, H. H., McGaughan, J., and Keehn, R. J.: Adjuvant chemotherapy in the surgical management of large bowel cancer. *Cancer 38: 1461–1467, 1976.*

9. Legha, S. S., Muggia, F. M., and Carter, S. K.: Adjuvant chemotherapy in lung cancer. *Cancer 39: 1415–1424, 1977.*

10. Long, R. L., Donegan, W. L., and Evans, A. M.: Extended surgical adjuvant chemotherapy for breast cancer. *Am J Surg 117: 701–704, 1969.*

11. Mathé, G., Tubianna, M., and Hayat, M.: Adjuvant

chemotherapy after radiotherapy in stage I and II Hodgkin's disease. In *Adjuvant Therapy of Cancer*, S. E. Salmon and S. E. Jones, Eds. North Holland Publishing Co., Amsterdam, 1977, pp. 517–528.

12. Pratt, C., Shanks, E., Hustu, D., et al.: Adjuvant multiple drug chemotherapy for osteosarcoma of the extremity. *Cancer 39: 51–57, 1977.*

13. Rosenberg, S. A., Kaplan, H. S., Glatstein, E., and Portlock, C. S.: The role of adjuvant MOPP in the radiation therapy of Hodgkin's disease: A progress report after eight years in the Stanford Trials. In *Adjuvant Therapy of Cancer*, S. E. Salmon and S. E. Jones, Eds. North Holland Publishing Co., Amsterdam, 1977, pp. 505–515.

14. Rubens, R. D., Bulbrook, R. D., Wang, D. Y., Knight, R. K., Hayward, J. L., Bush, H., George, D., Crowther, D., and Sellwood, R. A.: The effect of adjuvant che-

motherapy on endocrine function in patients with operable breast cancer. In *Adjuvant Therapy of Cancer*, S. E. Salmon and S. E. Jones, Eds. North Holland Publishing Co., Amsterdam, 1977, pp. 101–107.

15. Salmon, S. E.: Kinetic rationale for adjuvant chemotherapy of cancer. In *Adjuvant Therapy of Cancer*, S. E. Salmon and S. E. Jones, Eds. North Holland Publishing Co., Amsterdam, 1977, pp. 15–28.

16. Schabel, F. M.: Surgical adjuvant chemotherapy of metastatic murine tumors. *Cancer 40: 558–568, 1977.*

17. Sutow, W. W.: Adjuvant therapy in Wilm's tumor, rhabdomyosarcoma, osteosarcoma and other childhood neoplasms. An overview. In *Adjuvant Therapy of Cancer*, S. E. Salmon and S. E. Jones, Eds. North Holland Publishing Co., Amsterdam, 1977, pp. 345–356.

6

Clinical trials in cancer: General concepts and methodologies

Franco M. Muggia, M.D.

Major developments in therapeutic trials followed the early successes with chemotherapy in choriocarcinoma and the hematologic malignancies. During the 1950s and 1960s the National Cancer Institute established a chemotherapy program to develop and evaluate new anticancer agents. Shortly thereafter, a number of intramural and extramural clinical studies were launched to test new therapies. Although many of the tools were available for extending these trials to other malignancies, for many years the compartmentalization of medicine and the widespread notion that drugs were unlikely to cure cancer delayed the performance of therapeutic experiments needed to test and achieve this goal.[2]

I will discuss the phases of clinical trial involved in the study of a new treatment and describe the pertinent methodologies that we employ. I hope to leave you with the concept that well-designed therapeutic trials represent experiments performed at the bedside that will allow the testing of solidly based therapeutic hypotheses. Like any other scientific experiments, they are expected to answer specific questions but often lead to the generation of new hypotheses.[1]

The initial study has the major objective of establishing the tolerance of a schedule at increasing doses and provides the basis for selecting a mode of administration in the second phase of trial. It is often coupled with an initial pharmacologic evaluation. The Division of Cancer Treatment has de-

fined the second phase trial as a "screen" for efficacy against a variety of tumors. These initial trials provide the information on which to base the "pass, fail or hold" policy necessary before conducting more extended studies. Subsequently, the value of the agent in the treatment of a specific malignancy is defined relative to other treatments using concurrent or historical controls. After activity is identified, drugs are usually incorporated into combination regimens and pilot studies are carried out to define patient tolerance and seek any preliminary encouraging activity. The optimal treatment may then be tested in a combined modality study. In this instance, the overall treatment strategy, rather than a specific treatment regimen, is under consideration since the actual antitumor effect may be a composite of local therapy and systemic adjuvant treatment.

Combination chemotherapy deserves an additional comment in this scheme of treatment evaluation. The incorporation of drugs into combination regimens has been strictly empiric, based primarily on the activity of each drug alone and the pattern of toxicity (Table 1). Antitumor activity, convincingly demonstrated with large numbers of patients and reproducible in different studies, has justified the incorporation of an agent into a combination with other active drugs. In addition, minimizing of overlapping toxicities and the ability to deliver high doses of individual drugs in intermittent regimens were most important in the original design of successful combinations like MOPP, COP, and CMF. In the future, as more active drugs are identified, their incorporation into combinations might be based on: *a*) the degree of activity relative to other drug regimens; *b*) whether the drug is a new chemical entity, with a new mechanism of action, or is an analog possessing

From the Office of the Cancer Therapy Evaluation Program, Division of Cancer Treatment, National Cancer Institute, Bethesda, Maryland.

Reprinted from Cancer Clinical Trials 1: 139–144, 1978.

TABLE 1

Incorporation of Drugs into Combination Therapy

Usual Criteria
1. Drug activity as single agent
2. Minimal overlapping toxicity
3. Different mechanism of action

Additional Criteria
1. Less toxic analog of active drug
2. Strategy requires secondary combination
3. Preclinical, biochemical, pharmacologic
   rationales

advantages for combination over the parent; c) whether the treatment strategy includes a need for new combinations to supplement a primary treatment combination; and d) various considerations arising from other biochemical, preclinical, or pharmacologic rationales.

Clinical trial methodology

The methodology of phase II trials requires particular attention because the data obtained influence all subsequent strategies in testing a new treatment. However, it should be stressed that the initial "screen" for efficacy provides only one answer, i.e., a *pass* calling for subsequent studies, a *fail* discouraging further trial, or a *hold* when no decision can be reached and additional phase II and III testing is required. Randomization is often included in these trials to improve the ability to reach this decision and *not* necessarily to provide comparative data on efficacy. The methodology for comparative studies is quite similar, but emphasizes different statistical considerations and additional study endpoints such as duration of response and patient survival.

In the last few years, phase II trials have employed protocols designed to evaluate the activity of a drug regimen against a *specific* tumor. Hopefully, increasing reliance on these "disease-specific" protocols will overcome some of the shortcomings of the "broad" phase II studies of the late 1950s and 1960s. The latter will still be useful to encourage studies in rare tumors. However, in these early trials, inconclusive determinations of the activity of a drug against many tumor types often resulted from giving the drug to a large number and variety of patients with advanced cancer. Although they were true screens for drug efficacy,

some of these studies prematurely discouraged interest in a new drug or perpetuated use of an agent based on questionable results. Examples of inadequate evaluation are numerous. For example, few tumors were studied with glutamine antagonists, which are now being reinvestigated. Screening for drug activity in certain diseases was totally neglected. In ovarian cancer, alkylating agents and drug combinations assembled from experience with other neoplasms were repeatedly employed as treatment with little attempt to determine their relative efficacy. Since 1972, phase II trials targetted specifically to evaluate drug activity in ovarian cancer have led to the identification of efficacious nonalkylating drugs, including *cis*-diaminedichloroplatinum, hexamethylmelamine, 5-fluorouracil, and adriamycin. Drug combinations based on these agents are finally proving superior to treatment with mustard derivatives, with growing expectation of a curvative potential.

Each type of malignancy poses unique problems in the assessment of drug activity. These problems vary as more is learned about a disease, as staging and diagnostic procedures are developed, and as new therapeutic strategies are introduced. The following review of general concepts used in the evaluation of "efficacy" trials will further illustrate these complex problems.

Study design

Gehan, in 1961, first stressed that the determination of chemotherapeutic activity against a certain malignancy requires an adequate sample for study. If one wishes to reject a new drug having <20% true therapeutic effectiveness, an observation of no responses among 14 consecutive patients would allow rejection with a probability of error (false negative) of <0.05. These statistical considerations were partly responsible for introducing disease-specific studies to replace broad phase II studies. It should be noted, however, that such considerations apply to homogeneous populations and that patients with "signal" tumors suitable for such trials are hardly ever homogeneous in terms of important prognostic factors such as prior therapy, performance status, histologic type, site of metastatic disease, etc. Statistical considerations of sample size must therefore be adjusted according to the importance of the prognostic variables. For example, it is generally agreed that separate phase

II studies are necessary for small cell carcinoma of the lung, and, conceivably, a study entering a few patients with each of the non-small cell types will yield inadequate answers.

Various designs are used for these studies. Randomization may be employed to ensure a comparable patient entry into two new different drug regimens. Dynamic randomization procedures can be included to increase patient entry when responses are reported. Comparison with a standard regimen has been favored to safeguard against discarding drugs as "inactive" because of the unconscious inclusion of patients with exceptionally poor outlook. However, this design is attractive only when standard regimens are in themselves only slightly active. Unfortunately, no study design excludes the possibility of "false negative" evaluation due to unknown factors such as cross-resistance with drugs that patients have previously received. This is becoming an increasingly difficult problem, since chemotherapy is incorporated more and more into standard treatment regimens.

Patient characteristics

Most trials include an estimate of performance status as originally described by Karnofsky[3] and later simplified by the Zubrod-ECOG scale.[5] Although this assessment of a patient's functional capabilities would appear to be quite crude, it has shown striking correlations with survival and even with response rates.

Other important patients characteristics include status of prior cytotoxic therapy, age grouping, site of metastatic disease, and the nature of the lesion being assessed for antitumor response (Table 2). These variables assume greater or lesser importance depending on the disease under study. For example, performance status and histologic cell type affect response rate, as well as survival, in patients with *lung cancer*. In *breast cancer* and *malignant melanoma*, the site of metastases has been recognized as an important variable. Age has been identified as a determinant of response rate in many trials with *acute leukemia*. The presence of measurable lesions may be indicative of a more advanced and unresponsive state in patients with *gastric* and *pancreatic* cancers. Finally, exposure to prior chemotherapy is a frequently invoked factor affecting the response rate in most neoplasms.

TABLE 2
Phase II Trials: Patient Characteristics

1.	Status of prior therapy
2.	Age grouping
3.	Performance status: 0–1, 2–3
4.	Site of disease: visceral, nonvisceral
5.	Indicator lesion: measurable, evaluable

Ethical considerations arise regarding the study of new antitumor agents in patients with advanced cancer who have not been treated with other drugs known to be "active." Since no chemotherapeutic agent is considered active in *pancreatic cancer*, use of an investigational drug as the first systemic approach to therapy should pose no dilemma and untreated patients should be preferentially entered into phase II studies. Conversely, established efficacy of combination chemotherapy regimens in patients with disseminated *breast cancer* leads to virtual exclusion of previously untreated patients from any study of the therapeutic potential of a new drug. Other clinical situations are not so clear-cut. In *colon cancer* or *malignant melanoma* the most effective systemic chemotherapy, although benefitting up to one-third of the patients, has not convincingly affected survival. Selection of the most favorable cases allows prompt recognition of drug efficacy while minimizing the number of patients exposed to the new treatment if it is ineffective. One must reemphasize that therapeutic intent is an axiomatic requirement of all clinical trials, including phase I. The patient is suitable for study because the protocol is considered to provide an optimal possibility for benefit. Ethical objections to this type of clinical investigation often overlook the fact that use of known ineffective standard therapies, or no treatment at all, poses an equal ethical dilemma. The best safeguard in facing these moral questions is understanding the scientific rationale for the new treatment, together with the circumstances for its use, and meeting the needs of the patient.

Definitions of response and duration of effects

Antitumor activity in man has been primarily defined by measuring objective tumor regression. Reproducible measurement of regression by physical examination or x-ray has correlated well

TABLE 3

Phase II Trials: Definitions of Response in Measurable (Bidimensional) Disease

Complete regression	(CR):	All disease
Partial regression (PR):		Decrease >50% products of diameter and perpendicular, sum all lesions[a]
Often interim reports indicate:		
Minor regression[b] (MR):		Decrease >25–49%
Stable disease[b]	(SD):	Decrease <25% or increase <25%

[a] Only within same system and similar access to measurement. To qualify, the definition must apply after two courses of treatment or 1 month.
[b] These should not be included in any category until they definitely qualify for PR, CR, or progression.

TABLE 4

Common Criteria for Treatment Failure

1. Appearance of new lesions
2. Progressive growth (>25% increase in area)
3. Severe toxicity with cumulative, irreversible or unpredictable manifestations
4. Death from disease, with or without toxicity[a]
5. Symptomatic deterioration, stable objective measurements[b]
6. Symptomatic deterioration, after partial response.[b]

[a] "Early death" should be defined if excluded from analysis.
[b] Must document decline in performance status or weight loss, or increase in specific symptoms, and exclude drug toxicity or other complications (not applicable until patient has received minimum prescribed course of therapy).

with symptomatic benefit, improvement in biochemical parameters, and extension of survival time in responding patients as compared to nonresponders. However, with the exception of hCG measurement in gestational choriocarcinoma, correlation with any one of these determinations is quite imperfect. Therefore, assessment of tumor regression has employed a vast number of methods and has been variably defined. At present, most investigators rely on a 50% reduction in the product of the two largest perpendicular diameters of a measurable tumor as an objective tumor regression (Table 3). Other major problems requiring attention include: *a*) the assessment of response when many organ systems are affected and many indicator lesions are present, *b*) extension of these definitions to conditions where bidimensional measurable tumors are rare, and *c*) incorporation of a time element into the data reporting. Not only do serial measurements made over a period of time confer greater accuracy to the measurements, but the kinetics of tumor growth or regression may have biologic implications requiring further study.

The overall definitions usually are applicable to one or more of the five possible categories used in evaluating tumor response, as modified from those of the Breast Cancer Task Force[1]: (I) bidimensional disease; (II) unidimensional disease (e.g., liver, mediastinum); (III) disease without discretely measurable criteria, where improvements must be discerned by photographs, scans, or x-rays; (IV) disease assessible only by serial chemistries, tumor markers, or nonspecific scan findings; and (V)

functional manifestation of disease amenable to quantitation. Phase II trials should include only patients having disease measurable by categories I and II. However, in conditions like prostatic carcinoma, criteria of response may have to include other categories because uni- or bidimensionally measurable disease is distinctly unusual. The reliability of these measurable findings decreases as one considers parameters that are less directly related to tumor manifestations.

It has been useful, particularly in studies of patients with malignant lymphoma and, more recently, with testicular, ovarian, and small cell lung cancers, to define complete regression (CR) as opposed to a partial regression (PR) where persistence of disease can be demonstrated after an arbitrary time of induction therapy. Some studies in these rapidly growing, responsive tumors indicate a very favorable survival curve for complete regressions, but minimal or no survival benefit for those with only partial responses.

Another key definition is that of *treatment failure*, which is not easily defined except when a new tumor appears. However, in many instances of progressive disease, one must rely on increases in tumor size or on other less definable changes (Table 4). Time to treatment failure may be a useful alternative to documentation of response in conditions such as prostatic cancer and various gastrointestinal malignancies where bidimensionally measurable tumors are rare.

Methods of assessing response and toxicity

The methods of assessing response are unique for each disease. As mentioned previously, measurements of bidimensional tumors are most reliable, followed by unidimensional measurements and by the less direct methods of assessing tumor regression. In some diseases, accurate assessment of response must await implementation of new diagnostic techniques and a reawakening of interest in surgical staging. Better diagnostic procedures will increase the accuracy of current studies and, most importantly, allow a determination of response in earlier and hopefully more responsive stages of disease. In addition, early detection of treatment failure, as may be accomplished by peritoneoscopy in ovarian cancer, will permit discontinuation of ineffective therapy before chances for other treatment are fully compromised.

An essential part of any trial is assessment of toxicity, which routinely includes hematologic and other biologic effects. Specialized studies may be required for nephrotoxicity, ototoxicity, neurotoxicity, and cardiopulmonary toxicities. In addition, an estimate of the severity of these acute manifestations and the complications that occurred are important in the interpretation of results. A numerical scale from *0 to 4* is often used with *1* representing mild, *2* moderate, and *3* severe toxicity. Classification *4* is reserved for severe toxicity associated with a complication. Chronic organ dysfunction and complications, such as secondary neoplasias, also assume an increasingly greater importance in trials associated with prolonged survival.

Reporting format

A report of a clinical trial should include all the items discussed above. Breakdown of the results in terms of pertinent prognostic factors, such as prior therapy, is needed. The methods of assessment and the category of indicator lesions should be stated. The number of patients entered and the number declared evaluable should be reported. Reasons for excluding patients from the trial must be described. Under each category of response, the individual duration is expressed in months from the onset of treatment.

Reporting of toxicity should include, as a minimum, the nadirs of white cell or ganulocyte counts and platelet counts, as well as the total number of patients experiencing such hematologic toxicity. In addition, all other severe toxicities should also be reported.

The actuarial or life-table method is preferred for reporting the survival experience of groups of patients. The most appropriate zero time for calculations is the date of onset of treatment. Crude survival should be used with small numbers of patients, and with rapidly growing tumors and short trials. The median survival is often used to summarize the experience of a group of patients. This may be appropriate when the majority of the group has reached the 50% mark. Its principal usefulness is to give a rough estimate of a curve, but it is inappropriate as a comparison of two therapies.

In adjuvant studies, or in studies that are following patients in complete remission, the most important measurement is disease-free survival. This endpoint, like survival, is plotted by the actuarial method. Such a determination may provide a better assessment of the efficacy of an adjuvant treatment than would survival, because secondary cures may be achieved by other treatment after relapse; for example, in osteogenic sarcoma salvage may occur from resection of pulmonary metastases rather than from the adjuvant treatment itself.[4]

Conclusions

The last three decades have seen the birth and implementation of antitumor chemotherapy, first in advanced disease trials and more recently in combined modality approaches at earlier stages of disease. Clinical trials, initially exclusively concerned with advanced disease, have increasingly dealt with the integration of chemotherapy with irradiation or surgery. These studies have forced a reevaluation of long held concepts of local therapy; indeed, it is surprising that since the Halsted radical mastectomy was introduced, the extent of surgery needed, even following very early detection of the tumor, was never questioned.[1] As two or more therapeutic modalities are combined, a multiplicity of questions arise that require answers through carefully monitored therapeutic trials. Hence, there has been a recent growth of this type of studies. I have described some of the ingredients necessary for successful clinical trials and their proper interpretation.

In summary, the introduction of antitumor chemotherapy has been followed closely by the development of methodology for prospectively evaluating new treatments in man. Not only has the efficacy of chemotherapy been demonstrated, and the concept of cure by drugs been established, but also other treatment modalities can now be prospectively evaluated.

Clinical trials are not to be considered solely as the clinical testing of a new treatment which has been developed in the laboratory, but also constitute experiments to provide the answers to a hypothesis. Concepts such as combination chemotherapy, the presence of pharmacologic sanctuaries, adjuvant chemotherapy of micrometastases, induction-consolidation and maintenance, late intensification, and fixed crossover to noncross-resistant combinations have all arisen as hypotheses for testing in clinical trials.

References

1. *Breast Cancer: Suggested Protocol Guidelines for Combination Chemotherapy Trials and for Combined Modality Trials.* Breast Cancer Task Force Treatment Committee, National Cancer Institute. DHEW Publication No. (NIH) 77-1142.

2. DeVita, V. T., Jr.: The evolution of therapeutic research in cancer. *New Engl J Med 298: 907–910, 1978.*

3. Karnofsky, D. A., Abelmann, W. H., Craver, L. F. and Burchenal, J. H.: The use of the nitrogen mustards in the palliative treatment of carcinoma with particular reference to bronchogenic carcinoma. *Cancer 1: 634–656, 1948.*

4. Muggia, F. M., and Louie, A. C.: Five years of adjuvant treatment of osteosarcoma: More questions than answers. *Cancer Treat Rep 62: 301–305, 1978.*

5. Zubrod, C. G., Schneiderman, M., Frei, E., III, et al.: Appraisal of methods for the study of chemotherapy of cancer in man: Comparative therapeutic trial of nitrogen mustard and triethylene thiophosphoramide. *J Chron Dis 11: 7–33, 1960.*

Introduction

7

L. Gimeno Alfós, M.D.

The treatment of lung cancer continues being a problem at the present time as it was 20 years ago, this, in spite of the fact that we are now beginning to make some progress, at least on a better understanding of histology, tumor kinetics, behavior, and therapeutic responses. In some countries, such as the United States and England-Wales, it is the primary cause of death from cancer. It has also showed an increase in Spain, representing a 12% of all cancers, second after breast cancer.

Smoking and lung cancer

Parallel to increased frequency there has been an escalation of the vice of cigarette smoking, which is being increasingly taken up by women. We shall soon reach figures in this country equal to the Anglo-Saxon countries, with 22% of all lung cancers corresponding to women. In this relationship between smoking and lung cancer, we have a history of 20 years to cover. However, factors other than tobacco must also be considered. It is an evident factor but in small cell undifferentiated lung cancer, it is less obvious as the only cause in adenocarcinoma and in large cell cancers. With regard to epidermoid cancer, there is a relationship between the incidence and intensity of smoking. However, with high intensity of smoking, the squamous form may possibly yield to redevelopment of small cell lung cancers. Urban air pollution, industrial exposure, and genetic predispositions have been suggested as contributory factors.

If we analyze the crude survival rate at 5 years of an institution 20 years ago, we find it was equal or less than 6% of all the patients. If we observe their survival in relation to the different types of therapy employed, in a monodimensional scale, we find that surgery was what contributed to a greater survival. Even at the present time, surgery alone constitutes the best way of overcoming lung cancer. The problem is that scarcely 25% of the patients who are seen in an institution can undergo radical operation, and out of this selected group, the best figures barely reach about 20% survival. Therefore, even today we are faced with this 5%–6% of the total survivals seen in an institution.

In the next chapter we will review pathology, staging, and prognostic factors in order to set up the basis for an integrated therapeutic approach which can be extended to patients not cured by surgery. Examples of such approaches are found in the subsequent papers.

Marqués del Puerto, 10, Bilbao-B., Spain.

Pathology, role of staging and prognostic factors

8

L. Gimeno Alfós, M.D.

A major problem in lung cancer is the fact that definitively we are making our diagnosis too late. Lung cancer, although unicentric and focal in its origin, has a tendency to rapid local invasion, and systemic generalization, variable in degree according to pathology. If we compare the number of cells in relation to the size and weight of tumors, we see that the tumor of 1 cm diameter (which is when it can be visible radiographically) represents an enormously large cell number, in fact 10^9. Although this diameter of 1 cm seems to be small, still the quantity of cells represents a very high number. Even in this form of state, depending upon its dynamic pattern, there will have been a spreading of cells to the regional lymphatics and to the distant areas. This explains the tendency toward metastases of the lung cancer, which depends on histopathology, and let us say, on its growth characteristics or dynamic pattern. We should conceive this tumor, when we confront it today, not only as a loco-regional tumor, but also as a tumor with systemic projections.

Prognostic variables

Next, we summarize the main prognostic variables in lung cancer, which are conditioning in one way or another the survival and therapeutic response in this particular type of tumor. These are:

1) Histology
2) Dynamic pattern
3) Stage (extent of disease)
4) Performance status
5) Age
6) Weight loss (>6% of body weight)

7) Central nervous system (CNS) involvement
8) Immunologic status of host

Briefly, we shall review some of the aspects of these prognostic variables along this paper.

Histology, nomenclature and natural history

Throughout this section on lung cancer, we shall deal with the possibilities of the different types of therapy: surgery, radiotherapy, chemotherapy, and immunotherapy, in order to potentiate the loco-regional therapeutic response. In the possible control of the disease and the establishment of an "integrated therapy," I have said that there is a different pattern of loco-regional invasion and systemic generalization in relation to the histopathology.

Today we admit that probably we are dealing with three cancerous diseases of the lung, distinguished by the different histopathologies. We endorse the World Health Organization's classification (Table 1), observing[1] that the various pathological types have different biological and dynamic characteristic, manifested by differing rates and pattern of metastases, and varying sensitivity to cytotoxic agents either physical (radiation) or chemicals. Each has a characteristic incidence and survival statistics as well.

a) Squamous cell (epidermoid) carcinoma. Whether well or poorly differentiated, this is the most common histologic type of lung cancer (40–60%); overall, it has also the most favorable prognosis. These tumors tend to arise centrally in the surface epithelium of lobar, segmental, or subsegmental bronchi. Here the cancer apparently remains localized for a long time; thus efforts at early diagnosis could be of value; roentgen detection, however, is often delayed until pneumonia,

Marqués del Puerto, 10, Bilbao-B., Spain.

TABLE 1

WHO Classification of Lung Cancer[1]

I. Squamous cell Carcinoma
II. Small cell anaplastic carcinoma
   1. Fusiform
   2. Polygonal
   3. Lymphocyte-like (oat-cell)
   4. Others
III. Adenocarcinoma
   1. Bronchogenic
     a. Acinar
     b. Papillary
   2. Bronchio-alveolar
IV. Large cell carcinoma
   1. Solid tumors with mucin
   2. Solid tumors without mucin
   3. Giant cell
   4. Clear cell

atelectasia, or air-trapping distal is associated with the tumor. Extension of tumor generally occurs along and through the bronchus to regional lymphonodes. The relatively favorable prognosis for patients with epidermoid carcinoma are attributed to the lower indicende of regional lymph node and distant metastases at the time of diagnosis than in other histologic types.

b) Small cell anaplastic carcinoma group. The second most common histologic type of primary lung cancer (25–35%) bears some similarity to lymphoma in its histologic appearance, as well as in its associated lymphadenopathy, early systemic involvement, and relative radio- and chemo-sensitivity. Submucosal, lymphatic, and vascular invasion are common; widespread dissemination is generally present at the time of diagnosis, and survival is poor regardless of apparent stage. Polypeptide hormones, normally secreted by argentaffin ectodermal precursor cells, are frequently elaborated by these tumors, and cause ectopic hormonal syndromes.

c) Adenocarcinoma. Here we also include the bronchio-alveolar form, represents the third most common histologic type (10–25%). These tumors tend to occur in the lung periphery, and to extend submucosally in the bronchus, spreading generally very early, and are notoriously difficult to cure by local treatment. Broncho-alveolar carcinoma occurs in the lung periphery, especially in the vicinity of scars, as sheets of highly differentiated columnar cells that grow in the air spaces of the lung, using the alveolar walls as scaffolding. Submucosal, endobronchial, endolymphatic, and early hematogenous spread are common. This form of cancer may present in the form of solitary peripheral nodules, the so-called "coin-lesion."

d) Finally we have the *large cell undifferentiated carcinoma*, the fourth most common type of primary lung cancer (about 10%), where we have subvarieties: solid tumor with mucin and without mucin, giant cell, and clear cell tumors. They have many similarities to adenocarcinoma, occurring in the lung periphery and survival by stage is often similar to that for adenocarcinoma.

In relation to the natural history offered by the histological groups, we can think that the epidermoid is the tumor which has got the least systemic tendency, while the adenocarcinoma and the carcinoma of the large cells are similar with high loco-regional and systemic aggressiveness. And finally, there is carcinoma of the small cells, which is anaplastic and has got a "*sui generis*" personality, similar to systemic tumors, such as infantile tumors and lymphomas, with a great tendency to generalization, almost from the moment that the patient has been diagnosed.

These histopathological divisions, which show the possibility that we are contemplating three different aspects of one and the same disease, are, likely the expression of the morphological variation of different dynamic patterns.

Extensive growth characteristics of human tumors have been published by Malaise and coworkers, and others.[2,3] If we look at the figures of the different kinetic parameters, we see that the groups of lymphomas and embryonal tumors, with growth fractions of 90% and with a doubling time of 27–28 days, most resemble some small cell tumors (with a mean doubling time of 33 days). The epidermoid or squamous-cell cancers show growth fractions of about 25% and a mean doubling time of 58 days; specifically in the case of lung cancer, a mean of 103 days has been reported.[2] The adenocarcinoma has a very low growth fraction of 6% and a very long doubling time of 83 days, being in the case of lung cancer even longer with a mean value of 187 days. We can infer from these studies that there are differences in growth patterns between the small cell anaplastic cancers, the epidermoids, and the gorup of the adenocarcinomas.

We can conceive three dynamic patterns or

categories of lung cancer: fast (small cell), medium (epidermoid), and slow (adenocarcinoma), based on its kinetic parameters. There may be conditioning of their natural history and therapeutic responses. In general the worst symptoms occur in patients with tumors with the most rapid doubling-times ("fast tumors"), such as the small cell carcinoma, which is rarely resected, has the fastest doubling time and the poorest prognosis untreated. The implication is clear that patients with more rapidly growing tumors do worse and are usually smaller than tumors with slower doubling times ("slow tumors": adenocarcinoma) when initially found. Slower growing tumors infer a better prognosis, but rapid growth, as in small cell carcinoma, may infer a greater responsiveness to non-surgical therapy.

On the other hand, there is a good correlation between sensitivity to cytotoxic agents (radiation and chemicals) and dynamic pattern. Breur[4] has related the radiosensitivity of human tumors of doubling times; there was a strong correlation between a low D_{37} and a short doubling time (DT); patients, in general, who had embryonal tumors had the lowest D_{37}. This approach is interesting and may be applicable to the calculation of cell kill. These studies suggest that accurate dose response calculations in human cancer is possible if kinetic determinations become more sophisticated than doubling-time measurements. The value of measuring DTs is clear, and yet it is a crude parameter

at best, but it tells us nothing about rates of proliferation and death of cells and response to treatments of cell subpopulations.

Human studies to ascertain cell cycle times using classic radioautographic means have been few; some studies have been performed on tumors of patients that were previously evaluated for doubling times. These studies have necessitated injection of the labeled tritiated thymidine (3 HTdR), into patients intravenously or intralesionally, and, of necessity, most patients studied have had readily accessible metastatic lesions. Therefore, cell cycle calculations of skin metastases alone for solid tumors, such as in lung cancer, may not be sufficient as a basis to plan treatment designs. Radioautography is a time-consuming process and requires a substantial delay between biopsy and completion of kinetics determinations. Moreover, with the methods presently available, the technical and ethical problems are such that only a few tumors can be studied.

In relation to that concept, we have reported a clinical approach[5] over 200 tumoral cases, that have been studied with Gallium-67, and the uptake pattern assessed by gamma camera. (Table 2). Cases were grouped by their dynamic pattern: systemic (leukemia), systemic-like (lymphoma and embryonal tumors), localized solid (carcinomas) and intermediates (melanoma, sarcoma, and adenocarcinoma). Positive scintigraphy was consistent with tumors of high proliferative rate and great

TABLE 2

^{67}Gallium Uptake and Dynamic Pattern

Tumor Character	Histology	Labeling[a] Index (%)	Growth[a] Fraction (%)	Location	Cases	^{67}Gallium Uptake Positive No.	%	^{67}Gallium Uptake Negative No.	%
Systemic	Acute leukemia		93/20		2	—	—	2	—
Systemoid	Embryonic	30	90	Primary	12	12	100	—	—
	Lymphoma	29	90	All stages	63	62	98.4	1	1.6
Solid	Carcinoma	8.3	25	Lung primary	22	13	59.0	9	40.9
				Lung metastases	14	9	64.2	5	35.7
				Breast	15	4	26.6	11	73.3
				Head and neck	35	19	54.2	16	45.7
				Abdomen pelvis	19	10	52.6	9	47.3
Intermediate	Melanoma	5.1	25	Lung metastases	6	5	83.3	1	16.6
	Sarcoma	3.8	11	Lung metastases	8	5	62.5	3	37.5
	Adenocarcinoma (gastrointestinal)	2.1	6	Primary	4	1	25.0	3	75.0
Total					200				

[a] Literature results.[2]

growth fraction, showing evidence of a relationship between degree of positiveness and proliferation. A higher incidence of negative scintigraphy has been observed in tumors with low proliferative rate and small growth fraction, as well in those with cumulative dynamic pattern and with higher cell loss. Negative scintigraphy was evident after cytotoxic treatment (radio and chemotherapeutic) in tumors of high proliferative rate, and in relation with the depression of the proliferative compartment. Our studies support the hypothesis that gallium incorporation in tissues is related to, if not dependent on, partly with the size of the proliferative compartment. In the lung cancer group the figure of 59% positives is constituted mainly by the anaplastics (10 small cell, 1 large cell, and 2 undifferentiated epidermoids, with none of the anaplastics in the negative group). If we look at the upper limit of Table 2, where we have the systemic tumors, such as lymphomas and embryonal tumors, then we see that they reach values of positivity of 100% and 98.4%. This brings it to about the same positivity rate for small cell cancers.

Staging

These apparently dynamic differences must be considered in relation to the natural history and the prognostic implications of stage. When we analyze the mediastinic extension of each type, differences exist on the loco-regional dominant tendency when this is evaluated by means of mediastinoscopy (Goldberg, et al.[6]). In the epidermoid, mediastinal spread is found in only 16%, and dominantly ipsilateral (70%). Evidence of mediastinal tumor and lymph node involvement is documented in over 65% of patients with each other categories of tumor histology; furthermore, the pattern of bilateral mediastinal involvement was more evident in patients with all other tumor types compared to those with well-differentiated squamous cell carcinoma. It seems apparent that the degrees of differentiation represented by the four histological groups does indeed suggest a different biologic character, conditioning a different loco-regional aggressiveness.

If we study the production of metastasis, information on disease distribution at onset can be obtained by analyzing series of patients with inoperable disease. In patients with extensive (nonregional) lung cancer, deemed inoperable at time of diagnosis, the epidermoid shows a metastatizing tendency to liver (8%) and bone (16%) much lower than small cell carcinoma (40% and 72%, respectively), also being superior in brain, thorax, and skin (20%, 36%, and 36% versus 8%, 20%, and 16%).[7] Systemic involvement at clinical presentation may be approximated from studies showing extent of involvement in patients dying shortly after lung resection (Matthews, et al.)[8]; 35% of patients of such study had persistent disease at autopsy, whereas, in epidermoid cancer, persistent disease was found in 33% (distant metastasis and local disease occurring in equal numbers), in small cell carcinoma and adenocarcinoma persistent disease was found more often (70% and 43%, respectively) and was only exceptionally localized to regional sites. The frequency of metastatic involvement at autopsy varies with histologic cell type, being in general most prevalent in small cell carcinoma and least in epidermoid carcinoma, with adenocarcinoma and large cell undifferentiated carcinoma showing an intermediate tendency to disseminate,[7,9] confirming the systemoid character with "fast" dynamic pattern of the small cell cancer.

On the other hand, if all patients with lung cancer at the time of diagnosis are included and studied with sensitive diagnostic procedures, distant metastasis should be detectable in at least one fourth of patients considered to have regional and localized disease only.[7] A systemic search for metastatic involvement in both operable and inoperable candidates, at time of diagnosis, is, consequently, mandatory.

Today, we most employ the classification used by the American Joint Committes for Cancer Staging and End Results Reporting, accordingly to the "Task Force on Carcinoma of the Lung" report.[10]

Patients with undifferentiated small cell carcinoma have such a poor prognosis regardless of the demonstrable anatomic extent of their cancer that a TNM classification is not meaningful at this time. This reiterates the opinion that the cases should be classified by cell type. However, the relationship between survival and anatomic extent is quite similar for the epidermoid, adeno, and large cell carcinomas, and, therefore, a single set of definitions of the various categories of T, N, and M has been developed. In fact, these have been grouped into a single set of stages (see below).

All patients should have a Clinical Classification.

Those patients having a thoracotomy should have, in addition, a Surgical Evaluative Classification; the additional information obtained by complete examination of the therapeutically resected specimen, plus all other available data, should be used to assign a Postsurgical Treatment Classification.

The data in this report are based on the Clinical Classification. Each case must be assigned the highest category of T, N, and M that describes the full extent of disease in that particular case.

T: Primary tumors

T0: No evidence of primary tumor.

Tx: Tumor proved by the presence of malignant cells in bronchopulmonary secretions but not visualized roentgenographically or bronchoscopically.

T1: A tumor that is 3.0 cm or less in greatest diameter surrounded by lung or visceral pleura and without evidence of invasion proximal to a lobar bronchus at bronchoscopy.

T2: A tumor more than 3.0 cm in greatest diameter, or a tumor of any size, which, with its associated atelectasis or obstructive penumonitis, extends to the hilar region. At bronchoscopy the proximal extent of demonstrable tumor must be at least 2.0 cm distal to the carina. Any associated atelectasis or obstructive pneumonitis must involve less than an entire lung, and there must be no pleural effusion.

T3: A tumor of any size with direct extension into an adjacent structure such as the chest wall, the disphragm, or the mediastinum and its contents; or demonstrable bronchoscopically to be less than 2.0 cm distal to the carina; any tumor associated with atelectasis or obstructive pneumonitis of an entire lung or pleural effusion.

N: Regional lymph notes

N0: No demonstrable metastases to regional lymph nodes.

N1: Metastases to lymph nodes in the ipsilateral hilar region (including direct extension).

N2: Metastases to lymph nodes in the mediastinum.

M: Distant metastases

M0: No distant metastases

M1: Distant metastases such as in scalene, cervical, or contralateral hilar lymph nodes, brain, bones, liver, etc.

Stage grouping in carcinoma of the lung

Occult carcinoma

Tx, N0, M0: An occult carcinoma with bronchopulmonary secretions containing malignant cells but without other evidence of the primary tumor or evidence of metastases to the regional lymph nodes or distant metastases.

Invasive carcinoma

Stage I: T1–N0–M0; T1–N1–M0. A tumor that can be classified T1 without any metastases or with metastases to the lymph nodes in the ipsilateral hilar region only, or a tumor that can be classified T2 without any metastases to nodes or distant metastases.

Stage II: T2–N1–M0. A tumor classified as T_2 with metastases to the lymph nodes in the ipsilateral hilar region only.

Stage III: T3 any N or M; N2 any T or M; M1 any T or N. Any tumor more extensive than T2, or any tumor with metastases to the lymph nodes in the mediastinum or with distant metastases.

The Clinical Classification should be based on the anatomic extension of the disease, detectable by the examinations prior to any treatment, including thoracotomy (medical history, physical examination, assessment of the patients respiratory function, routine and special radiology, bronchoscopy and esophagoscopy, mediastinoscopy and thoracoscopy, mediastinotomy and thoracentesis, including nuclear medicine studies and others used to demonstrate the presence of extrathoracic metastases). The problem for the evaluation of the loco-regional extension is complicated, since by means of radiology and bronchofibroscopy, we can establish the location of the primary tumor and even have parameters for the operability or nonoperability according to its situation more or less distant of the carina. Mediastinoscopy which can give us a picture of the loco-regional extension of the disease with biopsies; this, however, involves certain risks which can limit the routine application of this technique.

With regard to the systemic process and the

definition of M, we should examine all the organs that are usually affected by lung cancer, by using nuclear scanning techniues, sonography, computerized transmission–emission tomography and conventional radiology: 1) Detection of bone metastases, including bone marrow study, skeletal X-rays, and bone scanning. 2) Detection of central nervous system metastases: brain scanning, electroencephalography, spinal fluid examination, and even arteriography. 3) Detection of liver metastases by means of liver scanning, and even liver biopsy and peritoneoscopy, or laparotomy. 4) Detection of adrenal metastases by means of adrenal scanning and adrenal venography. 5) Detection of other metastatic sites (less frequent): retroperitoneal lymph nodes (Lymphangiography), kidneys (urography), and eye (fluorescein angiography).

The application of protocol to search for metastatic involvement and knowledge of useful procedures is likely to play a major role in optimizing the treatment of patients with lung cancer. The advances made in Hodgkin's disease suggest some applicability to lung cancer. The use of conventional radiology, sonography, computarized transmission tomography, and nuclear scanning techniques, including "negative defect" forms or "positive effect" ones with tumor-seeking markers ([67]Gallium, ^{111}In-Bleomycin, radiolabeled antitumor organo-metallic complexes, etc.) detected either gammagraphically or by computarized emission tomography, should be sufficiently exploited in this disease. Study with [67]Gallium is easy and comfortable to practice and it can show the dynamic pattern of lung cancer, in well-differentiated tumors, it is often negative.

The use of "*markers*" (hormones, fetal antigens, polyamines, and others), found to be produced by or in association with malignant cells, may aid in the delineation of genetic and biochemical changes that occur as cells undergo the malignant degeneration and in the detection of metastatic disease. In addition, marker substances may help describe growth characteristics of tumors and the estimation of tumor response to treatment and the rational timing of chemotherapy. These "markers" have significance to both the researcher and oncologists in the diagnosis and location of the cancer as well as in evaluation of all forms of treatment. They have not yet been integrated into staging.

The survival curves for patients with lung cancer give evidence, as stated before, that the prognosis is related to the extent of the disease (stage), and to the cell type. Survival rates at 2 years for lung cancer,[10] we see that in epidermoid carcinoma, in stage I, when it is operable, survival rate is 46.6%, going to 39.8% in stage II, also when within the limits of operability, and finally it dropping to 11.5% for stage III, figures which are superior to the adenocarcinoma, show a similar 45.9% for stage I, but are clearly inferior in stage II (14.3%) and in stage III (7.9%); large cell carcinoma shows similar figures that adenocarcinoma (42.8% for stage I, 12.9% for stage II, and 12.9% for stage III). Small cell carcinoma shows the poorest values, with 6.0% for stage I and 5.0% and 3.8% for stages II and III, confirming the opinion that any patiert with this cell type has a poor prognosis regardless of the TNM classification or the stage grouping.

Therapeutic implications

There are certain factors which depend upon the host and therapeutic inventions, and not only of the histology, primary site, state of involvement and dynamic pattern, such as age, sex, coexisting pathology, immunological deficiency. Dependent on treatment, the major causes of failure may be categorized as noncontrol of the primary tumor and loco-regional extent, noncontrol of metastatic systemic spread, host failure secondary to preexisting or iatrogenic factors, or any combination of these causes. Surgery can cure lung cancer in a substantial number of properly selected patients. However, we must understand the role and limitations of surgery, as a loco-regional tool. Radiotherapy is another loco-regional method of controlling local cancer of the lung, but less frequently than surgery. Chemotherapy for disseminated disease has been tried with limited success. The effect of chemotherapy, as an adjuvant treatment, is controversial. Immunotherapy has not still found its proper place, but exploration is on-going as adjuvant. We are still measuring response to systemic therapy in weeks, and, what is important nearly 90% of patients have disseminated disease at the time of presentation. If major therapeutic advances are to be made, we will have to find ways to optimize therapy. Nevertheless, the clinical value of integrated approaches has already been amply demonstrated,[11] and several attempts will be described in the subsequent papers.

Examples of integrated cancer therapy in 300

TABLE 3

Inoperable Lung Cancer. Radiotherapy versus Radiochemotherapy (1.962–1974)

L. G. ALFÓS, Hospital de Basurto, Bilbao, Spain (Historical Series)

Treatment	Mean Survival Time in Months			
	Epidermoid	Small Cell	Adenocarcinoma	Large Cell
No treatment	1.6	1.1	3.2	2.6
30 cases	(21)	(4)	(4)	(1)
1962–67				
RT[a] Alone	6.4	3.2	4.3	5.1
105 cases	(70)	(27)	(6)	(2)
1968				
RT + Mono − ChT[b]	4.6	2.2	2.3	—
15 cases	(8)	(4)	(3)	
1969–74				
RT + Poly − ChT	18.1	8.1	8.0	8.7
150 cases	(81)	(42)	(18)	(9)
Total	(180)	(77)	(31)	(12)
(300)				

[a] RT = Radiotherapy.

[b] ChT = Chemotherapy.

cases of inoperable cancer of the lung, treated between 1962–1974 ("historical series") are presented in Table 3, and assessed as a function of the "mean survival time" (MST) in three series: radiotherapy alone (1962–67: 105 cases); radiotherapy plus monochemotherapy (1967–68: 16 cases); and radiotherapy plus polychemotherapy (1969–74: 150 cases). Tele-cobaltherapy was always used, including the primary and mediastinal, and supraclavicular lymphatic drainages in continuity, up to 4000–5000 (mediastinum-primary) and 4000 rads in 5–4 weeks (5 fractions per week of 200 rads) respectively; positive supraclavicular fossa was boosted with 1000–1500 rads. Monochemotherapy was carried out with 5 fluoruracil daily, in intravenous flush preirradiation up to the dose of 4000 rads. Polychemotherapy was always intermittent by pulses and constituted by vinblastine + L-phenyl-alanine-mustard (L-PAM) + 5-fluorouracil (5-FU). Radiotherapy was given between an opening cycle (VBL + L-PAM + 5-FU) and another closing one (VBL + L-PAM), following thereafter with intermittent cycles for up to 3 years. The additive effect of chemotherapy has modified the radiation dose, reducing the mediastinum dose to 3500 rads; this "modifying dose factor" (MDF) leads to the concept of "radiotherapeutic chemoequivalent" (RCE) which intends to express in

RETs the chemotherapy effect. The "mean survival time" of the radio-polychemotherapy group is almost three times that of the other groups. These results encourage further exploration of combined approaches.

References

1. Kreyburg, L.: *Histological Typing of Lung Tumors.* World Health Organization, Geneva, 1967.

2. Malaise, E. P., Chavaudra, N., and Tubiana, M.: The relationship between growth rate, labelling index and histological type of human solid tumours. *Eur J Cancer 9: 305–312, 1973.*

3. Strauss, M. J.: The growth characteristics of lung cancer and its application to treatment design. *Sem Oncol 1 (3): 167–164, 1974.*

4. Breur, K.: Growth rate and radiosensitivity of human tumors. II. Radiosensitivity of human tumors. *Eur J Cancer 2: 173–188, 1966.*

5. Gimeno, Alfós, L., Curto, L. M., and Marcos, F. Deteccion del cancer por radionúclidos. *Gaceta Med Bilbao 72: 1076–1082, 1975.*

6. Goldberg, E. M., Shapiro, C. M., and Glicksman, A. S.: Mediastinoscopy for assessing mediastinal spread in clinical staging of lung carcinoma. *Sem Oncol 1(3): 205–215, 1974.*

7. Muggia, F. M., and Chervu, L. R.: Lung cancer: Diagnosis in metastatic sites. *Sem Oncol 1(3): 217–228, 1974.*

8. Matthews, M. J., Kanhouwa, S., Pickren, J. et al.: Frequency of residual and metastatic tumors in patients undergoing curative surgical resection for lung cancer. *Cancer Chemother Rep Part 34: 63–67, 1973.*

9. Selawry, O. S., and Hansen, H. H.: Lung Cancer. In *Cancer Medicine*, J. F. Holland and E. Frei III, Eds.

Philadelphia, Lea & Febiger, 1973, pp. 1473–1518.

10. Carr, D. T., and Mountain, C. F.: The stagings of lung cancer. *Sem Oncol 1(3): 229–234, 1974.*

11. Johnson, R. E.: Symposium Theme: A conceptual approach to integrated cancer therapy. *Cancer 35: 1–4, 1975.*

Results of surgical therapy for lung carcinoma

F. Paris

with the collaboration of J. Padilla, V. Tarazona, E. Blasco, A. Canto, J. Pastor, and A. G. Zarza

A SERIES OF 300 PULMONARY RESECTIONS in patients with lung carcinoma is presented. Total survival rate of the series since the operation, including surgical mortality, was 33% at 3 years and 24% at 5 years.

The survival rate and surgical criteria were correlated, having better results when standard surgery was performed. The authors emphasize that the surgical figures of the series are of great value as the surgical indications were large and nonselective, with 85% of resectability in the thoracotomies.

This is a report of our experience in the surgical treatment of lung carcinoma, which includes 300 pulmonary resections performed in a series of 823 patients with lung carcinoma seen by us up to January 20, 1978.

In Table 1, the operability rate and resectability rate are shown. The oncological and/or functional evaluation excluded the operability of 468 patients (57%). Of 355 patients (43%) submitted to thoracotomy, lung resection was performed on 300 (85%), while it was considered not feasible ("explored only") on the remaining 55 (15%).

In Table 2, the type of operations performed are shown. According to their amplitude, the resections have been classified as pneumonectomy (44%) or as partial resections (56%). Following the surgical terms used by Chamberlain[2] and Abbey Smith,[1] the resections were defined as follows: *a) standard resection*, when the tumor is confined to the lung and surgical specimen consisted only of pulmonary structures. We include among this group not only the standard lobectomies or pneumonectomies but also the enlarged lobectomies with sleeve resection of the bronchus or pulmonary artery; *b) extended resection*, when the tumor was spread beyond the lung and extrapulmonary structures were removed with the specimen: mediastinal lymph nodes, trachea, pericardium, atrium, intrapericardial vessels, esophagus, chest wall or diaphragm; *c) noncurative resection*, when the tumor removal was incomplete, leaving some tumor or involved nodes in the

From Thoracic Surgery Service, Centro Hospitalario "La Fe," Valencia.
Reprinted from Cancer Clinical Trials 2: 71-76, 1979.

TABLE 1

Lung Carcinoma (20-1-78)

Patients seen in Thoracic Surgery Service	823
Explored patients	355/823 = 43%
Resections from the explored patients	300/355 = 85%
Resections from all the patients	300/823 = 36%

TABLE 2

Resections for Lung Carcinoma

Type of Resection (by Amplitude)		Surgical Criteria	
Pneumonectomy	133 = 44%	Standard resection	149 = 50%
Lobectomy	123 = 41%	Extended resection	117 = 39%
Enlarged lobectomy		Noncurative resection	34 = 11%
Sleeve resection	26 = 9%		
Segmentectomy	18 = 6%		

operative field, after excision of the major specimen, or when histological invasion of the line of section was demonstrated. In our series, surgery was standard in 50% of the cases, extended in 39% and noncurative in 11%.

Tables 3 and 4 outline the studies we carry out for preoperative assessment and our criteria of surgical contraindications, respectively. We must point out that in doubtful cases, if the possibility of resection is judged remote but no definite contraindication is found we prefer to explore, leaving for the operation the definitive evaluation of the resectability of the tumor. We adopt a greater surgical aggressivity in young patients with good cardiorespiratory reserves, although it does not mean that age by itself is considered as a criterion for contraindication, since in our series patients up to 74 years of age are operated on. The high percentage of extended resections in our series and the resectability rate of 85%, from the patients explored, place our unit among those which are not looking for selectivity.

The functional respiratory evaluation by conventional tests has been completed with the use of radioactive isotopes as tracers in the study of lung function. Combined perfusion and aerosol scanning

were performed. To study pulmonary perfusion Indium 113-m tagged to ferric hydroxide was administered. To study pulmonary ventilation we have used Technetium 99-m pertechnectate administered through a nebulizer. For the recording of the distribution of radioactivity we have used a gamma camera with computers to obtain digital information allowing quantification. In borderline patients with a low cardiorespiratory reserve, we have used hemodynamic studies following Le Brigand's[4] and Ratson-Britkers's[5,6] schemes, by determining the pressure in the pulmonary artery in basal condition, during exercise and after blocking the artery of the lung to be removed.

Oncologic evaluation has been directed to discover distant dissemination when clinical assessment or laboratory studies pointed out this possibility. In this situation we have turned to the scanning of bone, brain and liver, and recently to the computed tomography.

Mediastinoscopy and/or hilioscopy (anterior mediastinotomy) are two important aids in the study of patients with lung carcinoma reducing the number of exploratory thoracotomies, but in our opinion excessive use of these techniques is as unwise as too infrequent use. Our policy is to use mediastinoscopy only if there is clinical or radiological evidence or at least suspicion of upper mediastinal involvement. If the nodes are negative

TABLE 3

Preoperative Assessment

Cardiorespiratory Reserves
  Clinical examination, respiratory function tests, electrocardiography.
  Perfusion and aerosol lung scanning.
  Eventual hemodynamic studies blocking pulmonary artery.
Oncologic Evaluation
  Clinical examination, routine x-ray, tomography.
  Laboratory test: SMAC, bronchoscopy.
  Elective mediastinoscopy bassed on radiology.
  Scanning or computed tomography if suspicion of distal metastasis.

TABLE 4

Contraindications

Low cardiorespiratory reserve: sleeve lobectomy?
Distant dissemination, supraclavicular involved node, high mediastinal node.
Low mediastinal positive node if anaplastic or perinodal invasion.
Involvement of cava, esophagus, or pleural surface; recurrent paralysis.
Tracheal involvement: extended surgery + plastic procedures?

TABLE 5

Operative Mortality Rate for 300 Resections for Lung Carcinoma

Mortality of all resections	23/300 = 8%
Pneumonectomy	16/133 = 12%
Partial resection	7/167 = 4%
Standard resection	6/149 = 4%
Extended resection	16/117 = 14%
Noncurative resection	2/34 = 6%

TABLE 6

Histology and Survival since Resection

	≥3 Years	≥5 Years
Squamous	31/92 = 34%	15/53 = 28%
Large cell	10/30 = 33%	3/22 = 14%
Adenocarcinoma	10/28 = 36%	5/17 = 29%
Bronchiolar cell	2/4 = —	1/1 = —
Small cell	2/12 = 17%	0/7 = 0%
Unspecified	0/3 = —	0/1 = —
Total	55/169 = 33%	24/101 = 24%

we explore. In patients with ipsilateral, low located, mediastinal positive nodes, we consider the operability when the involvement is intranodal and the histologic type is favorable: squamous and adenocarcinoma. A poor-risk patient with a positive mediastinoscopy is considered to be inoperable. If there is perinodal growth or if positive nodes are present in anaplastic tumors or the nodal involvement is contralateral or high ipsilateral, the patient is not submitted to thoracotomy.

With respect to therapy, surgery has been applied alone when there were no positive mediastinal nodes; neither chest wall nor other extrapulmonary structures were involved.

We have indicated radiotherapy in various instances: 1) Prior to surgery in tumors involving the chest wall, including superior sulcus tumors, and in some cases of large tumoral mass—the dose administered was 3000 rads. 2) Postoperative radiotherapy was used if mediastinal node invasion or parietal infiltration were found when operating. If postoperative histologic study demonstrated an oat cell carcinoma, coadjuvant polychemotherapy was used. Patients with local postoperative recurrence were treated with associated radiotherapy and polychemotherapy and only with polychemotherapy when there existed generalized metastasis.

Postoperative deaths, occurring in the month following the operation, are shown in Table 5. The total percentage was 8%. It was higher (12%) in the cases of total resections than in partial resection (4%), as well as in extended resections (14%) compared with standard resections (4%).

All the patients have been followed up, by clinical and radiological evaluation, every 3 months during the first year and twice a year afterwards. When a local recurrence or metastasis was suspected, a more careful study was performed. Survival rate has been evaluated by calculating the percentage of surviving patients among those who

had been operated 3 and 5 years before, including all those who died during surgery or in the immediate postoperative period. With this direct method the 3-year survival rate, for all the resections performed, was 33% and the 5-year rate was 24%.

In Table 6, survival has been related to the histologic type of the tumor. With this purpose the Pathology Department has reviewed the histologic diagnosis recorded in daily routine. This revision was done because the microscopic diagnosis of the degree of anaplasia may sometimes present serious difficulties. Renault,[7] following Reid and Carr,[9] points out the problems regarding the separation of squamous and anaplastic large cell carcinoma. In our series there does not exist a difference in the 3-year survival rates between patients with squamous carcinoma, adenocarcinoma and large cell carcinoma, but in the 5-year survival rates the large cell carcinomas show a lower survival (14%) than the others. In our series, patients showing a postoperative histology of "oat cell" do not survive 5 years, nevertheless, we have two of 12 patients that have survived 3 years. The comparison of 5-year survival rate after resection between patients with non-anaplastic tumors (squamous, adenocarcinoma, and bronchiolar cell) and patients with anaplastic tumors (large and small cell) was significant 30% and 10%, respectively ($p < 0.05$).

According to the loco-regional spread of the tumor, the cases have been classified following the definition of T, N, and M categories suggested by the American Joint Committee of Cancer Staging and End Results Reporting and modified by Renault et al.[8]: a) T_1—a tumor that is 3.0 cm or less in greatest diameter surrounded by lung or visceral pleura which does not affect the main bronchus. b) T_2—a tumor more than 3.0 cm in greatest diameter or a tumor of any size which invades the visceral pleura or which has associated atelectasis or ob-

TABLE 7

Survival ≥ 3 Years and T-N-M

	N_0	N_1	N_2	N_3	Total	
T_1	6/9	—	0/3	0/1	6/13	(46%)
T_2	33/56	5/30	4/23	1/12	43/111	(38%)
T_{3-1}[a]	1/5	2/11	0/6	0/3	3/25	(12%)
T_{3-2}[b]	2/12	1/5	0/2	0/1	3/20	(15%)
Totals	42/82	8/46	4/34	1/17	55/169	(33%)
	(51%)	(17%)	(12%)			

[a] Tumor extended into mediastinal structures.
[b] Tumor extended into parietal pleura, chest wall, or diaphragm.

structive pneumonitis, extending to the hilar region; at bronchoscopy the proximal extent of demonstrable tumor must be within a lobar bronchus or at least 2.0 cm distal to the carina. c) T_3—a tumor of any size with direct extension into an adjacent structure such as the parietal pleura or chest wall, the diaphragm or the mediastinum and its contents, or demonstrable bronchoscopically to involve a main bronchus less than 2.0 cm distal to the carina.

The letter N defines the regional invasion. a) N_0—no demonstrable metastasis to regional lymph nodes; b) N_1—involved nodes in the peribronchial or hilar region; c) N_2—low-level mediastinal ipsilateral involved nodes (subcarinal and nodes of the azigos or esophagus); d) N_3—high-level mediastinal involved nodes, contralateral involved nodes.

The letter M stands for distal metastasis. The various combinations of T-N-M form the three stages of lung carcinoma. In Stage I are included cases T_1-N_0 or N_1 and T_2N_0; Stage II contains the cases T_2-N_1 and in Stage III the remaining combinations.

TABLE 8

Survival ≥ 5 Years and T-N-M

	N_0	N_1	N_2	N_3	Total	
T_1	3/6	—	0/3	0/1	3/10	(30%)
T_2	15/33	2/17	2/15	0/1	19/66	(29%)
T_{3-1}[a]	1/3	0/7	0/3	0/3	1/16	
T_{3-2}[b]	0/6	1/1	0/1	0/1	1/9	(8%)
Total	19/48	3/25	2/22	0/6	24/101	(24%)
	(40%)	(12%)	(9%)	—		
		(11%)				

[a] Tumor extended into mediastinal structures.
[b] Tumor extended into parietal pleura, chest wall or diaphragm.

TABLE 9

Surgical Stage of Disease and Survival

	Survival since Resection	
	≥3 Years	≥5 Years
Stage I	39/65 = 60%	18/39 = 46%
Stage II	5/30 = 17%	2/17 = 12%
Stage III	11/74 = 15%	4/45 = 9%

In Tables 7 and 8 the relationship between the categories of T-N-M and the survival rates are shown. The 3-year survival rate is about 51% for patients without lymph node invasion, decreasing this percentage to 17% and 12% for cases classified as N_1 and N_2, respectively ($p < 0.01$ between N_0 and N_1 and between N_0 and N_2). A similar difference is observed comparing the survival rate of patients with tumors T_1 or T_2 and patients with tumors T_3 ($p < 0.01$). The 5-year survival rate in cases N_0 was 40%, decreasing to 12% for N_1 and 9% for N_2 ($p < 0.05$ between N_0 and N_1, $p < 0.001$ between N_0 and N_2). A significant difference in postoperative 5-year survival rate is also observed ($p < 0.05$) between patients with tumors T_1 and T_2 and patients with T_3.

In Table 9, postoperative survival rate is considered according to tumoral staging. For Stage I the 3-year survival rate was 60%, decreasing to 17% and 15%, respectively, for Stages II and III. The differences in the percentages were significant between Stages I and II as well as between stages I and III ($p < 0.001$). The 5-year survival rate was 46% in Stage I, 12% in Stage II, and 9% in Stage III ($p < 0.05$ between Stages I and II, $p < 0.01$ between I and III).

In Table 10, surgical criteria and survival rate are correlated. The year survival rate was 46% in patients submitted to standard resections and 21% in those who needed extended surgery ($p < 0.01$). The 5-year survival rates were 37% and 12%, respectively ($p < 0.01$).

TABLE 10

Surgical Criteria and Survival

	Survival since Resection	
Type of Resection	≥3 Years	≥5 Years
Standard resection	43/94 = 46%	20/54 = 37%
Extended resection	12/57 = 21%	4/34 = 12%
Noncurative resection	0/18 = 0%	0/13 = 0%
All types	55/169 = 33%	24/101 = 24%

TABLE 11

Size of Carcinoma and Survival

Size of carcinoma (cm)	Survival since Resection	
	≥3 Years	≥5 Years
≤3 cm	8/14 = 57%	4/14 = 29%
>3–5 cm	19/60 = 32%	11/40 = 27%
>5–7 cm	23/65 = 35%	6/26 = 23%
>7 cm	5/30 = 17%	3/21 = 14%

In Table 11, data for tumoral size and survival rate are compared and a significant difference between patients having tumors of 3 cm in greatest diameter and those with tumors more than 7 cm was observed as emphasized by Soorae and Abbey Smith.[10] Finally, in Table 12 survival rate of patients with tumors involving the chest wall is described.

In conclusion, although the prognosis of lung carcinoma is very severe, postoperative results are not discouraging, especially when they are compared with other kinds of treatment, even knowing that the results published by surgeons correspond only to a small number of patients in whom the tumor was removed. There remain yet a number of patients in whom surgery alone is not the most efficient treatment; we would do well to look for a better associated therapy.

Survival figures, in our series, have an important value for us, since our indications have been large and nonselective cases with 85% of resectability when exploring and only 50% of standard resections. As Le Brigand[3] says, the first strategy in lung carcinoma therapy shall be to reduce the number of patients who are seen in very late stages, which has led the physicians towards pessimism. Surgeons are obligated to give their results in order to create an atmosphere of confidence and some optimism leading to a greater effort towards an early diagnosis. There will be aggressive tumoral forms to which we can do very little, but there will exist others in which the patient's future will depend on the orientation provided by the first physician who visited them.

Summary

The authors present a series of 300 pulmonary resections in patients with lung carcinoma. The tumors have been classified according to the hystologic type and to the T-N-M code; the operations according to the amplitude of resected lung and the surgical criteria (standard, extended, noncurative resection). The total survival rates of the series since the operation, including surgical mortality, were 33% at 3 years and 24% at 5 years.

The comparison of 5-year survival rates between patients with nonanaplastic tumors (squamous, adenocarcinoma and bronchiollar cell carcinoma) and anaplastic tumors (large and small cell) was significant 30% and 10%, respectively.

In Stage I, the survival was of 60% at 3 years and 46% at 5 years, decreasing to 17% and 12%, respectively, in Stage II and to 15% and 9% in Stage III. The survival rate and surgical criteria were correlated, yielding better results when standard surgery was performed. With respect to the size of the tumor there is a significant difference in 3-year survival rates between the tumors with a maximum of 3 cm of diameter and those of more than 7 cm.

Finally, the authors emphasize that the surgical figures of the series presented are of great value as the surgical indications were large and nonselective cases, with 85% of resectability in the thoracotomies.

TABLE 12

Survival and Chest Wall Invasion

Type of Invasion	Survival since Resection	
	≥3 Years	≥5 Years
Sulcus Superior, Pancoast	1[a]/4	0/2
Non Apical	2[b]/16	1/9
Total	3/20 (15%)	1/11 (9%)

[a] Dead after 3 years.
[b] Still alive.

References

1. Abbey Smith, R.: Pre-operative assessment, techniques and results of surgery for bronchial carcinoma. In *Surgery of the Lung. The Coventry Conference*, R. E. Smith and W. G. Williams, Eds., Butterworth, London, 1974.

2. Chamberlain, J. M., McNeill, J. M., Parnassa, T. M., and Edsall, J. R.: Bronchogenic carcinoma. An agressive Surgical Attitude. *J Thorac Surg* 38:727, 1959.

3. Le Brigand, H.: Place de la chirurgie et recherche d'une stratégie thérapeutique. *Rev Fr Mal Resp (Suppl 2)* 5: 67, 1977.

4. Le Brigand, H., Vayre, P., Noviant, I., Coutelle, R., Ranson-Britker, B., Semperleiva, A., David, Ph., Luizy, J., and Le Plaideur, J.: Les indications "limites" du traitement chirurgical dans la tuberculose pulmonaire. Le probléme fonctional. *Rev Tuberc Pneumol 31: 919, 1967.*

5. Ranson-Britker B.: La prevision du risque operatoire en chirurgie thoracique. *Bull Physiol Pathol Resp 2: 15, 1966.*

6. Ranson-Britker, B., Bouchar, F., and Bechtel, P.: Valeur pronostique du cathéterisme cardiaque droit avant pneumonectomie chez les insuffisant respira-toires. *Presse Med 24: 907, 1960.*

7. Renault, P.: Valeur pronostique des structures. Le code T. N. M. *Rev Fr Mal Resp (Suppl 2) 5: 45, 1977.*

8. Renault, P., Merlier, M., and Lange, J.: La codification T. N. M. apliquée aux cancers bronchopulmonaires operés. *Rev Fr Mal Resp 3: 59, 1975.*

9. Reid, J. D., and Carr, A. H.: The validity and value of histological and cytological classifications of lung cancer. *Cancer 14: 673, 1961.*

10. Soorae, A. S., and Abbey Smith, R.: Tumor size as a prognostic factor after resection of lung carcinoma. *Thorax 32: 19, 1977.*

Adjuvant systemic therapy of lung cancer

10

Franco M. Muggia, M.D. [a]

William P. McGuire, III, M.D. [b]

MOST PATIENTS WITH LUNG CANCER subjected to surgical resection are likely to have residual tumor burdens which lead to clinical relapse and death. Unfortunately, none of the systemic therapies for squamous cell, large cell and adenocarcinoma of the lung have demonstrated curative potential either in the advanced disease or in the surgical adjuvant setting.

Interest in clinical trials of adjuvant therapy in lung cancer have been rekindled by three factors: 1) reports indicating the value of immunotherapy, 2) preliminary encouraging experience with new chemotherapy programs, and 3) methodologies including stage- and cell type-specific clinical trials leading to better interpretation of results. These concepts have stimulated new treatment protocol studies within the NCI-sponsored Lung Cancer Study Group, and clinical cooperative groups.

Experimental foundations for the use of adjuvant chemotherapy in the treatment of cancer have been extensively delineated in the work of Skipper and Schabel and their co-workers at the Southern Research Institute.[17,21] The potential of systemic therapy is a function of the body burden of tumor and may be greatly enhanced by local cytoreductive therapeutic modalities. A major consideration in applying these concepts to lung cancer is that the presentation of this disease is generally in a very advanced state. In the small cell type, regional and systemic extension of tumor are recognized in the majority of patients.

In the other cell types of lung cancer, the situation is somewhat different, but not radically so. Eighteen percent of patients who die in the postoperative period after "curative" resections are found at autopsy to have distant metastases.[13] Even in the most favorable selection of Stage I lung cancer, 40% of the patients have recurrent disease at distant sites within 5 years of surgical resection. This pattern of relapse, coupled with assumptions of constant growth and a 20-day doubling time, led Skipper (Fig. 1) to estimate the usual residual body burden (i.e., tumor at distant sites) at presentation. This calculation indicated the presence of 10^6–10^{11} residual cells in two-thirds of the patients following curative resection of a primary squamous cell cancer. Therefore, even in this most favorable subgroup, a maximum of one-third might be considered amenable to control solely by immunologic means.[17] In the vast majority of patients, adjuvant therapy is actually directed to an "early" phase of advanced lung cancer. With these limitations in mind, the current methodology, basis, and prospects for adjuvant systemic therapy in lung cancer will be reviewed.

Division of Cancer Treatment, National Cancer Institute, Bethesda, Maryland.
Reprinted from Cancer Clinical Trials 1: 235–241, 1978.

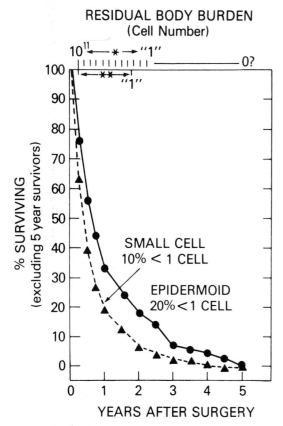

RESIDUAL BODY BURDEN
(Cell Number)

FIGURE 1. Lung, epidermoid; survival after surgery (failures only). Selawry and Hansen data adapted from Skipper.[19,20] * Twenty-day doubling time; ** 15-day doubling time.

Dissection of a lung cancer adjuvant protocol

In the design of an adjuvant study in lung cancer, it is important to consider the background and objectives, relevant prognostic factors and patient selection, presently available treatments, study parameters of evaluation, and statistical requirements.

Background and objectives

The use of adjuvant systemic therapy is justified in instances where a high risk of recurrence can be identified, satisfactory local or systemic therapy is available, and the short- and long-term morbidity of such therapy is significantly less than the chance of succumbing to recurrent disease. Most prior adjuvant chemotherapy studies in lung cancer have been inadequate by current standards because they used short-term treatment, inadequate doses, and drugs poorly active in advanced disease.[10] No benefit has been documented in randomized studies, and one study actually indicating a detrimental effect of cyclophosphamide has been reported.[4] As these shortcomings are recognized, additional adjuvant trials seem desirable, but with randomization as an essential feature in study designs.

Prognostic factors in patient selection

A most valuable development in clinical trials has been the refinement of methodologies required to provide reliable and interpretable results. An effort must be made to ensure that populations are balanced in terms of prognostic factors influencing response and survival. Histology, disease stage, and performance status are the prominent prognostic factors that have been identified in lung cancer and, at present, they are the most frequently used in such trials.[5]

Although possessing characteristic clinical features and patterns of tumor growth, patients with various histologic cell types appear to have a similar prognosis when undergoing resection of Stage I lesions. In Stage II disease, the results favor squamous cell carcinoma over large cell or adenocarcinoma. When the disease extends beyond regional metastases, all types share a poor outlook that may be inferior to that of patients with small cell carcinoma of the lung. A pathologic diagnosis may also determine relative susceptibility to a drug regimen, although this has not been established with certainty except in the small cell type, which is most responsive to cyclophosphamide and a number of other drugs. However, one must be aware of the lack of uniformity in classifying lung tumors, which is partly related to the varying degree of differentiation of the various cell types and also to the presence of mixed histologies.

Staging based on the TNM classification (Table 1) is a key ingredient of any adjuvant trial and demands that the extent of disease be fully documented by pathologic staging. Determination of the extent of disease at surgery includes assessment of subsegmental, hilar, subcarinal, paratracheal and other mediastinal lymph nodes; careful pathologic examination of tumor margins completes the staging. The survival of patients with Stage I and II tumors undergoing resection has been reported

TABLE 1

Lung Cancer: TNM Stages Included in Adjuvant Trials

Stage	TNM Classification	Findings
0	TX N0 M0	Malignant cells in secretions
I	T1 N0 M0	Tumor <3 cm, surround by lung or visceral pleura without invasion proximal to lobar bronchus
	T2 N0 M0	Tumor >3 cm, no effusion or total atelectasis
	T1 N1 M0	Nodes in ipsilateral hilar region
II	T2 N1 M0	
III (resectable)	T3 N0 M0 T3 N1 M0	Tumor of any size with total atelectasis, pleural transudate or exudate, chest wall or mediastinal invasion, within 2 cm of carina
	T any N2 M0	Nodes in subcarinal, paratracheal region

in detail by Mountain et al.[15] With the incorporation of careful mediastinal dissection into the initial surgical approach, survival following surgical resection of pathologic Stage I tumors of all types is not as unfavorable as previously believed.[12] Thus, proper interpretation of the results of an adjuvant trial must take into account the extent of surgical staging.

Finally, performance status, defined by the scale originally described by Karnofsky et al.[9] or by that subsequently simplified by Zubrod et al.[24] (Table 2), has been an easily determined prognostic factor correlating with survival independent of stage and cell type. However, its value is limited in surgical adjuvant trials since patients entered are likely to manifest minimal, if any, functional impairment.

Treatment programs

The efficacy of chemotherapy for cell types other than small cell carcinoma has been disappointing. Drug combinations have yielded encouraging results in preliminary studies, but an advantage over the single agents has not been clearly demonstrable. Moreover, they are more difficult to use in cooperative trials. For these reasons, there has been a reluctance to undertake surgical adjuvant studies employing drug combinations.[10]

On the other hand, additional adjuvant trials with single agents do not seem warranted at this time for several reasons: *a*) one of the best designed trials indicated that cyclophosphamide may have

TABLE 2

Performance Status Scale

Karnofsky et al.[9]		ECOG—Zubrod et al.[24]	
Normal, no complaints	100	0	Normal activity
Able to carry on normal activities; minor signs or symptoms of disease	90	1	Symptoms, but nearly fully ambulatory
Normal activity with effort	80		
Cares for self. Unable to carry on normal activity or to do active work.	70	2	Some bed time, but needs to be in bed less than 50% of normal daytime
Required occasional assistance, but able to care for most of his needs	60		
Requires considerable assistance and frequent medical care	50	3	Needs to be in bed more than 50% of normal daytime
Disabled; requires special care and assistance	40		
Severely disabled; hospitalization indicated though death not imminent	30	4	Unable to get out of bed
Very sick; hospitalization necessary; active supportive treatment necessary	20		
Moribund	10		
Dead	0		

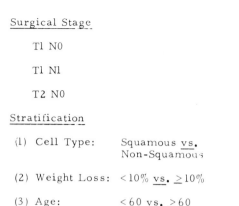
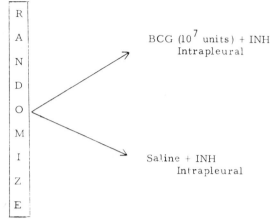

FIGURE 2.   Stage I carcinoma (resectable). Abbreviation: (INH) isoniazid.

been detrimental to survival after surgical resection[4]; b) no single drug has yielded results clearly superior to cyclophosphamide[10]; and c) published cumulative response rates to cyclophosphamide have gradually declined, mostly as a result of published series that used stricter assessment of chemotherapy responses (Table 3). These findings have raised doubts as to the true efficacy of such chemotherapy.

More recently, immunotherapy alone or combined with chemotherapy has been reported to be of benefit in specific subsets of patients with lung cancer. Specifically, use of intrapleural BCG[14] (Table 4) or BCG by scarification,[16] has indicated a short-term survival advantage for the treated group versus a group of Stage I patients undergoing only surgical resection. These beneficial effects were not apparent in Stage II patients, but another immunotherapeutic agent, levamisole, appeared to benefit this specific subset of patients when compared with the control group.[2] Another study demonstrated encouraging results through the use of a tumor-associated antigen cell extract in

Freund's adjuvant with or without methotrexate in comparison to concurrent but nonrandomized controls.[22] The surgical adjuvant effect of new chemotherapies, immunotherapy, and a combination of the two needs to be tested in carefully designed prospective clinical trials.

Current trials sponsored by the National Cancer Institute (NCI) are focusing on the role of immunotherapy in Stage I patients (Fig. 2). This trial, which is analogous to McKneally's study,[14] is a double-blind comparison to placebo and uses intrapleural Tice strain BCG given within 10 days of surgery in a dose of 1×10^7 colony-forming organisms, followed 2 weeks later by INH. The six participating institutions have entered 100 patients in the first 8 months; all cell types except small cell are being entered.

On the other hand, adjuvant trials in Stages II and III disease differ according to whether squamous cancer (Fig. 3) or the adenocarcinoma and large cell types (Fig. 4) are being entered. In squamous cell carcinoma, combined radiotherapy and levamisole will be included and compared to

TABLE 3

Lung Cancer: Cumulative Single-Agent Response to Cyclophosphamide

Reference	Year	No. Responding/ Total	%
Livingston and Carter[11]	1970	168/509	33
Selawry[18]	1973	189/814	23
Wasserman et al.[23]	1975	303/1513	20

TABLE 4

Effect of Adjuvant BCG in BCG in Stages I and II Lung Cancer[a]

Stage	Treatment	Patients	Recurrences
I	BCG + INH	30	2 ⎱ P = 0.009
I	INH	33	11 ⎰
II	BCG + INH	22	13
II	INH	15	8

[a] Adapted from McKneally et al.[14] Median follow-up = 617 days.

Surgical Stage

    T2 N1

    T3 NX

    TX N2

Stratification

(1) Stage: II vs. III

(2) Weight Loss: $<10\%$ vs. $\geq 10\%$

(3) Age: <60 vs. ≥ 60

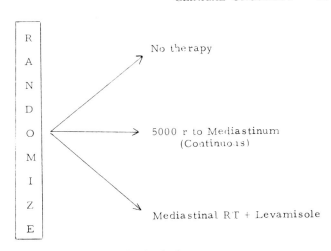

FIGURE 3.   Resectable Stage II/III squamous cell carcinoma. Abbreviation: (RT) radiotherapy.

radiotherapy alone and to no additional treatment. Radiotherapy alone has been considered helpful in controlling mediastinal disease,[6] and levamisole has reportedly been beneficial when combined with irradiation in breast cancer. Since the prognosis of the other two cell types is quite inferior to squamous carcinoma at comparable stages, the protocol plan is to compare the effect of combination chemotherapy versus combination immunotherapy employing intrapleural BCG and levamisole. The addition of levamisole will test whether restoration of T-cell function by this agent will counteract the lack of effectiveness of intrapleural BCG in Stages II and III lung cancer, as reported by McKneally et al.[14]

The basis for the combination chemotherapy to be used requires additional comment. Recent publications have pointed out the value of several regimens, some including radiotherapy, in advanced lung cancer. Most of these have been pilot programs including alkylating agents and adriamycin,[3] yielding data that are not very different from those of its predecessors,[1,8] which were usually disappointing in subsequent comparative trials. It remains to be seen whether these combinations and the CAP regimen (cyclophosphamide, adriamycin,

Surgical Stage

    T2 N1

    T3 NX

    TX N2

Stratification

(1) Stage: II vs. III

(2) Postop. Arrhythmia: Yes vs. No

(3) Weight Loss: $<10\%$ vs. $\geq 10\%$

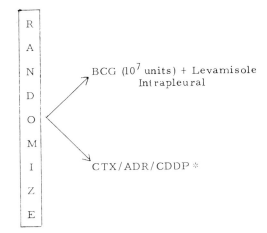

    * CTX   (450 mg/m^2)

      ADR   (40 mg/m^2)   All day 1 q 3 wks.

      CDDP (40 mg/m^2)

FIGURE 4.   Resectable Stage II/III adenocarcinoma/large cell carcinoma. Abbreviations: (CTX) cyclophosphamide; (ADR) adriamycin; (CDDP) cis-diamminedichloroplatinum.

cis-diamminedichloroplatinum) will prove to be consistently superior and provide benefit in the adjuvant setting. The experience with this regimen at the Mayo Clinic has been thoroughly reported,[7] and it does indicate its activity against all nonsmall cell types of lung cancer, with a convincing advantage in terms of response rate and survival compared to dianhydrogalactitol, an investigational alkylating agent.

Shortcomings of both adjuvant chemotherapy and immunotherapy in the more advanced stages should be readily apparent. A sizable number of these patients probably have large tumor cell burdens which will require regimens with a curative potential in advanced disease. At present, however, none of the newer regimens appears to have this degree of activity. Nevertheless, it seems justified to explore their efficacy in the more favorable circumstances of the surgical adjuvant setting.

Study parameters and statistical considerations

Evaluation of lung cancer adjuvant studies requires careful adherence to patient entry requirements, some uniformity of surgical techniques and review of pathologic specimens. The disease-free interval and survival from the date of randomization constitute the basis for analysis. Disease-free interval is established by either presumptive or proven evidence of local or distant recurrence.

From a statistical point of view, adjuvant trials in lung cancer should be able to yield reliable answers within a relatively short time. Even in the most favorable stages, we are dealing with a common disease and a dramatic death rate. In Stage I, if the 2-year survival were to increase from 60 to 80% with a new treatment option, less than 100 patients per arm would be required for the difference to have an adequate level of significance and power. A smaller number of patients would be required in more advanced stages, if a treatment were to improve the 1-year survival from 40 to 60%.

These figures should encourage the sequential testing of hypotheses in therapeutic trials, since answers with a reasonable degree of statistical support may be expected within a relatively short time. One can anticipate the subsequent step in Stage I trials to be an evaluation of another immunotherapeutic approach alone or combined with the preceding one, and eventually the testing of some form of chemotherapy that is successful in the more advanced stages. Combinations of chemotherapy and immunotherapy, as well as new chemotherapy regimens, appear to be the next logical step in Stages II and III undergoing resection. In squamous carcinoma, once the role of radiotherapy is defined, the addition of other modalities can be anticipated.

Conclusions

The curative potential of chemotherapy or immunotherapy in the adjuvant setting is limited by the realization that most patients undergoing surgical resection for lung cancer actually have a sizable residual tumor burden. Moreover, none of the systemic therapies now available for squamous cell, large cell and adenocarcinoma of the lung have curative potential in the advanced disease setting.

Nevertheless, three developments have rekindled interest in adjuvant trials in lung cancer: *a*) refinements in clinical trial methodologies as compared to past studies, indicating a reasonable certainty of providing distinct answers to therapeutic hypotheses being tested; *b*) the suggestion of a beneficial effect of immunotherapy in recent adjuvant lung cancer trials; and *c*) the availability of new chemotherapy programs with reproducible activity superior to single agents in advanced disease.

We have begun testing these concepts in prospective studies within a newly formed Lung Cancer Study Group composed of six institutions, and within some of the clinical cooperative groups sponsored by the National Cancer Institute.

References

1. Alberto, P., Brunner, K., Martz, G., and Senn, H. J.: Traitment du cancer bronchique per combination simultance ou sequentielle de methotrexate, cyclophosphamide, procarbazine et vincristine. In *10th International Cancer Congress*, Houston, 1970, p. 469.

2. Amery, W. K.: Double-blind levamisole trial in resectable lung cancer. *Ann NY Acad Sci 277: 260–268, 1976.*

3. Bitran, J. D., Desser, R. K., DeMeester, T. R., Colman, M., Evans, R., Billings, A., Griem, M., Rubenstein, L., Shapiro, C., and Golomb, H. M.: Cyclophosphamide,

adriamycin, methotrexate and procarbazine (CAMP)—Effective four-drug combination chemotherapy for metastatic non-oat cell bronchogenic carcinoma. *Cancer Treat Rep 60: 1225–1230, 1976.*

4. Brunner, K. W., Marthaler, T., and Muller, W.: Effects of long-term adjuvant chemotherapy with cyclophosphamide (NSC-26271) for radically resected bronchogenic carcinoma. *Cancer Chemother Rep (Part 3) 4: 125–132, 1973.*

5. Cohen, M. H., and Selawry, O. S.: Bronchogenic carcinoma: Prognostic factors and criteria of response. In *Cancer Therapy: Prognostic Factors and Criteria of Response*, M. J. Staquet, Ed. Raven Press, New York, 1975, pp. 185–197.

6. Deeley, T. J.: The treatment of carcinoma of the bronchus. *Br J Radiol 40: 802, 1967.*

7. Eagan, R. T., Ingle, J. N., Frytak, S., Rubin, J., Kvois, L. K., Carr, D. T., Coles, D. T., and O'Fallon, J. R.: Platinum-based polychemotherapy versus dianhydrogalactitol in advanced non-small cell lung cancer. *Cancer Treat Rep 61: 1339–1345, 1977.*

8. Hansen, H. H., Muggia, F. M., Andrews, R., and Selawry, O. S.: Intensive chemotherapy and radiotherapy in patients with non-resectable bronchogenic carcinoma. *Cancer 30: 315–324, 1972.*

9. Karnofsky, D. A., Abelmann, W. H., Craver, L. F., and Burchenal, J. H.: The use of the nitrogen mustards in the palliative treatment of carcinoma with particular reference to bronchogenic carcinoma. *Cancer 1: 634–656, 1948.*

10. Legha, S. S., Muggia, F. M., and Carter, S. K.: Adjuvant chemotherapy in lung cancer, review and prospect. *Cancer 39: 1415–1424, 1977.*

11. Livingston, R. B., and Carter, S. K.: *Single Agents in Cancer Chemotherapy.* IFI/Plenum, New York, 1970, pp. 36–38.

12. Martini, N., and Beattie, E. J.: Results of surgical treatment in stage I lung cancer. *J Thorac Cardiovasc Surg 74(4); 499–505, 1977.*

13. Matthews, M. J., Pickren, J., and Kanhouwa, S.: Who has occult metastases? In *Perspectives in Lung Cancer*, T. E. Williams, Jr., H. E. Wilson, and D. S. Yohn, Eds. S. Karger, Basel, 1977.

14. McKneally, M. F., Maver, C., Kausel, H. W., and Alley, R. D.: Regional immunotherapy with intrapleural BCG for lung cancer: Surgical consideration. *J Thorac Cardiovasc Surg 72: 333–347, 1976.*

15. Mountain, C. F., Carr, D. T., and Anderson, W. A. D.: A system for the clinical staging of lung cancer. *Am J Roentgenol Rad Ther Nucl Med 120: 130–138, 1974.*

16. Pouillart, P., Palangie, T., Huguenin, P., Morin, P., Gautier, H., Lededente, A., Baron, A., and Mathe, G.: Attempt at immunotherapy with BCG of patients with bronchus carcinoma: Preliminary results. In *Adjuvant Therapy of Cancer*, S. E. Salmon and S. E. Jones, Eds. North-Holland, Amsterdam, 1977, pp. 225–235.

17. Schabel, F. M., Jr.: Concepts for systemic treatment of micrometastases. *Cancer 35: 15–24, 1975.*

18. Selawry, O. S.: Monochemotherapy of bronchogenic carcinoma with special reference to cell type. *Cancer Chemother Rep (Part 3); 4: 177–188, 1973.*

19. Selawry, O. S., and Hansen, H. H.: Lung cancer. In *Cancer Medicine*, J. Holland and E. Frei, Eds. Lea and Febiger, Philadelphia, 1973, pp. 1473–1518.

20. Skipper, H.: Southern Research Institute Booklet, 1975.

21. Skipper, H. E., and Schabel, F. M., Jr.: Quantitative and cytokinetic studies in experimental tumor models. In *Cancer Medicine*, J. Holland and E. Frei, Eds. Lea and Febiger, Philadelphia, 1973, pp. 629–650.

22. Stewart, T. H., Hollinshead, A. C., Harris, J. E., Ranan, L., Belanger, R., Crepeau, A., Crook, A. F., Hirte, W. E., Hooper, D., Klaassen, D. J., Rapp, E. F., and Suchs, H. J.: Specific active immunochemotherapy in lung cancer: A survival study. *Can J Surg 20(4); 370–377, 1977.*

23. Wasserman, T. H., Comis, R. L., Goldsmith, M., Handelsman, H., Penta, J. S., Slavik, M., Soper, W. T., and Carter, S. K.: Tabular analysis of the clinical chemotherapy of solid tumors. *Cancer Chemother Rep (Part 3) 6: 399–419, 1975.*

24. Zubrod, C. G., Schneiderman, M., Frei, E., III, et al.: Appraisal of methods for the study of chemotherapy of cancer in man: Comparative therapeutic trial of nitrogen mustard and triethylene thiophosphoramide. *J Chron Dis 11: 7–33, 1960.*

Notes

a. Associate Director, Cancer Therapy Evaluation Program.

b. Head, Medicine Section, Clinical Investigations Branch, Cancer Therapy Evaluation Program.

11

Low dose BCG adjuvant therapy in resectable cases

A. Brugarolas*

Introduction

Adjuvant immunotherapy after surgical excision of non-small-cell carcinoma of lung is a novel approach undergoing extensive clinical investigations. Preliminary results appeared to suggest that immunomodulation with several agents such as levamisole, Bacillus Calmette-Guerin (BCG), and possibly certain tumor extracts might have contributed to the improvement in recurrence free survival in surgically resectable bronchogenic carcinoma.[1-4] Most of these trials, however, were based in small series, and final conclusions are awaiting confirmation in large double blind multicentric randomized studies.

The rationale supporting the use of adjuvant immunotherapy was based in the optimal treatment hypothesis of residual tumor left after a complete resection: that is, an immunologic reaction might be developed by the host bearing a small tumor burden against the remnant tumor cells, and cure might result.[5]

On the other hand, immunologic reconstitution might have had a general effect in patients with advanced cancer of the lung because immunosuppression was considered a frequent event and it was related to survival.[6,7] Anergic patients converting to positive tuberculin reaction were found to have an improved survival.[8]

During the past 5 years, patients with resectable lung cancer were given adjuvant low dose BCG in an attempt to investigate the effects of minimal immunotherapy, and the results were compared to those obtained in a small group of patients from the same institution who refused BCG therapy. Preliminary results were presented elsewhere.[9] Updated analysis of these results has been done, and the results are presented.

Material and methods

Selected patients met the following criteria: 1) Pathology proven non-small-cell lung cancer, that is Types I, III, and IV of the W.H.O. Classification.[10] 2) Stages I, II, and resectable III disease according to the American Joint Committee for Staging of Lung Cancer recommendations.[11] 3) And complete macroscopic resection of all visible tumor.

Patient consent was obtained.

BCG technique. 0.75 mg lyophilized Pasteur BCG (1.5 mg = 8×10^7 BCG) was administered by the skin escarification method every 2 weeks for 3 months, and every month for 1 year. At the end of this period BCG dose was individualized according to the local reaction obtained, and subsequent doses ranged from 0.15 to 0.75 mg Pasteur BCG. The first BCG administration was given within 1 month of surgery.

In case of fever, unexplained malaise, enlarged regional lymph nodes, and abnormally elevated liver enzyme profile, BCG treatment was discontinued and therapy with INH 450–600 mg daily was initiated and continued for 3 months.

Results

From 1973 to 1978, 78 patients with lung cancer underwent a complete macroscopic resection of the tumor. Fifty-nine patients accepted BCG treatment postoperatively, and 19 patients refused therapy with BCG. This analysis included the complete series.

There were 75 males and three females, and their ages ranged from 35 to 73 years. The char-

* Hospital General de Asturias with the collaboration of F. Alvarez de Linera, M. Gracia Marco, J. L. Alvarez Cofiño, F. Gosalvez Jordá, J. M. Buesa, J. Naya, A. J. Lacave, Oviedo, Spain.

TABLE 1

Patients Characteristics According to Treatment Given

	Number of patients Postoperative treatment	
	BCG	No BCG
Patients	59	19
Male/female	56/3	19/0
Median age	58	59
Stage I	32 (55%)	14 (73%)
II	12 (20%)	2 (10%)
III	15 (25%)	3 (15%)
Pathology:		
Epidermoid	34 (57%)	9 (48%)
Adenocarcinoma	11 (19%)	5 (26%)
Large cell— anaplastic	14 (24%)	5 (26%)
Surgical procedure:		
Pneumectomy	20 (34%)	9 (47%)
Lobectomy	31 (52%)	9 (47%)
Other	8 (14%)	1 (6%)

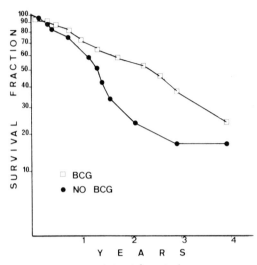

FIGURE 1.   Actuarial survival curves.

acteristics of the patients can be seen in Table 1. As it is shown, a small proportion of patients were in pathologic stage III. There was a similar distribution of patients according to the major prognostic factors, and patients not treated with adjuvant BCG represented a well-matched control except for the relatively small group size.

At the time of this analysis there were 40 deaths; 27 (46%) in the BCG treated group of patients, and 13 (68%) in the untreated group of patients. In addition, four patients in the BCG treated group were alive with recurrent disease at the time of this report. There were 28 patients alive (47%) with no evidence of disease in the BCG treatment group, and six patients alive (32%) with no evidence of disease in the untreated group.

The overall median survival time (MST) was in excess of 352 days for the BCG treated group of patients, and in excess of 263 days for the untreated group of patients. When only patients with a minimum follow up of 1 year were included, MST was in excess of 665 days for patients receiving BCG, and 478 days for patients not receiving BCG. Median time to relapse was 260 days and 150 days for the BCG treated and untreated groups of patients respectively.

Actuarial survival time was calculated for both groups of patients. Early on there was a slight difference in favor of BCG treated patients, but any

difference was fading out at the 3–4-year end point (Fig. 1).

Survival was analyzed according to the pathologic stage of the disease (Table 2). Approximately one-half of patients with stage I disease died. Survival rate was the same in stage I disease among BCG treated and untreated patients. In pathologic stages II and III more patients and longer follow-up was required for proper evaluation.

The site of first recurrence was the object of a detailed analysis in 31 patients treated with BCG and in 13 patients without BCG treatment. Early recurrence was noticed in five of 31 patients (16%) from the BCG group and in two of 13 patients (15%) from the non-BCG group.

Recurrence within the chest occurred in 17 patients (54%) treated with BCG postoperatively, and in seven patients (53%) not treated with BCG.

TABLE 2

Survival According to Treatment and Stage of the Disease

Stage of Disease	Adjuvant Therapy	Alive Patients		Dead Patients	
		No.	MST[a] (days)	No.	MST[a] (days)
I	BCG	17 (53%)	338+	15 (46%)	540
I	no BCG	7 (50%)	400+	7 (50%)	436
II	BCG	8 (66%)	793+	4 (33%)	217
II	no BCG	0		2 (100%)	478, 612
III	BCG	6 (40%)	353+	9 (60%)	305
III	no BCG	1	55+	2 (66%)	109, 484

[a] MST = median survival time.

Distant metastases in the liver, bone, and other sites occurred in 8 patients receiving BCG (25%) and in four patients (30%) not receiving BCG. Central nervous system metastases were found in eight patients treated with BCG and in four patients without BCG.

Discussion

The series of this report were not strictly comparative since this was not designed as a randomized trial, but patients who refused BCG therapy provided a concomitant simultaneous intramural control for the evaluation of results. As a general statement it was concluded that low-dose BCG therapy as given to these patients would probably have had no effect in the ultimate cure rate in stage I patients. A very modest increase in the expected median time to relapse might be suggested in the more advanced stages of the disease, but this would not be conclusive from the small series of patients studied.

Several reports from the recent literature have claimed a prolongation in the recurrence free interval, but more prolonged follow-up was required to define the influence of treatment in the final cure rate.

Amery in the final results analysis of a trial comparing levamisole and placebo found that adequately treated patients demonstrated a significant improvement in the short-term disease-free survival. At 2 years, survival was 87% in 40 patients receiving 2.1–3.8 mg/kg daily levamisole, and 60% in 52 control patients.[12]

Wright reported the preliminary results of a second multicentric trial comparing adjuvant BCG, adjuvant BCG, and levamisole, and placebo in resectable non-small-cell lung cancer. At the time of the report, with a median follow up time of 8 months, a trend to higher relapse rate was found for the placebo group of patients, but the differences were not significant.[13]

On the other hand, high-dose adjuvant BCG therapy in stage I squamous cell carcinoma of lung was the object of a randomized trial by Pouillart, et al.[14] Final analysis of this study demonstrated no differences in survival among BCG and control patients.[15]

McKneally, in a follow-up report of the original series comparing intrapleural BCG followed by INH and placebo, have shown a significant im-

provement in the recurrence-free survival at all end points of the evaluation of the study. At $2\frac{1}{2}$ years, actuarial survival curves showed 90% disease-free survival for BCG patients and 50% survival for control patients. The results obtained in the control group were comparable to a retrospective historical control population from the same institution.[16] These favorable results might have been achieved because of the particular method of BCG administration in this study. Final confirmation in a large multicentric trial is of utmost importance.

References

1. Study Group for Bronchogenic Carcinoma: Immunopotentiation with levamisole in resectable bronchogenic carcinoma. *Br Med J 3: 461–464, 1975.*

2. McKneally, M. F., Maver, C., and Kausel, H. W.: Regional immunotherapy of lung cancer with intrapleural BCG. *Lancet 1: 377–379, 1976.*

3. Stewart, T. H. M., Hollinshead, A. C., and Harris, J. E.: Immunochemotherapy of lung cancer. *Proc AACR & ASCO 17: 305, 1976.*

4. Takita, H., Han, T., and Brugarolas, A.: Adjuvant immunotherapy in bronchogenic carcinoma. *Proc XI Intern Cancer Cong 4: 710, 1974.*

5. Mathé, G.: Immunopharmacology and immunotherapy of residual disease in cancer patients. In *Recent Advances in Cancer Treatment,* H. J. Tagnon and M. J. Staquet, Eds. Raven Press, New York, 1977, pp. 87–120.

6. Brugarolas, A., and Takita, H.: Immunological status in lung cancer. *Chest 64: 427–430, 1973.*

7. Hersh, E. M., Lurie, P. M., Takita, H., Ritts, R., and Zelen, M.: Immunocompetence and prognosis in lung cancer. *Proc AACR & ASCO 17: 58, 1976.*

8. Israel, L., Mugica, J., and Chahinian, P.: Prognosis of early bronchogenic carcinoma. Survival curves of 451 patients after resection of lung cancer in relation to the results of preoperative tuberculin skin test. *Biomed 19: 68–72, 1973.*

9. Brugarolas, A., Alvarez de Linera, F., Lacave, A. J., Gosalvez, F., Alvarez Cofiño, J. L., Buesa, J. M., and Gracia, M.: Inmunoterapia con BCG en el cancer de pulmon resecado. *Oncol 80* (In press).

10. Kreyberg, L.: Histological typing of lung tumors. W.H.O., Geneva, 1967.

11. Mountain, C. F., Carr, D. T., and Anderson, W. A. D.: A system for the clinical staging of lung cancer. *Am J Roentgenol Rad Ther Nucl Med 120: 130–138, 1974.*

12. Amery, W. K.: Final results of a multicentric placebo controlled levamisole study of resectable lung cancer. *Cancer Treat Rep 62: 1677–1683, 1978.*

13. Wright, P. W., Hill, L. D., Peterson, A. V., Pinkham, R., Johnson, L., Ivey, T., Bernstein, I., Bagley, C., and Anderson, R.: Preliminary results of combined surgery

and adjuvant BCG plus levamisole treatment of resectable lung cancer. *Cancer Treat Rep 62: 1671–1675, 1978.*

14. Pouillart, P., Palangie, T., Huguenin, P., Morin, P., Gutier, H., Lededente, A., Baron, A., and Mathé, G.: Adjuvant nonintrapleural BCG. In *Lung Cancer Progress in Therapeutic Research*, F. Muggia and M. Rozencweig, Eds. Raven Press, New York, 1979, pp. 477–481.

15. Pouillart, P., presented at the 1978 Annual Plenary Meeting of the European Organization for Research on Treatment of Cancer, Paris, 1978: Adjuvant therapies and markers of postsurgical minimal residual disease.

16. McKneally, M. F., Maver, C. M., and Kausel, H. W.: Intrapleural BCG immunostimulation in lung cancer. *Lancet 1: 593, 1977.*

12

"Radical" radiotherapy in the treatment of inoperable lung cancer

D. Gonzalez Gonzalez

Inoperable lung cancer, still limited to the thorax, has generally been treated by irradiation, 5000–6000 rad in 5–6 weeks to the primary tumor and the regional lymph nodes. This approach has been in some cases considered as a "radical" treatment. But the results are in general very disappointing. In 1973, we reviewed 182 cases of inoperable lung cancer, treated in our department of radiotherapy: 43 patients had extended and 139 limited disease at the moment of diagnosis. As can be observed in Figure 1, about 80% of the patients with extended disease died within the 4 months post-treatment. The patients with limited disease received a tumor dose of 5600 rad in 5 weeks (mediastinum 4000 rad in 4 weeks). Figure 2 shows the actuarial survival of this group of patients: 27%, 12%, and 2%—1, 2, and 4 years survival respectively. Table 1 presents a survey of some series in the literature.[1–7] The poorer results in our series are probably due to a negative selection because we included all the pathological types while the other series shown in Table 1 only included squamous cell carcinomas. This pitfall can be found in Figure 3 where the actuarial survival of the squamous cell carcinoma is compared with that of the small cell carcinoma: 7% and 2%, 4-year survival, respectively. When the patients were classified according to the UICC staging system, Figure 4, the results were more favorable in Stage I. However, the 4-year survival was in general poor: 7% in Stage I, 2% in Stage III (M_0), and 0% in Stage III (M_1). This subdivision of Stage III in M_0 (tumor less than 2 cm from the carina) and M_1 (distant metastases) was done because both types of patients are Stage III in

the UICC classification but, as observed in Figure 4, the prognosis is very different.

From the results discussed up till now, it is clear that this concept of "radical" radiotherapy is an optimistic one. As a matter of fact, some randomized studies have shown that more or less similar results as the above can be achieved with placebo.[8]

There are two essential reasons for explaining the dismal results obtained with radiotherapy:

a) failure in control of the primary tumor and eventually in the control of the regional metastases (mediastinum);
b) although the control of the primary is achieved, the final prognosis is dependent on the existence of distant metastases, which are not detectable with the normal diagnostic procedures.

Table 2 shows the rate of tumor control as referred to by different authors. In autopsy material, the percentage of tumor control varied between

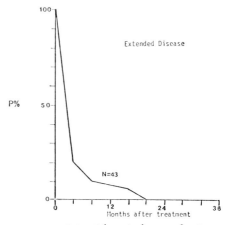

FIGURE 1. Actuarial survival curve of patients with extended disease.

Department of Radiotherapy, Wilhelmina Gasthuis, Amsterdam.

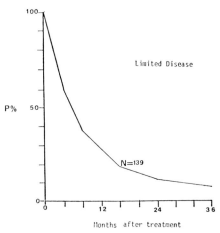

FIGURE 2. Actuarial survival curve of patients with limited disease.

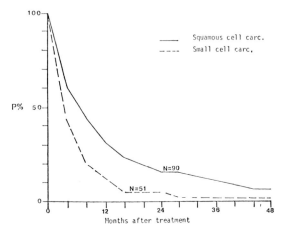

FIGURE 3. Actuarial survival curves of patients with squamous cell carcinoma or small cell carcinoma.

14% and 46%.[9–11] In material obtained after preoperative irradiation, the percentage of tumor control ranged between 0% and 54%.[5,12–15] These percentages of tumor control correspond to a heterogeneous group of lung cancer. Salazar, et al.[16] used as criteria of tumor response to radiation, the resolution of the tumor burden observed on x-ray film. In 80–90% of the patients with small cell carcinoma, there was a resolution of more than 50% of the tumor. The corresponding rate for squamous cell carcinoma was 30–60%. Adenocarcinoma of the lung showed the lowest response to irradiation: 25–30% of tumor resolution. In general, split-course regimens were more effective than continuous irradiation.

The other principal factor explaining the dismal results in inoperable lung cancer treated with radiotherapy, is the presence of distant metastases. Hansen, et al.[17] found 3.6% in the squamous cell

carcinoma, 19% in the adenocarcinoma, and 13% in the large cell carcinoma. Eagan, et al.[18,19] confirmed these findings with 47% of positive bone biopsies in patients with small cell carcinoma. These authors pointed out that, at the moment of diagnosis, 84% of the patients with small cell carcinoma, have blood-borne metastases. Table 3 shows the sites of metastases for the different histological types of lung cancer, as reported by Hansen.[20] Our own data are also presented. It is evident that some differences between the histological types exist, as can be demonstrated by the higher percentage of liver and bone metastases in the small cell carcinoma. These sites of metastases correspond quite well with autopsy findings[21] and with a recently published review by Komaki, et al.[22]

It is evident from the data presented up to now that progress in the treatment of lung cancer can only be expected if the rate of tumor control can be

TABLE 1

Results of Radiotherapy in Inoperable Lung Cancer
Limited Disease

| No. Patients | Survival (%) | | | Reference |
	1 Year	5 Years	10 Years	
347	40	6	—	1
284	30	6	—	2
513	36	6	—	3
103	59	9	7	4
150	40	3	—	5
277	30	6	—	6
188	37	3	—	7
139	27	2	—	Own series
		(4 years)		

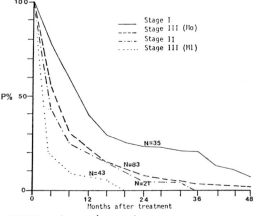

FIGURE 4. Actuarial survival curves according to UICC stages.

TABLE 2

Control Probability of the Primary Tumor

Reference	Tumor Control (%)	Remarks
Guttmann[4]	20 (20)[a]	Autopsy
Rissanen, et al.[9]	37 (38)	Autopsy
	14 (29)	
Bromley-Szur[10]	46 (66)	Autopsy
Bates, et al.[11]	0 (24)	Preoperative
Bloedorn, et al.[12]	54 (26)	Preoperative
Hellman, et al.[13]	29 (24)	Preoperative
Lawton[14]	50 (30)	Preoperative
Shields[15]	26.7	Preoperative

[a] ( ) = number of patients.

TABLE 4

"Radical" Radiotherapy in Lung Cancer

1. Extended field radiotherapy:	Primary
	Regional spread
	Brain
	Upper abdomen (liver + adrenals)
2. Total body irradiation (TBI) + Booster to the:	Primary tumor
	Regional spread
	Brain
	Liver
3. Two half-body irradiation (HBI) + Booster to the:	Primary tumor
	Regional spread
	Brain
	Liver

increased and/or the treatment of distant metastases can be carried out with success.

During the last years, two new approaches in the treatment of inoperable lung cancer are being assayed. The first strategy conceives the treatment of lung cancer as an integration of different therapeutic modalities: radiotherapy is mainly directed to the control of the primary tumor and its regional extension. Chemotherapy is integrated in the treatment with the object of eradicating the distant metastases. Furthermore, the cytostatic can contribute to increasing the control of the primary tumor. Because of the existence of sanctuarial areas (brain) for cytostatic drugs, irradiation of these territories is integrated in the whole treatment. Eventually immunotherapy could be added to the treatment schedule in order to increase the immunoresponse of patients with lung cancer which is known to be depressed in most of the cases and further will be compromised after radio- and chemotherapeutic treatments. Using these integrated approaches for the treatment of small cell carcinoma, Kent, et al.[23] achieved an 80% 1-year survival in patients with limited disease and a 94% complete remission. Hornback, et al.,[24] using a similar integrated treatment, obtained a 63% 1-year survival. In this last series, most of the cases had distant metastases at the moment of diagnosis. When these survival rates are compared with the results previously mentioned after local radiotherapy (11% 1-year survival) as well as with other published series,[25,26] it is obvious that this combined treatment modality, at least in the small cell carcinoma, offers interesting prospects for the future.

The second strategy being tried in several centers is what perhaps in the future could be more properly named "radical" radiotherapy. Table 4 shows the different methods being tested. The first policy

TABLE 3

Sites of Metastases in Patients with "Limited Disease" at Diagnosis

Pathology	No. of Patients	Liver (%)	Bone (%)	Brain (%)	Thorax[a] (%)	Lymphnodes[b] (%)
Squamous cell carcinoma	25	8	16	20	36	36
Small cell carcinoma	25	40	72	8	20	16
Adenocarcinoma	24	12.5	6	21	29	33
Large cell carcinoma	31	6.4	26	13	48	48
Total	105	16	39	25	34	34
					H. H. Hansen, 1974[20]	
Own series	113	37	31	20.4	—	24.5

[a] Extrathoraxic lymphnodes.

[b] Contralateral lung, pericard, mediastinum.

TABLE 5

"Radical" Radiotherapy in Lung Cancer

I. Extended Field

No. Cases	Treatment	Results	Remarks
24	—modified mantle (axillas excluded) —primary: 1733 rets —nodal areas: 718 rets —Brain + liver + adrenals: 766 rets	1 yr surv., 60% 20 months surv. 50%	Oat and undifferentiated carcinoma
		Marks, et al., 1976	

combines a loco-regional radiotherapy with a prophylactic irradiation of the sites where metastases occur more frequently. In the second and third policies, the whole body is irradiated either using a fractionated irradiation of the total body (TBI) or dividing the body into two halves and giving one single fraction to each half with a recovery interval in between (HBI). The mechanism of action of the TBI is not yet known; however, this type of treatment has been effective in patients with disseminated non-Hodgkin's lymphoma. In general, this treatment is given in fractions of 10–20 rad up to a total dose of 100–200 rad. From a radiobiological point of view, it is difficult to expect a direct high cell lethality with these fractionated doses. That is not the case when HBI is used and a single dose of 800 rad is administered. This single dose can be enough to sterilize micrometastases or at least to produce a considerable cell lethality (especially if the radiosensitivity of the tumor is expected to be high as it is in the case of small cell carcinoma).

We shall now present some provisional results with these irradiation policies. Marks, et al.[27] reported a series of 24 patients with undifferentiated carcinoma and small cell carcinoma treated with extended field techniques (modified mantle).

Apart from the primary and regional extension, the brain, liver, and adrenals were prophylactically irradiated. Table 5 shows the results of this treatment: 1-year survival of 60% and 20-month survival of 50%. These results compare quite well with those previously described in the "integrated" therapy.

In Rotterdam, Qasim[28] is doing a pilot study with TBI in patients with small cell carcinoma. Table 6 presents some preliminary results as well as the irradiation technique. The number of patients is too small to be able to draw conclusions. However, it seems that patients with limited disease respond well to this type of treatment.

The HBI was introduced by Fitzpatrick, et al.[29] as a form of treatment in patients with disseminated cancer of different origins. Recently, Rubin, et al.[30] have started systematic studies of this type of radiotherapy in lung cancer. The therapeutic scheme is shown in Table 7. Results have not yet been published.

Lung cancer remains a challenge for the oncologist. With the exception of a small percentage of

TABLE 6

"Radical" Radiotherapy in Lung Cancer

II. TBI + Booster

No. Cases	Treatment	Results	Remarks
11	—TBI: 10 rad/5 days a week Total: 100 rad/2 weeks	2 CR[a] 7 ED ⎞ 5 NR	Oat cell carcinoma
	—Booster: 4000 rad/4 weeks to the primary 2000 rad/2 weeks to the liver	3 GR 4 LD ⎞ 1 death	
		Qasim, 1977	

[a] CR = complete response; GR = good response; NR = no response; ED = early death; LD = late death.

TABLE 7

"Radical" Radiotherapy in Lung Cancer

III. HBI + Booster

Treatment	Remarks
—Primary + regional nodes: split-course: 250 rad × 10—2 weeks rest—250 rads × 10	Non-oat cell carcinoma 6–8 weeks between UHB and LHB
—Upper half-body (UHB): above iliac crest 800 rad single fraction	
—Low half-body (LHB): below iliac crest 800 rad single fraction	
Rubin, et al., 1977	

patients who can obtain benefit from radical surgery, the prognosis of this disease has been stationary for the last two decades and in general poor. The above-mentioned strategies seem to offer new prospects for the future.

Prospective controlled trials, carried out by groups of experts, can change the actual status quo in this disease and perhaps open new horizons in the future.

References

1. Abramson, N., et al.: Radiation therapy in carcinoma of the lung. The short-course method. XIIIth Int. Congress of Radiology, Madrid, Spain, 1973.

2. Caldwell, W. L., et al.: Indication for and results of irradiation of carcinoma of the lung. *Cancer 22: 999–1004, 1968.*

3. Deeley, T. J., et al.: Treatment of inoperable carcinoma of the bronchus by megavoltage x-rays. *Thorax 22: 562–566, 1967.*

4. Guttmann, R. J.: Radical supervoltage therapy in inoperable carcinoma of the lung. In *Carcinoma of the Bronchus*, Deeley, Ed. Butterworths, London, 1971.

5. Guttmann, R. J.: Results of radiation therapy in patients with inoperable carcinoma of the lung whose status was established at exploratory thoracotomy. *Am J Roentgenol 93: 99–103, 1965.*

6. Perez Tamayo, R., et al.: The place of radiotherapy in the treatment of bronchogenic carcinoma. *Mo Med 66:876–880, 1969.*

7. Lee, R. E.: Radiotherapy of broncogenic carcinoma. *Sem Oncol 1: 245–252, 1974.*

8. Durrant, K. R., et al.: Comparison of treatment in inoperable bronchial carcinoma. *Lancet 715–719, 1971.*

9. Rissanen, P. M., et al.: Autopsy findings in lung cancer treated with megavoltage. *Acta Radiol (Ther) 7: 433–442, 1968.*

10. Bromley-Szur, L. L.: Combined radiotherapy and resection for with 66 patients. *Lancet 2: 937–941, 1955.*

11. Bates, M., et al.: Treatment of oat cell carcinoma of bronchus by preoperative radiotherapy and surgery. *Lancet: 1134–1135, 1974.*

12. Bloedorn, F. G.: Rational and benefit of preoperative irradiation in lung cancer. *JAMA 196: 340–341, 1966.*

13. Hellman, S., et al.: Sequelae of radical radiotherapy of carcinoma of the lung. *Radiology 82: 1055, 1964.*

14. Lawton, R., et al.: Preoperative irradiation in the treatment of clinically operable lung cancer. *J Thorac Cardiovasc. Lung 51: 745–750, 1966.*

15. Shields, T.: Preoperative radiation therapy in the treatment of bronchial carcinoma. *Cancer 30: 1388–1393, 1972.*

16. Salazar, O. M., et al.: The assesement of tumor response to irradiation of lung cancer: Continuous versus split-course regimes. *Int J Radiat Oncol 1: 1107–1118, 1976.*

17. Hansen, H. H., et al.: Staging of inoperable patients with bronchogenic carcinoma with especial refrerence to bone marrow examination and peritoneoscopy. *Cancer 30: 1395–1401, 1972.*

18. Eagan, R. T., et al: Small cell carcinoma of the lung. Staging, paraneoplastic symdromus, treatment and survival. *Cancer 33: 527, 1974.*

19. Eagan, R. T., et al.: Combination chemotherapy and radiation therapy in small carcinoma of the lung. *Cancer 32: 371–379, 1973.*

20. Hansen, H. H.: In lung cancer. *Sem Oncol 1: 217–228, 1974.*

21. Muggia, F. M., et al.: Lung cancer: diagnosis in metastatic site. *Sem Oncol 1: 217–228, 1974.*

22. Komaki, R., et al.: Irradiation of bronchial carcinoma—II. Pattern of spread and potential for prophylactic irradiation. *Int J Radiat Oncol 2: 441–446, 1977.*

23. Kent, C. H., et al.: Total therapy for oat cell carcinoma of the lung. *Int J Radiat Oncol 2: 427–432, 1977.*

24. Hornback, N. B., et al.: Oat cell carcinoma of the lung. Early treatment results of combination radiation therapy and chemotherapy. *Cancer 37: 2658–2664, 1976.*

25. Tucker, R. D., et al.: Clinical trial of cyclophosphamide and radiation therapy for oat cell carcinoma of the lung. *Cancer Chem Rep Part 3: 159–160, 1973.*

26. Nixon, D. W., et al.: Combination chemotherapy in oat cell carcinoma of the lung. *Cancer 36: 867–872, 1975.*

27. Marks, S. A., et al.: Extended field radiotherapy for carcinoma of the Bronchus. *Int J Radiat Oncol 1 (Suppl): 74, 1976.*

28. Qasim,: Personal communication, 1977.

29. Fitzpatrick, P. J., et al.: Half body radiotherapy. *Int J Radiat Oncol 1: 197–208, 1976.*

30. Rubin, Ph., et al.: Systemic radiation for the treatment of micrometastasis in non-oat cell lung cancer. *Int J Radiat Oncol 2 (Suppl): 115, 1977.*

13

Chemotherapy as a palliative treatment of primary lung cancer

P. Alberto

CHEMOTHERAPY OF PRIMARY LUNG CANCER has benefited considerably from the experience gained in the combined use of chemotherapy for other malignancies. Yet the results obtained so far remain unsatisfactory. Small cell cancer is one of the human tumors which is very sensitive to the cell-killing effect of antitumor agents. Improved combined treatment schedules, including a chemotherapy–radiotherapy approach, can probably improve more consistently the survival of small cell tumor patients. For non-small cell types, the first priority in further therapeutic research should be placed on the development and clinical screening of new potentially active agents rather than on combinations of limited value.

Chemotherapy of lung cancer is characterized by a large number of agents with limited antitumor activity. Table 1 summarizes the agents for which some activity in human lung cancer was demonstrated and gives a rough estimation of the response rate to be expected, either for the histological tumor types taken separately or for lung cancer in general. It is worth noticing that no single agent has an overall response rate superior to 20%, that small cell carcinoma is more responsive than other cell types, and that even for the most responsive cell type the response rate remains less than or equal to 50%. To this it must also be added that the duration of remissions is generally disappointingly short and that the benefit of chemotherapy is often compromised by the intensity of toxic side effects. This probably explains why single-drug chemotherapy of lung cancer is generally considered of little use, or possibly detrimental to the patients. It is one of the most urgent objectives

TABLE 1

Chemotherapy of Lung Cancer: Estimation of Response Rate in Single-Drug Therapy

Agent	Epidermoid	Small Cell	Large Cell	Adenocarcinoma	Total
Mechloretamin	20	40	30	20	30
Cyclophosphamide	20	40	30	20	30
Adriamycin	20	40	30	20	20
Mitomycin C	20	20	20	20	20
VP 12-213	—	50	—	—	—
Methotrexate	20	40	20	20	20
CCNU	20	20	20	20	20
Procarbazine	20	30	30	20	20
Vincristine	20	40	20	20	20
Hexamethylmelamine	20	30	20	20	20
cis-DDPlatinum	20	—	—	—	—

Reprinted from Cancer Clinical Trials 2: 157–163, 1979.

TABLE 2

Polychemotherapy of Lung Cancer: Combinations with Two Agents

Agents	Schedule (mg/m^2)	No. of Patients	% Response				Authors
			Epidermoid	Adenocarcinoma	Large Cell	Small Cell	
CPA CCNU	700 q3w 70 q6w	218	—	12	—	45	ECOG
CPA MTX	1100 q3w 20 biw	41	—	6	—	38	VALG
HN2 MTX	15 q3w 20 biw	34	10	—	7	—	VALG
CPA ADM	750 q3w 50 q3w	100	—	—	—	>50	M. D. Anderson
ADM VP16	40–45 q4w 70–75 × 3		—	—	—	>50	Mayo

in the future development of chemotherapy to improve the therapeutic effectiveness of single agents in the treatment of primary lung cancer. Combination chemotherapy, or polychemotherapy, is presently the only possible approach to the treatment of disseminated lung cancer. The purpose of this paper is to summarize most of the best known polychemotherapy schedules, to analyze their results in a comparative way, and to draw a few conclusions.

Tables 2–5 summarize commonly used combinations with two, three, four and more than four agents. In all cases the agents combined have different mechanisms of action, a basic requirement in the pharmacological background of polychemotherapy. Unfortunately, the majority of these combinations do not fulfill another important theoretical prerequisite for polychemotherapy, which is that the dose-limiting toxicity should not be identical for the combined agents. It is a fact that

TABLE 3

Polychemotherapy of Lung Cancer: Combinations with Three Agents

Agents	Schedule (mg/m^2)	No. of Patients	% Response				Authors
			Epidermoid	Adenocarcinoma	Large Cell	Small Cell	
HN2 CCNU MTX	10 q3w 5.0 q6w 10 biw	27	6	—	10	—	VALG
CPA CCNU MTX	500 q3w 50 q6w 10 biw	51	—	38	—	56	VALG
CPA CCNU MTX	1000 q3w 100 q6w 15 biw	38	—	—	—	96	VALG
HN2 ADM CCNU	8 q4w 40 q4w 65 q8w	107	14	—	—	—	SWOG "NAC"
CPA ADM C-DDP	400 q4w 40 q4w 40 q4	41	44	43	17	—	Mayo "CAP"

TABLE 4

Polychemotherapy of Lung Cancer: Combinations with Four Agents

Agents	Schedule (mg/m^2)	No. of Patients	% Response				Authors
			Epidermoid	Adenocarcinoma	Large Cell	Small Cell	
CPA	70 d						
PCZ	70 d	130	28	54	50	62	SAKK
MTX	25 w						
VCR	1.3 w						
CPA	700 q4w						
CCNU	70 q4w	49	—	—	—	83	Finsen
MTX	2 × 20 q4w						
VCR	1.5 w						
CPA	800 q4w						
MeCCNU	100 q4w	73	37	11	—	87	M. D. Anderson "COMB"
BLM	15–30 biw						
VCR	0.75 biw						

myelosuppression represents the major dose-limiting toxicity for the majority of the agents used.

Combinations with two agents (Table 2) are often made of an alkylating drug and a drug of another pharmacological category. Cyclophosphamide is the most commonly used agent, probably because it is well tolerated and also because of the large experience of combination treatment with this agent in other malignant diseases such as malignant lymphomas, Hodgkin's disease, and breast cancer. In a large study by the Veterans Administration Lung Group, the alkylating agent used was cyclophosphamide for adenocarcinoma and small cell carcinoma, whereas nitrogen mustard was preferred for epidermoid cancer and large cell tumors. This was based on the assumption that there is a difference of activity of various alkylating agents in the four main cell types of lung cancer. Such a difference, however, has not been clearly demonstrated so far. The combination of adriamycin and VP 16-213 gives very encouraging results for small cell cancer in a series from the

TABLE 5

Polychemotherapy of Lung Cancer: Combinations with More than Four Agents

Agents	Schedule (mg/m^2)	No. of Patients	% Response				Authors
			Epidermoid	Adenocarcinoma	Large Cell	Small Cell	
ADM	40 q4w						
HN2	8 q4w						
CCNU	65 q8w	106	21	—	—	—	SWOG "BACON"
VCR	0.75 w						
BLM	30 w						
CPA	70 dx14						
PCZ	70 dx14						
ADM	25 q4w						
CCNU	60 q4w	30	—	—	—	60	SAKK
VCR	1.2 q4w						
MTX	25 q4w						
HU	6 × 1000 q4w						

TABLE 6

Polychemotherapy of Lung Cancer: Sequential vs. Simultaneous Combination

| Agents | Schedule (mg/m^2) | No. of Patients | % Response | | Large Cell | Small Cell | Author |
			Epidermoid	Adenocarcinoma			
MTX	25 w						
CPA	70 d	49	33	(^{2}/$_3$)	60	65	SAKK
PCZ	70 d						
VCR	1.3 w						
MTX	25 d 1, 8						
CPA	150 d 15–28	43	13	(^{1}/$_3$)	0	36	
PCZ	150 d 29–42						
VCR	1.3 d 43,50						

Mayo clinic. The same is true for the combination adriamycin–cyclophosphamide studied at the M. D. Anderson Cancer Institute in Houston.

A selection of combinations with three agents is presented in Table 3. In the VALG studies, the adjunction of a nitrosourea to the combination alkylating agent methotrexate increases the response rate in adenocarcinoma and small cell tumors, whereas no improvement is obtained in epidermoid and large cell cancers. A more intensive dosage of the same three-agent combination produces in a later study by the same group an impressive re-

sponse rate of 96% in small cell carcinoma, but at the cost of a more severe toxicity. The combination of cyclophosphamide, adriamycin and *cis*-platinum proposed by the Mayo Clinic Group under the nickname CAP is very interesting in terms of the high response rate obtained in epidermoid cancer. Another combination called NAC also seems very promising in a preliminary series at M. D. Anderson, whereas a further study by the South West Oncology Group gave a disappointing result of 14%.

A few well-known combinations with four drugs

TABLE 7

Polychemotherapy of Lung Cancer: Sequences of Combinations

| Agents | Schedule (mg/m^2) | No. of Patients | % Response | | Large Cell | Small Cell | Author |
			Epidermoid	Adenocarcinoma			
CPA	1100 q3w						
HN2	15 q3w	75	10	6	7	38	
MTX	20 biw						
Progression:							
CCNU	100 q6w	31	0	0	0	0	VALG
HU	2000 biw						
Progression:							
PCZ	100 d	6	0	0	0	0	
VCR	2 w						
CPA	500 q3w						
MTX	10 biw	78	6	38	10	56	
CCNU	50 q6w						
Progression:							VALG
VCR	2 w						
PCZ	70 d	33	0	7	0	15	
HU	1400 biw						

TABLE 8

Polychemotherapy of Lung Cancer: Single vs. Double Combination

Agents	Schedule (mg/m^2)	No. of Patients	% Response		Author
			Small Cell	(Complete Response)	
CPA	1000 q3w				
MTX	15 biw	38	96	(25)	VALG
CCNU	100 q6w				
CPA	1500 q4w ⎫				
MTX	15 biw ⎬ w1–6				
CCNU	100 q6w ⎭				
VCR	2 q3w ⎫	50	92	(56)	VALG
ADM	60 q3w ⎬ w7–12				
PCZ	100 d × 10 ⎭				
	q3w				

are illustrated in Table 4. In general, the response rate is superior to that observed with two- or three-drug schedules, for small cell tumors as well as for other cell types. The combination of cyclophosphamide, procarbazine, methotrexate and vincristine has been used by investigators of the Swiss Group for 10 years and is still considered equal or superior to all other regimens which have been compared to it. Combinations with more than four agents (Table 5) have rarely been investigated. The BACON program as proposed by M. D. Anderson Institute, particularly for epidermoid carcinoma, does not seem superior to other treatments. Similarly, a seven-drug regimen used in a still un-

TABLE 9

Polychemotherapy of Lung Cancer: Sequence of Phase-Nonspecific–Phase-Specific Combinations

Agents	Schedule (mg/m^2)	No. of Patients	% Response		Author
			Small Cell	(Complete Response)	
CPA	70 d				
PCZ	70 d	30	73	(33)	SAKK
MTX	25 w				
VCR	1.3 w				
ADM	30 q8w				
CCNU	70 q8w				
CPA	70 dx7 q8w				
PCZ	70 dx7 q8w				
Alternating with:		65	62	(17)	
MTX	25 wx2 q8w				
VCR	1.3 wx2 q8w				
HU	3 × 1000 wx2 q8w				
ADM	30 q4w				
CCNU	70 q4w				
CPA	70 dx7 q4w				
PCZ	70 dx7 q4w	30	60	(23)	
MTX	25 q4w				
VCR	1.3 q4w				
HU	3 × 1000 q4w				

published study by the Swiss Group did not give better results than the aforementioned four-drug combination.

All previously discussed polychemotherapy programs were based on simultaneous combinations, either pulsed or continuous. Another approach to multiple-drug treatment concerns the sequential application of single-drug or multiple-drug programs. Table 6 illustrates a comparison of two regimens where the same four agents are used, in one case simultaneously, in the other sequentially. This study clearly shows that the simultaneous combination is superior, in terms of response rate, to the sequential combination, either for small cell cancer or for other cell types. Table 7 summarizes another study of sequential treatment, realized by the VALG. Here sequential combinations with two or three agents are used, each one being only initiated after primary or secondary failure of the preceding one. The most striking point is the ineffectiveness of the second and third combination after failure of the first one. There is no satisfactory explanation for this, aside from the well-known observation that chemotherapy is less active in pretreated than in non-pretreated patients.

Another sequential scheduling is exemplified in Table 8. In this VALG study a three-drug simultaneous polychemotherapy is compared to an alternation of two dissimilar three-drug regimens, each one being given for 6 weeks. The result of the alternating program seems to be better, particularly in terms of the rate of complete remissions. Table 9 shows a more sophisticated approach, in which an alternating program is used, the first part being made of phase-nonspecific agents, and the second part of phase-specific agents. This type of sequence is based on the assumption that each time the phase-nonspecific treatment reduces the tumor volume, the growth rate of the tumor increases and the tumor becomes more sensitive to the phase specific therapy. In the study shown here, the phase-nonspecific–phase-specific sequence has been compared to the standard four-drug treatment used since 1968 by the Swiss Group, and also with a simultaneous seven-drug combination including the same agents. The results do not suggest any superiority of the cycle-adapted sequence.

In conclusion, chemotherapy of primary lung cancer has benefited considerably from the experience acquired in the combined use of chemotherapy for other malignancies. Yet the results obtained so far remain unsatisfactory. For small cell carcinoma, the effects of combined chemotherapy on survival is still limited despite a high response rate. For the other cell types, chemotherapy, even combined, is of very limited effectiveness. Small cell cancer is one of the human tumors which is very sensitive to the cell-killing effect of antitumor agents. Improved combined treatment schedules, including a chemotherapy–radiotherapy approach, can probably improve more consistently the survival of small cell tumor patients. For non-small cell types, the first priority in further therapeutic research should be put on the development and clinical screening of new potentially active agents rather than on combinations of limited value.

References

1. Alberto, P., Brunner, K. W., Martz, G., Obrecht, J.-P., and Sonntag, R. W.: Treatment of bronchogenic carcinoma with simultaneous or sequential combination chemotherapy, including methotrexate, cyclophosphamide, procarbazine and vincristine. *Cancer 38: 2208–2216, 1976.*

2. Bunn, P. A., Jr., Cohen, M. H., Ihde, D. C., Fossieck, B. E., Jr., Matthews, M. J., and Minna J. D.: Commentary: Advances in small cell bronchogenic carcinoma. *Cancer Treat Rep 61: 333–338, 1977.*

3. Cavalli, F.: VP-16-213 Monotherapy for remission induction of small cell lung cancer: A randomized trial using 3 dosage schedules. *Cancer Treat Rep 62: 3, 1978.*

4. Cohen, M. H., Broder, L. E., Fossieck, B. E., Ihde, D. C., and Minna, J. D.: Phase II clinical trial of weekly administration of VP-16-213 in small cell bronchogenic carcinoma. *Cancer Treat Rep 61: 489, 1977.*

5. Cohen, M. H.: Lung cancer: A status report. *J NCI 55: 505–511, 1975.*

6. Eagan, R. T., Ingle, J. N., Frytak, S., Rubin, J., Kvols, L. K., Carr, D. T., Coles, D. T., and O'Fallon, J. R.: Platinum-based polychemotherapy versus dianhydrogalactitol in advanced non-small cell lung cancer. *Cancer Treat Rep 61: 1339–1345, 1977.*

7. Hansen, H. H.: Management of lung cancer. *Med Clin North Am 61: 979–989, 1977.*

8. Herman, T. S., Jones, S. E., McMahon, L. J., Lloyd, R. E., Heusinkveld, R. S., Miller, R. C., and Salmon, S. E.: Combination chemotherapy with adriamycin and cyclophosphamide (with or without radiation therapy) for carcinoma of the lung. *Cancer Treat Rep 61: 875, 1977.*

9. Jungi, W. F., and Senn, J. H.: Clinical study of the new podophyllotoxin derivative, 4'-demethylepipodophyllotoxin 9-(4,6-0-ethylidene-β-D-glucopyranoside) (NSC-141540; VP-16-213) in solid tumors in man. *Cancer Treat Rep 59: 737–742, 1975.* Legha, S. S.,

Muggia, F. M., and Carter, S. K.: Adjuvant chemotherapy in lung cancer: Review and prospect. *Cancer 39: 1415–1424, 1977.*

10. Livingston, R. B.: Combination chemotherapy of bronchogenic carcinoma I. Non oat cell. *Cancer Treat Rev 4: 153–165, 1977.*

11. Matthews, M. J., Kanhouwa, S., Pickren, J., and Robinette, D.: Frequency of residual and metastatic tumor in patients undergoing surgical resection for lung cancer. *Cancer Chemother Rep 41: 63–67, 1973.*

12. Riotton, G., Raymond, L., Obradovic, M., Roch, R., and Reiben, A.: *Cancer à Genève: Incidence et Mortalité 1970–1973.* Registre Genevois des Tumeurs, 1976.

13. Straus, M. J.: *Lung Cancer: Clinical Diagnosis and Treatment.* Grune & Stratton, New York, 1977.

14. Wasserman, T. H., Comis, R. L., Goldsmith, M., Handelsman, H., Pents, J. S., Slavik, M., Soper, W. T., and Carter, S. K.: Tabular analysis of the clinical chemotherapy of solid tumors. *Cancer Chemother Rep 6: 399, 1975.*

15. Yesner, R.: A unified concept of lung cancer histopathology. *Proc Am Soc Clin Oncol 18: 271, 1977.*

Conclusions

14

P. Alberto, M.D.

In a symposium predominantly attended by physicians interested in clinical oncology but not considering themselves (at least for the majority of them) as fully trained oncologists, conclusions need to cover problems of general medical importance. Many such problems were extensively treated during the session. Dr. L. Jimeno Alfós summarized the presently available methods of clinicopathological staging of primary lung tumors, and showed the prognostic significance of many clinical parameters including characteristics of the tumor and of the patient. In this problem of staging procedures and prognostic factors, I see two aspects of particular interest for non-oncologists. The first is the need for an extensive clinical staging in all patients with a diagnosis of lung cancer before the best possible curative or palliative treatment can be determined. The second is more theoretical and concerns the importance of an even distribution of all prognostic factors in patient groups to be compared for the relative effectiveness of various treatments. Unfortunately, it must be admitted that an important part of the differences, or of the absence of differences, observed in comparative clinical trials, are due to an uneven distribution of prognostic factors and not to the intrinsic value of the treatment programs compared.

Dr. F. Paris showed very clearly the dilemma faced by the lung cancer surgeon, squeezed between the restrictive staging requirements of a high standard surgical curative approach, and the temptation of a broader indication of surgical treatment. Curative surgery of lung cancer is characterized by a rate of failure of 70% or more. This justifies amply the large effort of combined treatment modality approach realized presently. Dr. D. Gonzales exposed the practical possibilities and the physical limits of radiotherapy. The combination of surgery and radiotherapy was extensively explored and, unfortunately, did not constitute a major improvement compared with surgery alone. The future of radiation treatment of lung cancer also probably lies in combined modality approach. In this respect, half-body radiation treatment as a potentially active systemic treatment deserves a special interest, particularly if its combination with chemotherapy is feasible.

Dr. F. Muggia stressed the major importance of adjuvant treatment for lung cancer. He also showed that this problem is far from being solved. If one considers postsurgical chemotherapy in particular, its value is intrinsically limited by the fact that surgery is poorly effective in the only cell type responsive to chemotherapy, whereas chemotherapy is hardly of any value for epidermoid carcinoma. Adenocarcinoma is presently the best candidate among lung tumors for a chemosurgical therapy. An effective chemotherapy of epidermoid cancer of the lung would certainly find a major place in adjuvant treatment.

From a practical point of view the role of chemotherapy is presently limited to the treatment of anaplastic tumors in an advanced stage. For this purpose only polychemotherapy is sufficiently effective. It can be hoped that further investigation of alternating combined schedules, or, possibly, of radiotherapy programs, will eventually improve the patients' survival. Previous experience with chemotherapy of other tumors suggests that cancer cure should be possible when response rates close to 100% have been achieved. For other cell types (the so called nonsmall-cell tumors) chemotherapy is still at its beginning. So is also immunology for all types and all stages of lung cancer.

Centre d'Onco, Hematologie des Policliniques et de l'Hôpital Cantonal, Geneve, Switzerland.

Breast cancer. Introduction

15

Jose G. Catalan Fernandez, M.D.

Breast cancer accounts for at least 25% of all female malignancies, and yet important aspects of its biology remain unknown.

From the first cellular alteration to an identifiable clinical stage, an estimated interval of at least 2 years will elapse. We are rarely able to detect a tumor less than 1 cm in diameter. Often what we call an early stage is already associated with metastatic disease.

Our treatment strategies, introduced at the turn of the century, are able to interfere with the natural course of the disease, but survival rates have not changed in the last thirty years, until perhaps the recent generation of adjuvant trials.

Surgery has offered various treatment modalities, from the most conservative approaches of tumorectomy and lobectomy to the very aggressive ultra-radical mastectomy. Whichever method we select, a proportion of cases will develop metastasis over a variable length of time.

Radiation therapy is also under constant evolution in regards to techniques, dosages, and the optimal moment in which it should be applied. In view of the results, which individually are not very encouraging even in the early stages, the most attractive issue for the near future might be therapeutic combination and strategy design.

Hormones and chemotherapy, which for some time were used only to treat advanced stages, are now being introduced as adjuvant treatments in the so-called early stages. Metastatic disease has traditionally been handled by the use of endocrine treatments, either additive or ablative and chemotherapy. In recent years, a wealth of information has been introduced on the use of these approaches. Hormone receptors offer the availability of a new prognostic index and the ability to predict response. New drugs have been introduced, such as androgens of low activity antiestrogens, inhibitors of adrenal cortical function and inhibitors of prolactin among many others. The possibility of replacing surgical adenalectomy and hypophysectomy by drug inhibition of the various endocrine glands might allow less aggressive technique of ablative therapy to be used in most patients. Chemotherapy has seen the introduction of new active drugs, and development of new combinations. Remission rates have plateaued at a 50–70% level. Several combinations of hormones and chemotherapy are being tested, which explore the theoretical benefits of both therapies used simultaneously.

Prognostic factors have also been enriched through the study quantification of hormonal receptors and biochemical markers, as well as the study of host-immunity. The following papers will transmit more of this new information.

Oncology Center of the Balearic Islands, Palma de Mallorca, Spain.

16

Surgical treatment of primary breast cancer

Roberto Saccozzi, M.D.

The criticism of Halsted's treatment of mammary carcinoma emerges from two points of view: first that this treatment has been considered incomplete and second that it is unduly and needlessly mutilating.

The diversity of these two criticisms in the result of two different philosophies regarding the natural history of breast cancer. The first, and more traditional, view sees the tumor as a local disease which later spreads further afield and therefore the surgeon must remove as much tissue as possible. The second sees it as a proliferation which, right from the start, bombards the whole organism with malignant cells, whose "take" depends mainly on immunologic factors. In this case, the surgeon's job is to control the take and growth of these cells with the aid of other procedures such as chemotherapy, immunotherapy or endocrine therapy rather than concern himself overmuch with the primary tumor.

Since it is difficult to establish which of these two philosophies is the more correct for each single tumor and since they probably both contain part of the truth, a third, more pragmatic, line of thought has evolved which sees the solution to the therapeutic problem in experimental terms without being unduly influenced by theoretical implications.

According to this approach, the answers to our questions can only emerge from a series of rationally designed clinical trials.

Our main starting point was that the old dictum "small tumor, large operation," was to be challenged with the new concept "small tumor, small operation" and "extensive tumor, extended operation."

The introduction of large-scale mass screening, more sophisticated diagnostic tools, and a systematic self-examination by women themselves resulted in an increased number of breast cancers of limited extent. For these reasons the traditional radical mastectomy seemed to be too mutilating a procedure and a more conservative surgery was introduced.

In June 1973 the National Cancer Institute of Milan started a randomized clinical trial in T_1N_0 cases, which allows for a comparison between the standard treatment, Halsted radical mastectomy, and a conservative surgery based on a quadrantectomy of the breast plus axillary dissection plus radiotherapy on the remaining breast. This operation consists in the resection of an entire quadrant of the breast together with the overlying skin and the corresponding portion of the fascial sheet of the pectoralis major. The axillary dissection is always performed, whenever possible, en-bloc and in continuity with the breast quadrant. Axillary dissection is intended to prevent recurrences due to

TABLE 1

Trial Design of Conservative Surgery

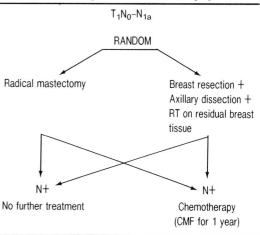

81

TABLE 2

Internal Mammary Involvement in 2023 Cases Operated on with Radical Mastectomy and Internal Mammary Dissection

Site	No. of Cases	No. with Internal Mammary Metastases	%
Outer quadrants	681	103	15.1
Inner quadrants	1020	257	25.2
Central quadrants	280	91	32.6
Whole gland	42	19	44.2
Total	2023	470	23.2

occult lymph node metastases which account for about 25% of T_1N_0 cases.

After surgery the patients receive 6000 rad to the residual breast tissue over 5–6 weeks starting 15 days after operation. According to the policy of the Institute all cases with positive nodes are treated with adjuvant combined chemotherapy with CMF for 1 year (Table 1).

At the end of October 1977, 437 cases were entered the trial: 214 of them have been submitted to radical mastectomy and 223 to quadrantectomy plus axillary dissection and radiotherapy. Till now two cases in the group of radical mastectomy and two in the group of conservative surgery had a recurrences in the loco-regional area. Thirteen cases, in the radical mastectomy group, and eight in the conservative group had distant metastases. The cosmetic results may be defined good in 65%. If the conservative protocol will result in the same recurrence-free survival rate as the one observed for

TABLE 3

Incidence of Internal Mammary Metastases According to Age

Age Group	No.	No. with Internal Mammary Metastases	%
30	31	14	45.2
31–40	283	106	37.4
41–50	699	161	23.0
51–60	672	137	20.4
61–70	324	50	15.4
70	14	2	14.3
Total	2023	470	23.2

TABLE 4

5-Year Survival in 1002 Cases Treated with Extended Mastectomy (with Removal of Internal Mammary Nodes) According to Regional Metastases

Regional Involvement	No.	5-Year Survival	%
No metastases	493	420	82.5
Axillary only	275	159	57.8
Internal mammary only	43	33	76.9
Axillary and internal mammary	191	62	32.4
Total	1002	674	67.3

radical mastectomy, limited surgery will find a definite place in breast cancer treatment.

For T_2 and T_3 cases and all N_1 cases no substitutes to radical mastectomy or to modified radical mastectomy were considered acceptable. However, for this group of patients the question of the value of internal mammary lymph node removal had to be solved.

From 1946 up to now, 2023 cases of breast cancer have been subjected to this procedure with minor technical variations, and 470 showed internal mammary involvement (Tables 2 and 3). Two important findings emerged in our series: first that internal mammary chain involvement is more likely in young women and decreases with age, and

TABLE 5

Design of the Trial of Chemotherapy plus Radiotherapy in T_{3b}–T_4 Cases without Distant Metastases (1973)

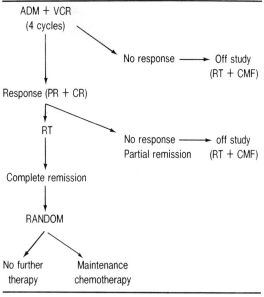

TABLE 6

Outline of the New Trial on Chemotherapy plus Radiotherapy versus Chemotherapy plus "Reductive" Surgery in T_{3b}–T_4 Cases (1976)

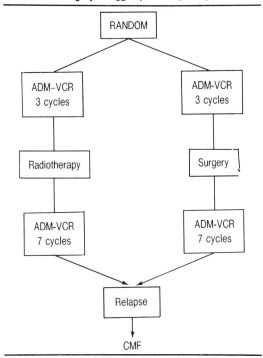

secondly that the 5-year survival rate (Table 4) is satisfactory in cases with internal mammary involvement without axillary metastases, thus

showing that internal mammary involvement in itself is not so ominous prognostic factor as was considered. However, the proper indication for internal mammary dissection was still not clear in our series until a cooperative clinical trial clarified the picture. This trial was conducted by five institutes in the world, and a total of 1580 cases were collected in 5 years. The overall 5-year results showed no statistical difference in the two series of cases (72% survival for extended mastectomy, 69% for radical mastectomy).[1]

Another attempt to search for new surgical techniques was conducted in cases with massive regional lymph node involvement without distant metastases. In these patients we started in 1962 a new type of operation which was defined superradical, since it leads to the simultaneous removal of the axillary, supraclavicular, internal mammary and mediastinal lymph nodes, that is, all the network of lymph vessels and lymph nodes connected with the breast. This operation was devised to evaluate what surgery alone would achieve in breast cancer when pushed to the limits of its possibilities hoping that, when radical removal was not obtained, the drastic reduction of cancer cells might be all the same beneficial to the patient. Till now, 162 cases have been submitted to this operation without operative mortality and with results which may be defined very encouraging. For 81 patients evaluable for 5-year survival the rate of 46.9% is in fact double than similar cases treated

TABLE 7

1978 Policy at the National Cancer Institute of Milan as Regards the Various Forms of Surgery According to Disease Extent

T_1N_0		Resection of the breast Axillary dissection Radiotherapy on the residual breast	⊤ a
T_2N_0		Modified radical mastectomy	
T_3N_0 $T_{1-2-3}N_1$		Radical mastectomy	In N+ cases adjuvant chemotherapy
T_3N_0 $T_{1-2-3}N_1$	inner quadrants	Radical mastectomy Internal mammary dissection	⊤ a
N_{2-3}		Superradical mastectomy	
T_4		Induction chemotherapy Radical mastectomy Maintenance chemotherapy	⊤ a

a ⊤ = Trial in progress.

with RT. However, no randomized trials were done for these cases and no strictly comparative data are therefore available for evaluation.

Finally, on the last problems of T_{3b}–T_4 cases, we started a new trial comparing the therapeutic program "induction chemotherapy-radiotherapy-maintenance chemotherapy" with the program "induction chemotherapy-reductive surgery-maintenance chemotherapy," where surgery is represented by radical mastectomy (Tables 5 and 6). The first results of this trial will be available in 3–5 years.

The results of the various trials have allowed us to identify different types of operation according to the extent of the disease (Table 7). This is obviously a provisional setting of the complex matter, but we believe that it may be an important step towards a more rational approach to breast cancer treatment, particularly with regards to the initial management of local disease.

Conservative treatments and more extended treatments must find their right place among the therapeutic indications of breast cancer and must respond to different needs.

Summary

Radical mastectomy should be replaced by a number of different types of operation either more conservative or more extended according to the extent of the disease. For cases T_1N_0 a new procedure consisting of the removal of a quadrant of the breast, with axillary dissection plus radiotherapy on the residual breast tissue is under evaluation. In cases T_2N_0 modified radical mastectomy is suggested as a procedure of choice, while T_3 cases and all N_1 cases should probably still be submitted to radical mastectomy. Extended and superradical mastectomies are limited to specially selected cases. All N+ cases are submitted to adjuvant chemotherapy (CMF). In locally advanced cases "reductive" surgery may be part of an aggressive chemotherapy program.

References

1.   Lacour, J., et al.: *Cancer 37: 206–214, 1976.*

17

Adjuvant chemotherapy

Studies of the NCI-Milano

M. De Lena

Introduction

The traditional surgical and/or radiotherapeutic approach in early breast cancer with positive axillary nodes can cure only a limited fraction of patients.[1,2] During the past two decades many trials employing adjuvant hormonal or cytotoxic therapy were carried out to improve the long-term results of primary treatment, but they were inconclusive or negative.[3,4] The critical review showed that the rationale of these studies was based on the assumption that treatment failure was due primarily to dissemination of cancer cells during surgical manipulation and, for this reason, the single cytotoxic agent was administered during the perioperative or short-term postoperative time. More recently, modern concepts about natural history of operable breast cancer,[1,2] growth kinetics of residual micrometastases,[5] and efficacy of cyclic combination chemotherapy have provided a more accurate baseline for the design of clinical trials.

This paper summarizes the results so far obtained with the adjuvant chemotherapy trials in breast cancer at the Istituto Nazionale Tumori of Milan with two CMF programs.

Results

The new generation of adjuvant studies was initiated few years ago. The study design included selection of patients at high risk of early relapse (N+), stratification and randomization after radical surgery, and administration of intermittent prolonged chemotherapy. The first studies were initiated by the NSABP group in September 1972[6] and by the Istituto Nazionale Tumori of Milan in

June 1973.[7] Patients with positive axillary nodes at the time of mastectomy were randomly allocated within 4 weeks from surgery to either no further treatment of melphalan for 2 years in the NSABP study (348 patients) or combination chemotherapy with cyclophosphamide, methotrexate, and fluorouracil (CMF) for 1 year in the Istituto Nazionale Tumori study (386 patients). Both studies have confirmed that prolonged cyclical adjuvant chemotherapy can statistically reduce the relapse rate compared to women treated only with surgery.

CMF programs at the Istituto Nazionale Tumori of Milan

The first adjuvant study with prolonged combination chemotherapy in operable breast cancer having histologically positive axillary nodes (T_{1-2-3a} $N+$), was started in Milan on June 1973. The details of this controlled trial, the dosage of the drugs, and the modality of administration have appeared in previous publications.[8–11]

In the control group no further treatment was given after radical mastectomy. By September 1975 a total of 386 patients (radical mastectomy or control group: 179; radical mastectomy plus CMF: 207) were considered evaluable for statistical analysis. Both groups were comparable in terms of T. extent, number of axillary lymph nodes (1–3, >3), and menopausal status.

The total failure time distribution at 4 years for both treatment groups has been published.[11,12] At 48 months from mastectomy the difference remains highly significant (34.4% vs. 52.7%). The advantage of CMF therapy is evident in the premenopausal patients (59.2% vs. 25.0%), independently of the number of lymph nodes involved. On the contrary, in postmenopausal women the difference was not statistically significant (47.6% vs. 43.8%).

Istituto Nazionale per lo Studio e la Cura dei Tumori, Milano.

Also, the overall survival was statistically improved by adjuvant chemotherapy. At 48 months 26.4% of the control group died from progressive cancer compared to 17.0% of CMF patients.

Gastrointestinal symptoms of nausea and anorexia were present in most patients. Marked leukopenia (WBC below 2,500 per mm^3) occurred only in 7% of the patients; platelets below 75,000 per mm^3 was observed in 19%. Nineteen percent of the patients had a very mild stomatitis and 30% had transient chemical cystitis. Loss of hair was observed in 69% of the patients, but in only 5% was it complete. Amenorrhea was induced in 71.6% of menstruating women, but it was temporary in 13.8% ($\leq$40 years: 42.9%; >40 years: 4.5%). The average percentage of optimal dose administered to patients who have completed 12 cycles (CTX 74%, MTX 90%, FU 80%) indicates that the prolonged CMF therapy was, generally, well tolerated.

It is important to note that all women were treated in the out-patient clinic and none had to be readmitted to the hospital because of severe toxicity.

More recently, we have closed the patient accrual of the second CMF program carried out in premenopausal patients.[11] The aim of this study was to determine the optimal length of adjuvant chemotherapy. For this reason, premenopausal patients classified as $T_{1-2-3a} N+$, were randomly treated with 6 or 12 cycles of CMF following radical mastectomy. A total of 326 women entered into the study (12 cycles: 161; 6 cycles: 165). At 36 months after surgery there is no statistical difference between the two groups in the relapse free survival (12 cycles: 84.5%; 6 cycles: 82.6%) or in the overall survival rates (86.2% and 85.1%, respectively).

Therefore, it is our opinion that a longer follow-up period is necessary to define better if 6 cycles of CMF are similar to 12 cycles in terms of therapeutic efficacy.

TABLE 1

Istituto Nazionale Tumori, Milano. Ongoing Study Protocols with Adjuvant Chemotherapy in Various Stages of Breast Cancer[a]

Pathological Stage	Type of Treatment	No. of Patients Entered into the Study	Preliminary Findings
T_1N+, M_0	® RM / CS + RT } + CMF, 12 cycles	50 37	3 patients in the RM and 1 in the CS + RT group relapsed (median time of observation: 23 months).
$T_{1-2-3a}N+ M_0$ (pre menopause)	RM + CMF, 12 cycles	96	Too early to evaluate.
$T_{1-2-3a}N+ M_0$ (post menopause) <65 years	RM → ® CMFP, 6 cycles → AV, 4 cycles (with intensification) / CMFP, 6 cycles → AV, 4 cycles (without intensification)	51 53	Too early to evaluate; however, no difference between the two groups at 27 months from beginning of the study (4 and 3 relapsed with and without intensification, respectively).
$T_{1-2-3a}N+, M_0$ (post menopausal) >65 yrs.	RM + { CMF, 12 cycles + Tamoxifen (20 mg/day for 1 year)	73	Too early to evaluate; however, 3 relapsed at 27 months from beginning of the study.
$T_{3b} - T_4N+, M_0$	® AV (3 cycles) + RT + AV (6–7 cycles) / AV (3 cycles) + RM + AV (6–7 cycles)	79 79	At 2 years no difference between the two treatment groups in RFS and overall survival.

[a] RM: Radical mastectomy; CS: conservative surgery; RT: radiation therapy; CMF: cyclophosphamide, methotrexate, 5-fluorouracil; P: prednisolone; AV: adriamycin, vincristine.

Current trials in adjuvant breast cancer in Istituto Nazionale Tumori of Milan

Table 1 summarizes the ongoing adjuvant trials in various stages of breast cancer.

In the first study (T_1 disease) patients are clinically N_{o-1a} and entered into the study after surgery which consists of radical mastectomy or of a large resection of the breast with axillary dissection (conservative surgery, CS). Radiotherapy (RT) to residual breast tissue is given only to patients treated with conservative surgery and consists of 5000 rad through two opposing tangential fields with high-energy radiation (^{60}Co). A booster of 1000 rad to the skin surrounding the scar with orthovoltage radiotherapy is also given.[12]

The second study was designed to better define the prognostic importance of bone scan, estrogen-receptor status, and hormone profile.

The third study was carried out with the intent to overcome selective drug resistance in postmenopausal patients under 65 years of age. For this reason, two non-cross-resistant combinations were administered sequentially for a total of 10 cycles. Furthermore, this study intends to test in postmenopausal women the mathematical hypothesis of tumor cell kinetics proposed by Norton and Simon. The comparison is made between progressive dose intensification versus a conventional dose schedule.

In the group of patients older than 65 years, a combination of chemo-hormone therapy was administered. This association was designed considering that in this group of patients it is not easy, for hematological reasons, to administer a high percentage of chemotherapeutic drugs. Furthermore, a high percentage of post menopausal women have positive estrogen receptors.

The last study was designed to compare the efficacy of two different local treatments (radiotherapy according to the Baclesse technique versus radical mastectomy) in locally advanced breast cancer. Patients with inflammatory carcinoma and with infraclavicular lymph node involvement were excluded. Of the five studies, this is the only one in which it is possible to state that there is no statistically significant difference between the two treatment groups in terms of relapse free and overall survival.[13] For this reason, a new study will be undertaken in a near future.

Comment

The new strategic approach for primary breast cancer raises a number of clinical problems. The first deals with the selection of patients who, at the present moment, can be considered as good candidates for prolonged systemic adjuvant therapy. The well-known data on natural history following radical mastectomy[1,2] indicate that the group with histologically positive axillary nodes is at high risk of early relapse.

Recently, Nime et al.[14] reported the results of a histopathologic study indicating that patients with histologically negative axillary lymph nodes but with tumor cells in the intramammary lymphatics vessels, represents a subgroup at high risk of relapse (43% compared to 4% of women who had no intramammary tumor emboli). If this important observation will be confirmed in a larger series, this sub-group of patients with N- will also be considered at high risk for early relapse in distant sites and then treated with adjuvant systemic therapy.

Present results would indicate that adjuvant chemotherapy appears indicated in all premenopausal women. A relation between drug-induced amenorrhea and the effect of adjuvant treatment was not demonstrated in the two CMF studies. In fact, in this first study, patients with drug-induced amenorrhea had a reduced incidence of relapse (26.7% vs. 43.8%), but this finding was not statistically significant ($P = 0.26$). Similar results in relapse free survival (RFS), were observed in the second CMF study (RFS in the 12-cycle-treated group: with amenorrhea 84.6%, without amenorrhea 73.6%, $P = 0.44$; RFS in 6-cycle-treated group, 86.1% and 68.8%, respectively, $P = 0.09$).

Moreover, the results of studies with some prophylactic castration are, at 4 years, inferior when compared in terms of RFS and total survival to the CMF adjuvant treatment.[15–17]

Probably other yet unidentified histological reasons (high incidence of tumor with low growth fraction, selective drug resistance, low drug doses, or endocrine factors), are responsible for the lower activity of adjuvant CMF in postmenopausal women.

In conclusion, many problems in the adjuvant chemotherapy for operable breast cancer remain open (selection of patient candidates to the systemic therapy, duration and type of optimal adjuvant treatment, role of hormonal therapy and of immunotherapy, role of adjuvant therapy in postmenopausal patients, risk of drug-induced second tumors, etc.). However, the preliminary results of the first two CMF studies have demonstrated that the combined modality approach for early breast cancer is correct. Prospective trials as well as rigorous clinical and statistical evaluation are the only means to overcome the present period of therapeutic uncertainty.

References

1. Fisher, B., Slack, N., Katrych, D., and Wolmark, N.: Ten year follow-up results of patients with carcinoma of the breast in a co-operative clinical trial evaluating surgical adjuvant chemotherapy. *Surg Gynecol Obstet* 140: 528-534, 1975.

2. Valagussa, P., Bonadonna, G., and Veronesi, U.: Pattern of relapse and survival following radical mastectomy. Analysis of 716 consecutive patients. *Cancer 41:* 1170-1178, 1978.

3. Bonadonna, G., Valagussa, P., and Veronesi, U.: Results of ongoing clinical trials with adjuvant chemotherapy in operable breast cancer. In J. C. Heuson, W. H. Mattheim, and M. Rozencweig, Eds., *Breast Cancer: Trends in Research and Treatment*, Raven Press, New York, 1976, pp. 239-258.

4. Tormey, D. C.: Combined chemotherapy and surgery in breast cancer: a review. *Cancer 36: 881-892,* 1975.

5. Schabel, F. M.: Rationale for adjuvant chemotherapy. *Cancer 39: 2875-2882, 1977.*

6. Fisher, B., Carbone, P., Economou, S. G., et al.: L-Phenylalanine mustard (L-PAM) in the management of primary breast cancer. A report of early findings. *N Engl J Med 292: 117-122, 1975.*

7. Bonadonna, G., Brusamolino, E., Valagussa, P., et al.: Combination chemotherapy as an adjuvant treatment in operable breast cancer. *N Engl J Med 294: 405-410,* 1976.

8. Bonadonna, G., Rossi, A., Valagussa, P., et al.: Adjuvant chemotherapy with CMF in breast cancer with positive axillary nodes. In S. S. Salmon and S. E. Jones, Eds., *Adjuvant Therapy of Cancer*, Elsevier/North Holland, Amsterdam, 1977, pp. 83-94.

9. Bonadonna, G., Rossi, A., Valagussa, P., et al.: The CMF program for operable breast cancer with positive axillary nodes. *Cancer 39: 2904-2915, 1977.*

10. Bonadonna, G., Valagussa, P., Rossi, A., et al.: Are surgical adjuvant trials altering the course of breast cancer? *Sem Oncol 5(4), 450-464, 1978.*

11. Rossi, A., Bonadonna, G., Tancini, G., et al.: Trials of adjuvant chemotherapy in breast cancer. The experience of the Istituto Nazionale Tumori of Milan. Second Breast Cancer Working Conference. Copenhagen, May 31 to June 2, 1979 (in press).

12. Veronesi, U.: Value of limited surgery for breast cancer. *Sem Oncol 5(4), 395-402, 1978.*

13. De Lena, M., Zucali, R., Varini, M., et al.: Combined modality approach in locally advanced breast cancer ($T_{3b} - T_4$). 70th Annual Meeting of the American Association for Cancer Research. New Orleans, May 16-19, 1979. Abstr. 693.

14. Nime, F. A., Rosen, P. P., Thaler, H., et al.: Prognostic significance of tumor emboli in intramammary lymphatics in patients with mammary carcinoma. *Am J Surg Pathol 1: 1-6, 1977.*

15. Radvin, R. G., Lewison, E. F., Slack, N. H. et al.: Results of a clinical trial concerning the worth of prophylactic oophorectomy for breast carcinoma. *Surg Gynecol Obstet 131: 1055-1064, 1970.*

16. Cole, M. P.: Suppression of ovarian function in primary breast cancer. In A. P. M. Forrest and P. B. Kunkler, Eds., *Prognostic Factors in Breast Cancer*. Livingstone, Edinburgh, 1968, pp. 146-156.

17. Meakin, S. W., Allt, W. E. C., Beale, F. A., et al.: Ovarian irradiation and prednisone following surgery and radiotherapy for carcinoma of the breast. *J Canad Med Ass 120: 1221-1229, 1979.*

18

Prognostic factors for the response to chemotherapy in advanced breast cancer

Marcel Rozencweig[a]

Maurice J. Staquet[b]

Daniel D. Von Hoff[a]

Jean-Claude Heuson[c]

Franco M. Muggia[a]

COMBINATION CHEMOTHERAPY is reportedly achieving increasing effectiveness in advanced breast cancer. A retrospective review of published information reveals that the status of prior cytotoxic treatment, probably performance status and/or type of metastatic involvement, and possibly age of the patient appear to be the most relevant factors modulating the response to combination chemotherapy. It is suggested that data reports should further detail results by potential prognostic factors in complete responders.

Breast cancer is the most frequent malignant disease of women in western countries.[26] It is characterized by an extreme variability of evolution, ranging from weeks to several decades.[12] It has the remarkable property of being hormone-dependent, at least in some cases,[17] and lends itself to very effective forms of therapy involving all types of oncologic treatments. These characteristics stimulate much interest and explain the large number of studies devoted to breast cancer, especially to variables of prognostic significance in this disease.

In a previous review,[23] prognostic factors have been analyzed essentially in relation to local treatment of the primary tumor and hormone therapy in advanced disease. Recent developments in the therapeutic approach to breast cancer presently allow a broadening of this previous analysis.

Increasing experience is accumulating with combination chemotherapy in advanced breast cancer.[5,24] Combination chemotherapy has generally been more effective than single-agent chemotherapy.[9,24] The present review will be restricted to prognostic factors for the response of breast cancer to combination chemotherapy. This retrospective analysis is based on a selection of published reports and involves variables that commonly affect results of chemotherapy as well as parameters of accepted relevance for hormone therapy.[23] Unless otherwise indicated, responses

[a] Division of Cancer Treatment, National Cancer Institute, Bethesda, Maryland.

[b] EORTC Data Center, Institut Jules Bordet, Brussels, Belgium.

[c] Department of Medicine, Institut Jules Bordet, Brussels, Belgium.

Reprinted from Cancer Clinical Trials 2: 165–170, 1979.

TABLE 1

ECOG—Zubrod Performance Status Score[29]

Performance Status	Score
Ambulatory	
Normal activity	0
Restricted activity	1
Bedridden	
<50%	2
>50%	3
100%	4

correspond to complete and partial responses as defined in the individual reports.

Performance status

Patient's physical condition or performance status reflects the degree of tolerance of the host to the aggressiveness and the extent of his disease which is somewhat related to the duration of its evolution. It represents an important predictor for survival of cancer patients,[8,27] but its impact on cancer chemotherapy has been less clearly established, perhaps as a result of the usual exclusion of patients with low performance status from large-scale clinical trials involving this treatment modality.

Various scoring systems have been devised to provide an easily measurable and reproducible estimate of the performance status[18,29] (Table 1). When considering response to chemotherapy of ambulatory versus nonambulatory patients with breast cancer, our cumulative data (Table 2) indicate that response rates are definitely higher among ambulatory patients in accordance to findings previously described by Zelen.[28] These data should be analyzed further according to the amount of chemotherapy given.

TABLE 2

Response Rate to Chemotherapy According to Performance Status

	Ambulatory	Nonambulatory
Ahmann et al.[1]	41/70	7/20
Bull et al.[7]	43/56	13/22
Kennealey et al.[19]	15/28	8/17
Total	99/154 (64%)	28/59 (48%)

TABLE 3

Decreased Response Rate to Chemotherapy after Prior Chemotherapy[3]

	ADM + VCR	CTX + MTX + 5FU
Primary Chemotherapy		
No. of patients	52	53
Response (%)	52 (8)[a]	47 (10)[a]
Secondary Chemotherapy		
No. of patients	23	15
Response (%)	35 (0)[a]	20 (0)[a]

[a] Rate of complete response listed in parentheses.

Prior chemotherapy

Prior chemotherapy has been widely recognized as a deleterious factor for response rates to subsequent chemotherapy. This effect of prior chemotherapy may be explained by cross-resistance of subsequent regimens, residual cumulative toxic effects, more advanced disease, or the emergence of cancer cells particularly resistant to chemotherapy.

There is a great deal of information available on this matter in a broad spectrum of tumor types, including breast cancer.[1,3,10] The reduction of response rate to chemotherapy following prior cytotoxic therapy is illustrated here with results achieved in a randomized trial comparing cyclophosphamide + methotrexate + 5-fluorouracil to adriamycin + vincristine with cross-over upon development of resistance to the first-line regimen.[3] In this trial, the cumulative response rate was 50% with primary chemotherapy versus 29% with secondary chemotherapy (Table 3).

Estrogen receptors

Conflicting results based on retrospective analyses have been recently published on the predictive value of estrogen receptors (ER) for the response to chemotherapy (Table 4). These data point to the caution required in interpreting data when arbitrary limits are chosen to define categories within continuous distributions.[16]

Kiang et al.[20] considered ER+, tissue ER over 3 fmol/mg protein. The response ratios in ER+ and ER− patients were 24 of 28 and 13 of 36, respectively ($p < 0.001$), suggesting that ER+ tumors were more likely to respond to chemotherapy than ER− tumors.

TABLE 4

Response Rate to Chemotherapy According to Status of Estrogen Receptors (ER)

	ER+	ER−	p
Kiang et al.[20]	24/28 (86%)	13/36 (36%)	<0.001
Lippman et al.[22]	3/25 (12%)	34/45 (76%)	<0.0001

Opposite findings were reported by Lippman et al.[22] Using another assay and a cutoff point of 10 fmol/mg protein, these authors obtained corresponding ratios of three of 25 and 34 of 45, respectively ($p < 0.0001$).

Disease-free interval

According to different authors, the free interval is defined as the time lapse between diagnosis or treatment of the relapse, inclusive or not of local recurrences. The length of this interval reflects the rapidity of evolution of the tumor, although it depends to some extent on the quality of follow-up and site of recurrence, either visible or hidden.

Disease-free intervals compared here are more than 1 year versus less than 1 year. This cutoff point at 1 year has been observed to be of strong relevance for hormone therapy.[23]

Shorter free intervals have been seen as favorable for the response to single-agent chemotherapy.[9] By pooling recent data, no particular trend in response rate could be detected according to this variable (Table 5).

If we suppose that free interval is a weak prognostic factor for chemotherapy, it might well be that its significance becomes blurred with highly active regimens. It is also worth noting that other investigators have found increasing response rates with more prolonged intervals when combining complete, partial, and minor responses.[14] Moreover, it has been proposed that shorter free intervals could be associated with shorter response duration.[7]

TABLE 5

Response Rate to Chemotherapy by Disease-Free and Postmenopausal Interval

	<1 Year	>1 Year
Free interval[1,4,7]	82/144 (57%)	84/134 (67%)
Postmenopausal interval[1,4]	32/54 (59%)	78/146 (53%)

Postmenopausal interval

Shorter postmenopausal intervals have also been suggested to be possible indicators of higher response rates, including complete, partial, and minor responses.[11] In another trial where stratification was carried out for postmenopausal intervals (less than 1 year, 1–5 years, 5–10 years, and greater than 10 years), patients with intervals longer than 10 years achieved lower response rates (complete and partial responses) than all the other postmenopausal categories, with figures of 12 of 31 (39%) versus 36 of 59 (61%), respectively ($p < 0.05$).[1] No trend could be detected among the series analyzed in this review as a function of intervals of more or less than 1 year (Table 5).

Postmenopausal interval is related to age. Hence, the actual predictive potential of this time interval may be difficult to assess since older patients are frequently excluded from study protocols involving aggressive chemotherapy.

Site of involvement

In the current literature on advanced breast cancer, the results are often expressed by categories of "dominant site of involvement" as originally reported in the classical studies of the Cooperative Breast Cancer Group. Patients are classified into the visceral category when there are visceral lesions, the osseous category when skeletal lesions exist without visceral involvement, and into the soft tissue category when only cutaneous, subcutaneous, mammary, or superficial lymphatic structures are involved. It is usually accepted that the visceral category carries the worst prognosis and the soft tissue category the best.

Interpretation of the prognostic value of involvement by organ is made difficult by the very definition of the categories of dominant site and criteria of response to treatment. Thus, in practice, soft-tissue lesions are often the sole objective criterion of evaluation in patients belonging to the osseous or even the visceral category. In addition, certain sites, such as pleura or internal mammary nodes, are classified differently in various protocols. In this text, "site" designates the organ *per se*, while "dominant site" refers to a category.

Among the series compiled in this review, there was surprisingly no difference in response rates between the various categories of dominant disease

TABLE 6

Response Rate to Chemotherapy According to Dominant Disease and Site of Involvement

	No. of Responses/No. of Patients (%)
Dominant disease[1,4,7,15]	
Soft tissue	65/102 (64)
Osseous	40/63 (64)
Visceral	101/168 (60)
Site of Involvement[4,8]	
Skin/Soft	95/163 (58)
Lymph nodes	56/92 (61)
Osseous	9/70 (13)
Lung/pleura	28/72 (39)
Liver	17/37 (46)

(Table 6). However, it must be kept in mind that these series include patients with relatively high performance status and, in addition, all regimens used produced high overall response rates ranging from 53 to 73%.[1,4,7,15]

When the analysis is restricted to complete remissions only,[7,15] the cumulative response rates for soft tissue, osseous and visceral categories are 14 of 28 (50%), one of 29 (3%), and eight of 76 (10.5%), respectively. Of note, in one of these series,[7] although the number of metastatic sites involved apparently did not influence the response rate, patients with one or two sites involved had a longer remission duration than patients with three or more sites of metastatic disease ($p < 0.01$).

When data are analyzed by organ involved, there is clearly a trend toward lower response rates in visceral organs as compared to soft tissue involvement, whereas responses of osseous lesions are definitely much rarer (Table 6). These findings further emphasize the predominant role of superficial lesions in the assessment of chemotherapy, whatever the category of dominant disease.

Discussion

Identification of variables that influence the response to therapy is essential for the selection of the most appropriate treatment in individual patients and for the design and analysis of clinical trials. Conceivably, investigation of prognostic factors can also provide some insight into the understanding of the natural history of a disease by pointing out key parameters for the outcome of this disease.

Multiple variables have been proposed as potential prognostic factors for the response of breast cancer to chemotherapy. Practically, it would not be advisable to take all these variables into consideration for stratification purposes because the efficiency of a trial decreases when the number of strata increases.[28] This would aggravate the lack of power because of small sample sizes commonly observed in randomized clinical trials.[24] Thus, it is important to identify the most powerful and relevant of these prognostic factors.[14]

Prognostic factors must also be selected with reference to the type of response to the therapy chosen. In breast cancer, combination chemotherapy is currently yielding high response rates in terms of complete and partial remissions. Hence, treatment is playing a prominent prognostic role in this disease and is progressively obscuring the impact of classic prognostic factors.

Strategies devoted to increasing the rate and the duration of complete remissions deserve the greatest consideration and should be based on careful analysis of currently available data. The rate of complete responses achieved in recent series roughly ranges from 10 to 20%. Thus, it might be premature to accurately define prognostic factors for the duration of these complete responses, whereas predictive parameters could be determined more easily for the very rate of complete responses. However, at this point only scanty data are available in relation to the occurrence of complete remissions.[7,15] In this respect, the category of dominant disease appears to have a strong discriminating potential.

It may be reasonably assumed that factors clearly affecting complete *and* partial response would also be of relevance for the rate of complete responses, whereas analyses dealing in addition with minor responses appear much less reliable. The status of prior chemotherapy has been most consistently reported as a variable of paramount importance for the overall response rate. The role of performance status (ambulatory versus nonambulatory) in favorable selections of patients must await further clarification. The intrinsic predictive value of the performance status, relative to extent of disease and type of metastatic involvement, also remains to be established. Estrogen receptors and disease-free interval have produced inconclusive results. Prolonged postmenopausal interval could be associated with lower response rates, perhaps in connection to an actual relationship between age and response to chemotherapy.[8] However, available data by age do not support this latter contention.[6]

An accurate knowledge of prognostic factors for achieving complete response to chemotherapy in advanced disease might conceivably help sharpen targets in the treatment of early disease.

It is still too early to draw firm conclusions on the role of current adjuvant chemotherapy, but the data so far show that adjuvant chemotherapy delays recurrence in premenopausal patients whereas no advantage has yet been detected with this treatment in postmenopausal women.[2,13] No clear explanation is readily available to account for this apparently differential effect of adjuvant chemotherapy according to menopausal status.[2,25] Further exploration of the possible value of estrogen receptors (ER) for predicting relapse-free intervals could conceivably shed some light on this problem.[21]

In the final analysis, our review points essentially to the need for additional information regarding prognostic factors. In view of the large number of clinical trials in advanced breast cancer, a routine reporting format tabulating separately complete and partial responders with no prior chemotherapy by performance status, dominant disease category, site of involvement, age, and disease-free and postmenopausal intervals could rapidly allow a clearer delineation of the respective prognostic value of these parameters. A standardization of this procedure would probably introduce some sterile rigidity in analyzing the data, but it would also avoid the retrospective selection of arbitrary cutoff points that lead to significant but invalid differences.

References

1. Ahmann, D. L., Bisel, H. F., Hahn, R. G., Eagan, R. T., Edmonson, J. H., Steinfeld, J. L., Tormey, D. C., and Taylor, W. F.: An analysis of a multiple drug program in the treatment of patients with advanced breast cancer utilizing 5-fluorouracil, cyclophosphamide, and prednisone with or without vincristine. *Cancer 36: 1925–1935, 1975.*

2. Bonadonna, G., Rossi, A., Valagussa, P., Banfi, A., and Veronesi, U.: The CMF program for operable breast cancer with positive axillary nodes: Updated analysis on the disease-free interval, site of relapse and drug tolerance. *Cancer 39: 2904–2915, 1977.*

3. Brambilla, C., De Lena, M., Rossi, A., Valagussa, P., and Bonadonna, G.: Response and survival in advanced breast cancer after two non-cross-resistant combinations. *Br Med J 1: 801–804, 1976.*

4. Brambilla, C., Valagussa, P., and Bonadonna, G.: Sequential combination chemotherapy in advanced breast cancer. *Cancer Chemother Pharmacol 1: 35–39, 1978.*

5. Broder, L. E., and Tormey, D. C.: Combination chemotherapy of carcinoma of the breast. *Cancer Treat Rev 1: 183–203, 1974.*

6. Brunner, K. R., Sonntag, R. W., Alberto, P., Senn, H. J., Martz, G., Obrecht, P., and Maurice, P.: Combined chemo- and hormonal therapy in advanced breast cancer. *Cancer 39: 2923–2933, 1977.*

7. Bull, J. M., Tormey, D. C., Li, S. H., Carbone, P. P., Falkson, G., Blom, J., Perlin, E., and Simon, R.: A randomized comparative trial of adriamycin versus methotrexate in combination drug therapy. *Cancer 41: 1649–1657, 1978.*

8. Canellos, G. P., Pocock, S. J., Taylor, S. G., III, Sears, M. E., Klaasen, D. J., and Band, P. R.: Combination chemotherapy for metastatic breast carcinoma. Prospective comparison of multiple drug therapy with L-phenylalanine mustard. *Cancer 38: 1882–1886, 1976.*

9. Carter, S. K.: Single and combination nonhormonal chemotherapy in breast cancer. *Cancer 30: 1543–1555, 1972.*

10. Davis, H. L., Jr., Ramirez, G., Ellerby, R. A., and Ansfield, F. J.: Five-drug therapy in advanced breast cancer. Factors influencing toxicity and response. *Cancer 34: 239–245, 1974.*

11. De Lena, M., Brambilla, C., Morabito, A., and Bonadonna, G.: Adriamycin plus vincristine compared to and combined with cyclophosphamide, methotrexate, and 5-fluorouracil for advanced breast cancer. *Cancer 35: 1108–1115, 1975.*

12. Devitt, J. E.: The enigmatic behavior of breast cancer. *Cancer 27: 12–17, 1971.*

13. Fisher, B., Glass, A., Redmond, C., Fisher, E. R., Barton, B., Such, E., Carbone, P., Economou, S., Foster, R., Frelick, R., Lerner, H., Levitt, M., Margolese, R., MacFarlane, J., Plotkin, D., Shibata, H., Volk, H. (and other cooperating investigators): L-phenylalanine mustard (L-PAM) in the management of primary breast cancer: An update of earlier findings and a comparison with those utilizing L-PAM plus 5-fluorouracil (5-FU). *Cancer 39: 2883–2903, 1977.*

14. George, S. L., and Hoogstraten, B.: Prognostic factors in the initial response to therapy by patients with advanced breast cancer. *J Natl Cancer Inst 60: 731–736, 1978.*

15. Heuson, J. C.: Current overview of EORTC clinical trials with tamoxifen. *Cancer Treat Rep 60: 1463–1466, 1976.*

16. Heuson, J. C., Longeval, E., Mattheiem, W. H., Deboel, M. C., Sylvester, R. J., and Leclercq, G.: Significance of quantitative assessment of estrogen receptors for endocrine therapy in advanced breast cancer. *Cancer 39: 1971–1977, 1977.*

17. Huggins, C.: Endocrine methods of treatment of cancer of the breast. *J Natl Cancer Inst 15: 1–27, 1954.*

18. Karnofsky, D. A., Abelmann, W. H., Craver, L. F., and Burchenal, J. H.: The use of the nitrogen mustards in the palliative treatment of carcinoma with particular reference to bronchogenic carcinoma. *Cancer 1: 634–656, 1948.*

19. Kennealey, G. T., Boston, B., Mitchell, M. S., Knobf, M. K., Bobrow, S. N., Pezzimenti, J. F., Lawrence, R., and Bertino, J. R.: Combination chemotherapy for advanced breast cancer—Two regimens containing adriamycin. *Cancer 42: 27–33, 1978.*

20. Kiang, D. T., Frenning, D. H., Goldman, A. I., Ascensao, V. F., and Kennedy, B. J.: Estrogen receptors in responses to chemotherapy and hormonal therapy in advanced breast cancer. *N Engl J Med 299: 1330–1334, 1978.*

21. Knight, W. A., III, Livingston, R. B., Gregory, E. J., and McGuire, W. L.: Estrogen receptor as an independent prognostic factor for early recurrence in breast cancer. *Cancer Res 37: 4669–4671, 1977.*

22. Lippman, M. E., Allegra, J. C., Thompson, E. B., Simon, R., Barlock, A., Green, L., Huff, K. K., Do, H. M. T., Aitken, S. C., and Warren, R.: The relation between estrogen receptors and response rate to cytotoxic chemotherapy in metastatic breast cancer. *N Engl J Med 298: 1223–1228, 1978.*

23. Rozencweig, M., and Heuson, J. C., Breast cancer: Prognostic factors and clinical evaluation. In *Cancer Therapy: Prognostic Factors and Criteria of Response*, M. J. Staquet, Ed. Raven Press, New York, 1975, pp. 139–183.

24. Rozencweig, M., Heuson, J. C., Von Hoff, D. D., Mattheiem, W. H., Davis, H. L., and Muggia, F. M.: Breast cancer. In *Randomized Trials in Cancer: A Critical Review by Sites*, M. J. Staquet, Ed., Raven Press, New York, 1978, pp. 231–272.

25. Rozencweig, M., Zelen, M., Von Hoff, D. D., and Muggia, F. M.: Waiting for a Bus: Does it explain age-dependent differences in response to chemotherapy of early breast cancer? *N Engl J Med 299: 1363–1364, 1978.*

26. Seidman, H.: Cancer of the breast: Statistical and epidemiological data. *Cancer 24: 1259–1262, 1969.*

27. Zelen, M.: Keynote address on biostatistics and data retrieval. *Cancer Chemother Rep (Pt 3) 4: 31–42, 1973.*

28. Zelen, M.: Importance of prognostic factors in planning therapeutic trials. In *Cancer Therapy: Prognostic Factors and Criteria of Response*, M. J. Staquet, Ed. Raven Press, New York, 1975, pp. 1–6.

29. Zubrod, C. G., Schneiderman, M., Frei, E., III, Brindley, C., Gold, G. L., Shnider, B., Oviedo, R., Gorman, J., Jones, R., Jr., Jonsson, U., Colsky, J., Chalmers, T., Ferguson, B., Dederick, M., Holland, J., Selawry, O., Regelson, W., Lasagna, L., and Owens, A. H., Jr.: Appraisal of methods for the study of chemotherapy of cancer in man: Comparative therapeutic trial of nitrogen mustard and triethylene thiophosphoramide. *J Chron Dis 11: 7–33, 1960.*

19

Chemotherapy of advanced breast cancer

Paul P. Carbone, M.D.

Thomas E. Davis, M.D.

AS THE RESULT of controlled clinical trials, fundamental concepts have changed regarding the biology of human breast cancer and leading to improvements in the clinical management of patients with the disease. Participation of patients in trials is quite consistent with the requirement that the treatment for any particular patient be individualized. The best clinical trials, like the best laboratory experiments, must ask important biological questions. Further improvements in the management of patients with breast cancer will depend on the continuation of these well-designed clinical trials.

Introduction

The chemotherapeutic approach to the treatment of breast cancer has undergone considerable change. Traditionally, treatment with single chemotherapeutic agents was employed only after the exhaustion of all potentially useful surgical, radiotherapeutic, and hormonal methods. More recently, combination chemotherapy has been shown to be more effective than the use of single hormonal agents for inducing tumor regression. This improved response rate with combination chemotherapy has led to a critical reappraisal of the relative roles of surgery, radiotherapy, hormonal therapy, and chemotherapy in the management of breast cancer. Combination chemotherapy has become the primary therapeutic modality for patients with disseminated disease either alone or in combination with hormonal manipulation. Early breast cancer has also become a prime target for a combined-modality approach to treatment with surgery and chemotherapy.

Prognostic factors in advanced breast cancer

The survival of patients with advanced breast cancer is influenced by the specific sites of metastatic involvement, the extent of the metastatic disease, the disease-free interval, the performance status, the menopausal status, and the presence or absence of hormonal receptors in the tumor. Patients with metastatic involvement of the liver or central nervous system have a very short median survival time of less than 6 months.[13] Patients with massive nodular pulmonary metastases or lymphangitic pulmonary disease also have very short survival times compared to patients with other sites

From the Department of Human Oncology, Eastern Cooperative Oncology Group, Madison, Wisconsin.

of involvement. Bone marrow involvement has been considered to be an unfavorable prognostic factor, but one recent study has demonstrated that bone marrow involvement is not associated with a poor prognosis in patients treated with combination chemotherapy.[34] Patients with local recurrences involving the skin, soft tissues, and lymph nodes have generally been considered to have a favorable prognosis. However, local recurrence is soon followed by evidence of more widely disseminated disease in most patients.[7,15] It has also been observed that for patients with metastatic involvement in sites other than the liver or central nervous system, mortality is more clearly associated with the number of sites of involvement rather than with the specific sites of involvement.[13]

In patients who relapse following primary surgical therapy, the survival subsequent to evidence of dissemination is strongly correlated with the disease-free interval following surgery. In one series of 725 recurrent cases, the median survival time varied from a low of 6 months for patients with a disease-free interval of less than 1 year to a high of 25 months for patients with an interval of greater than 5 years.[13] The performance status of patients with advanced breast cancer also has an important influence on response and survival. Ambulatory patients survive almost twice as long as patients who are not ambulatory.[51] Postmenopausal patients have a longer median survival time than premenopausal patients following relapse after surgical therapy.[23] This suggests that the disease may be

TABLE 1

Single-Agent Response Rates in Metastatic Breast Carcinoma[a]

Drug	No. of Patients Evaluated	No. of Patients Responding	Percent Response
Alkylating Agents			
Nitrogen mustard	92	32	35
Cyclophosphamide	529	182	34
Thiotepa	162	48	30
L-Phenylalanine mustard	86	20	23
Chlorambucil	54	11	20
Antimetabolites			
Methotrexate	356	120	34
5-Fluorouracil	1236	324	26
6-Mercaptopurine	44	6	14
Hydroxyurea	16	2	12
Cytosine arabinoside	64	6	9
Mitotic Inhibitors			
Vincristine	226	47	21
Vinblastine	95	19	20
Antibiotics			
Mitomycin-C	60	23	38
Adriamycin	221	81	37
Others (actinomycin-D, mithramycin, streptonigrin, bleomycin, daunomycin)	99	13	13
Synthetics			
Hexamethylmelamine	39	11	28
Dibromodulcitol	22	6	27
BCNU[b]	76	16	21
CCNU[b]	155	18	12
Imidazole carboxamide	29	2	7
MCCNU[b]	33	2	6
Procarbazine	21	1	5

[a] Modified from Broder and Tormey.[6] [b] Abbreviations: BCNU—1,3-bis(2-chloroethyl)-1-nitrosourea; CCNU—1-(2-chloroethyl)-3-cyclohexyl-1-nitrosourea; MCCNU—1-(2-chloroethyl)-3-(4-methylcyclohexyl)-1-nitrosourea.

TABLE 2

Representative Dosage Schedules and Major Toxicities of the Single Agents

Drug	Dosage Schedule	Major Toxicity
Nitrogen mustard	15–25 mg/m^2 I.V. q 3 wk	Nausea and emesis, myelosuppression
cyclophosphamide	500–800 mg/m^2 I.V. q wk 100–150 mg/m^2 P.O. daily	Nausea and emesis, myelosuppression hemorrhagic cystitis, alopecia
Thiotepa	0.1–0.25 mg/kg I.V. q wk	Myelosuppression
L-Phenylalanine mustard	6 mg/m^2 P.O. daily × 5 q 4–6 wk	Myelosuppression
Chlorambucil	0.1–0.2 mg/kg P.O. daily	Myelosuppression
Methotrexate	15–30 mg/m^2 I.M. or I.V. twice weekly	Nausea, stomatitis, enteritis, myelosuppression, hepatic fibrosis, pneumonitis
5-Fluorouracil	12 mg/kg I.V. daily × 5, then 6 mg/kg I.V. on day 7 and 9; 15 mg/kg I.V. weekly	Nausea, stomatitis, enteritis, alopecia, dermatitis, cerebellar ataxia
Vincristine	0.015–0.03 mg/kg I.V. q wk	Peripheral neuropathy, paralytic ileus, urinary retention, alopecia
Vinblastine	0.1–0.2 mg/kg I.V. q wk	Myelosuppression, peripheral neuropathy
Mitomycin-C	20 mg/m^2 I.V. q 6 wk	Nausea, myelosuppression
Adriamycin	60–75 mg/m^2 I.V. q 3 wk	Nausea, myelosuppression, cardiomyopathy, stomatitis, dermatitis, alopecia
Hexamethylmelamine	4–8 mg/kg P.O. daily	Nausea and emesis, myelosuppression, neuropathies
Dibromodulcitol	180–210 mg/m^2 P.O. daily × 10 q 4 wk	Nausea, meylosuppression
BCNU	100–150 mg/m^2 I.V. q 6 wk	Nausea and emesis, myelosuppression

somewhat more indolent in postmenopausal women.

Single-agent chemotherapy in breast cancer

Of all the major solid tumors, breast cancer is one of the most responsive to chemotherapy. A wide range of drugs with different mechanisms of action have produced objective clinical responses in patients with this disease. Table 1 shows the relative activity of single chemotherapeutic agents in advanced breast cancer. In general, the more active agents have produced objective regressions in 20–38% of patients. Representative schedules for the use of these drugs in clinical practice are listed in Table 2 along with their major toxicities.

Only a few clinical trials have directly compared the response rates of the various single agents in advanced breast cancer. However, the cumulative data in Table 1 suggest that the most effective single agents are cyclophosphamide, methotrexate, 5-fluorouracil, and adriamycin. Other agents have been investigated in smaller numbers of patients and with variable degrees of efficacy. The duration of response for most single agents has been reported

to be in the range of 4–8 months.[6] Complete responses are uncommon, occurring in not more than about 5% of patients treated with a variety of single agents.[10,52] The achievement of an objective response to therapy with a single agent appears to correlate with an improved survival. Patients responding to cyclophosphamide, methotrexate or 5-fluorouracil have been reported to survive more than twice as long as nonresponders.[20,27,50]

Combination chemotherapy in breast cancer

The superiority of drug combinations over single agents had been well documented in animal tumor models by the early 1950s.[26,47] About 10 years later, clinical trials in advanced testicular cancer and acute leukemia demonstrated that combinations of active single agents could produce improved therapeutic results in human neoplasms.[24,41] In subsequent years, the search for more effective drug combinations has led to great triumphs in the chemotherapy of advanced testicular carcinoma,[14,22] acute lymphocytic leukemia,[46] and Hodgkin's disease.[17] An exhaustive analysis of the laboratory and clinical aspects of combination chemotherapy for diseases other than human breast cancer is beyond the scope of this discussion; however, two recent reviews of the subject might be of interest to the reader.[18,36]

In general, the prerequisites for the development of successful combination chemotherapy programs have been: 1) the drugs employed in the combinations are active as single agents; 2) the drugs have independent mechanisms of action; and 3) the drugs have nonoverlapping toxicities, permitting the administration of effective doses of the individual agents. To a variable degree, these same conditions can be met in the chemotherapy of breast cancer. Several drugs are highly active when used as single agents in this disease. The most active drugs have independent mechanisms of action (i.e., alkylating agents, antimetabolites, and antibiotics). Although most of these drugs have in common the capacity to produce bone marrow depression, other toxicities associated with these agents do not necessarily overlap.

Greenspan was the first investigator to exploit the concept of combination chemotherapy in advanced breast cancer.[29] Utilizing a combination of Thiotepa and methotrexate, he reported an objective response rate of 60%. This represented a doubling of the anticipated response rate for either of the agents when used alone, and set the stage for future clinical trials.

In 1969, Cooper provided a major stimulus to the investigation of combination chemotherapy with the report of his experience utilizing a five-drug combination of cyclophosphamide, methotrexate, 5-fluorouracil, vincristine and prednisone.[12] He reported a 90% objective response rate in a group of 60 patients with advanced, hormone-resistant breast cancer. Carter has analyzed the results of 11 clinical trials involving 529 patients treated with the same five drugs as in Cooper's original report.[11] The cumulative response rate for these 529 patients was 47%.

Several randomized clinical trials have been designed to evaluate the five-drug regimen by eliminating one or more of the drugs and then comparing various three- or four-drug combinations with the original five drugs. Critical analysis of the data from these trials has suggested that: 1) regimens consisting of cytoxan, methotrexate plus 5-fluorouracil, or cytoxan, methotrexate plus prednisone, or cytoxan, 5-fluorouracil plus prednisone may be as effective as the five-drug com-

bination; 2) vincristine does not add to the therapeutic efficacy of these regimens; and 3) prednisone enhances the effectiveness of two- and three-drug combinations (i.e., cyclophosphamide and methotrexate; 5-fluorouracil and methotrexate). A study by the Central Oncology Group, comparing the five drugs of the Cooper regimen with the same combination minus prednisone,[45] showed a higher response rate for the five-drug combination with prednisone (62% versus 44%), but the difference was not statistically significant and survival was the same for the two treatment groups. More recently, treatment with a combination of cyclophosphamide, methotrexate and 5-fluorouracil with and without prednisone by the Eastern Cooperative Oncology Group,[3] showed that the use of prednisone was associated with an increased response rate (63% versus 48%).

There have been only a few randomized clinical trials directly comparing drug combinations to single agents. The Eastern Cooperative Oncology Group compared a combination of cyclophosphamide, methotrexate and 5-fluorouracil to L-phenylalanine mustard.[10] In this study, the combination regimen was significantly better than the single agent in terms of response rate (53% versus 20%), duration of response (25 versus 13 weeks), and survival. Two studies have compared drug combinations to adriamycin used as a single agent. The Southwestern Oncology Group compared two different dosage schedules of a five-drug combination to adriamycin.[33] The response rates for the weekly combination were superior to the response rate for adriamycin and the duration of response was longer for both of the combinations. In another study, a combination of cyclophosphamide, 5-fluorouracil, and prednisone was compared to adriamycin.[44] This study showed an increased rate and survival with the combination.

Prior chemotherapy decreases the response rate observed with these effective drug combinations. In one series, 11 of 16 patients with no prior chemotherapy responded to a modified version of Cooper's five-drug regimen, whereas only 13 of 25 patients with prior 5-fluorouracil therapy and seven of 33 patients with prior 5-fluorouracil and alkylating agent therapy responded.[16]

The role of adriamycin in combination chemotherapy

Adriamycin is probably the most effective single

agent in the treatment of advanced breast cancer.[53] Based on the results of randomized trials, the response rate with adriamycin as a single agent is nearly equivalent to that of certain combinations, although the duration of response with adriamycin would appear to be shorter.[33,44]

The response for several adriamycin and non-adriamycin combinations are listed in Table 3. Combinations of adriamycin plus vincristine[4] and adriamycin plus vincristine and methotrexate[19] have been shown to produce response rates that are equivalent to those achieved with effective combinations which do not contain adriamycin. However, two randomized clinical trials have demonstrated that combinations containing both adriamycin and an alkylating agent are superior to effective combinations which do not contain adriamycin.[9,48] Additional support for the use of adriamycin in combination with an alkylating agent has been provided by two nonrandomized trials.[30,35]

Adriamycin combinations have also been shown to be effective in patients who have previously received chemotherapy with other active agents. The combination of adriamycin plus vincristine has been reported to produce objective responses in

35% of patients who developed progression or relapse following treatment with cytoxan, methotrexate and 5-fluorouracil.[4] The combination of adriamycin plus dibromodulcitol has yielded a response rate of 46% in another series of patients with prior chemotherapy.[55] These results have suggested that the use of alternating cycles of non-cross-resistant combinations might improve the response of patients who have not received prior chemotherapy. However, the only reported trial to test this hypothesis has failed to demonstrate an improved response rate with the alternating combinations.[5]

Combined chemotherapy and hormonal therapy

Hormonal therapy is one of the most effective treatment modalities for patients with advanced breast cancer. Approximately one-third of all patients with disseminated disease will respond to either additive or ablative hormonal manipulation. Since chemotherapy and hormonal therapy have different mechanisms of action and entirely different spectra of toxicity, it would seem reasonable

TABLE 3

Response Rates with Selected Combination Chemotherapy Regimens

Reference	Regimen	Responses/ Total	% Responses
Ramirez et al.[45]	Cyclophosphamide 2 mg/kg P.O. daily Methotrexate 0.5 mg/kg I.V. weekly 5-Fluorouracil 10 mg/kg I.V. weekly Vincristine 0.002 mg/kg I.V. weekly Prednisone 45 mg PO daily × 15 then taper	30/48	62
Canellos et al.[10]	Cyclophosphamide 100 mg/m^2 P.O. day 1–14 Methotrexate 60 mg/m^2 I.V. day 1 and 8 5-Fluorouracil 600 mg/m^2 I.V. day 1 and 8 (Repeat cycles q 4 wks)	49/93	53
Brambilla et al.[4]	Adriamycin 75 mg/m^2 I.V. day 1 Vincristine 1.4 mg/m^2 I.V. day 1 and 8 (Repeat cycles q 3 wks)	27/52	52
Jones et al.[35]	Cyclophosphamide 200 mg/m^2 P.O. day 1–4 Adriamycin 40 mg/m^2 I.V. day 1 (Repeat cycles q 3–4 wks)	40/55	74
Gutterman et al.[30]	Cyclophosphamide 500 mg/m^2 I.V. day 1 Adriamycin 50 mg/M^2 I.V. day 1 5-Fluorouracil 500 mg/m^2 I.V. day 1 and 8 (Repeat cycles q 3–4 wks)	32/44	73

to combine these two treatment modalities in an attempt to achieve improved response rates and survival.

Oophorectomy has been the traditional therapy of first choice for premenopausal patients with recurrent breast cancer, resulting in objective response rates of approximately 30%.[40] The duration of palliative benefit is unpredictable, but is usually in the range of 10–14 months. Two published clinical studies have suggested that the use of chemotherapy as an early adjunct to oophorectomy is superior to the administration of chemotherapy at a later time, when patients have progressed or relapsed following castration. The first of these studies demonstrated that both the incidence of remission and the duration of survival were better in patients who received cyclophosphamide at the time of oophorectomy, as compared to patients who were initially treated by oophorectomy alone.[56] In the second study, patients who received combination chemotherapy at the time of oophorectomy experienced an improved response rate, survival-free interval and survival, when compared to patients who were treated with the same chemotherapy regimen after progression or relapse following castration.[1] A third study has suggested that premenopausal patients treated only with combination chemotherapy at the time of first recurrence do not fare as well as similar patients treated with the same drugs plus oophorectomy, in terms of response, progression-free interval, and survival.[8]

There is less information available regarding the combination of chemotherapy with adrenalectomy or hypophysectomy. A high remission rate of 85% has been reported in a small, nonrandomized series of 39 patients treated with chemotherapy and adrenalectomy.[32] In a much larger series of 238 patients, the use of 5-fluorouracil in combination with adrenalectomy was compared with adrenalectomy alone.[43] The combination of 5-fluorouracil plus adrenalectomy produced a significantly higher rate of objective response, although there was no difference in survival for responders in the two treatment groups.

Approximately 20–35% of patients with metastatic breast cancer will respond to additive hormonal therapy with estrogens, androgens, or progestagens.[2,37] However, there has been only one published study to suggest that additive hormonal therapy significantly enhances the effectiveness of chemotherapy.[28] In a randomized trial, physiologic

doses of premarin combined with 5-fluorouracil produced no improvement in response or survival as compared to treatment with 5-fluorouracil alone.[51] In two other randomized trials, the combination of diethylstilbesterol plus chemotherapy yielded no better results than hormonal therapy alone or chemotherapy alone.[8,38] Additional randomized trials have failed to demonstrate improved therapeutic results for the combination of adrogens or progestagens with chemotherapy.[8,25,42,49]

The antiestrogenic agents represent the newest development in the hormonal therapy of advanced breast cancer. These agents have been shown to have antitumor activity comparable to that of additive hormonal agents.[39] Because of its relative lack of toxicity, Tamoxifen is presently the most widely utilized antiestrogen in clinical studies. Two recent clinical trials have suggested that the therapeutic efficacy of combination chemotherapy might be enhanced by the concomitant administration of Tamoxifen. In the first trial which utilized Tamoxifen plus alternating cycles of two different drug combinations, the objective response rate in 55 patients was 73%.[31] The complete response rate of 24% was higher than has generally been reported for combination chemotherapy alone. In the second trial which included only patients who had progressed following previous chemotherapy, Tamoxifen plus a combination of adriamycin and dibromodulcitol was shown to be better than the combination of adriamycin and dibromodulcitol alone in terms of response rate (64% versus 36%) and time to treatment failure.[54]

Patients with a positive assay for estrogen receptors are known to have a much higher rate of response to hormonal therapy than patients in whom the assay is negative. Therefore, it will be very important to test the concept of combined chemotherapy and hormonal therapy in controlled clinical trials which will utilize the estrogen receptor assay as a criterion for patient selection and stratification.

Comments

Controlled clinical trials have provided much of the data on which this review of chemotherapy in breast cancer has been based. The results of these trials have changed our fundamental concepts regarding the biology of human breast cancer while leading to improvements in the clinical management of patients with this disease. The participation of patients in these controlled clinical trials is quite consistent with the requirement that the treatment for any particular patient should be individualized. The best clinical trials, like the best laboratory experiments, must ask important biological questions. At the same time, they must be designed to insure that patients will be selected on the basis of known prognostic variables and will be treated with the best available therapeutic options. Further improvements in the management of patients with breast cancer will depend on the continuation of these well-designed clinical trials.

References

1. Ahmann, D. L., O'Connell, M. J., Hahn, R. G., Bisel, H. F., and Lee, R. A.: Chemotherapy in premenopausal patients with advanced breast cancer undergoing oophorectomy. *N Engl J Med 297: 356–360, 1977.*

2. Ansfield, F. J., Davis, H. L., Jr., Ramirez, G., Davis, T. E., Borden, E. C., Johnson, R. O., and Bryan, G. T.: Further clinical studies with megesterol acetate in advanced breast cancer. *Cancer 38: 53–55, 1976.*

3. Band, P. R., Tormey, D. C., and Bauer, M.: Induction chemotherapy and maintenance chemo–hormono-therapy in metastatic breast cancer (Abstract). *Proc AACR ASCO 18: 228, 1977.*

4. Brambilla, C., DeLena, M., Rossi, A., Valagussa, P., and Bonadonna, G.: Response and survival in advanced breast cancer after two non-crossresistant combinations. *Br Med J 1: 801–804, 1976.*

5. Brambilla, C., Valagussa, P., and Bonadonna, G.: Sequential combination chemotherapy in advanced breast cancer (Abstract). *Proc AACR ASCO 18: 77, 1977.*

6. Broder, L. E., and Tormey, D. C.: Combination chemotherapy of carcinoma of the breast. *Cancer Treat Rev 1: 183–203, 1974.*

7. Bruce, J., Carter, D. C., and Fraser, J.: Patterns of recurrent disease in breast cancer. *Lancet 1: 433–435, 1970.*

8. Brunner, K. W., Sonntag, R. W., Alberto, P., Senn, H. J., Martz, G., Obrecht, P., and Maurice, P.: Combined chemo- and hormonal therapy in advanced breast cancer. *Cancer 39: 2923–2933, 1977.*

9. Bull, J. M., Tormey, D. C., Carbone, P. P., Falkson, G., Blom, J., Perlin, E., Li, S. H., and Simon, R.: A randomized comparative trial of adriamycin versus methotrexate in combination drug therapy. *Cancer (in press).*

10. Canellos, G. P., Pocock, S. J., Taylor, S. G., III, Sears, M. E., Klaassen, D. J., and Band, P. R.: Combination chemotherapy for metastatic breast carcinoma: Prospective comparison of multiple drug therapy with L-phenylalanine mustard. *Cancer 38: 1882–1886, 1976.*

11. Carter, S. K.: Integration of chemotherapy into combined modality treatment of solid tumors: VII. Adenocarcinoma of the breast. *Cancer Treat Rev 3: 141–174, 1976.*

12. Cooper, R. G.: Combination chemotherapy in hormone resistant breast carcinoma (Abstract). *Proc AACR ASCO 10: 15, 1969.*

13. Cutler, S. J.: Classification of extent of disease in breast cancer. *Semin Oncol 1: 91–96, 1974.*

14. Cvitkovic, E., Cheng, E., Whitmore, W. F., and Golbey, R. B.: Germ cell chemotherapy update (Abstract). *Proc AACR ASCO 18: 324, 1977.*

15. Dao, T. L., and Nemoto, T.: The clinical significance of skin recurrence after radical mastectomy in women with cancer of the breast. *Surg Gynec Obstet 117: 447–453, 1963.*

16. Davis, H. L., Jr., Ramirez, G., Ellerby, R. A., and Ansfield, F. J.: Five-drug therapy in advanced breast cancer: Factors influencing toxicity and response. *Cancer 34: 239–245, 1974.*

17. DeVita, V. T., Jr., Serpick, A. A., and Carbone, P. P.: Combination chemotherapy in the treatment of advanced Hodgkin's disease. *Ann Intern Med 73: 881–895, 1970.*

18. DeVita, V. T., Jr., Young, R. C., and Canellos, G. P.: Combination versus single agent chemotherapy: A review of the basis for selection of drug treatment of cancer. *Cancer 35: 98–110, 1975.*

19. Eagen, R. T., Ahmann, D. L., Edmonson, J. H., Hahn, R. G., and Bisel, H. F.: Controlled evaluation of adriamycin (NSC 123127), vincristine (NSC 67574), and methotrexate (NSC 740) in patients with disseminated breast cancer. *Cancer Chemother Rep 6: 339–342, 1975.*

20. Eastern Cooperative Group in Solid Tumor Chemotherapy: Comparison of antimetabolites in the treatment of breast and colon cancer. *JAMA 200: 770–778, 1967.*

21. Eastern Cooperative Oncology Group: Results of analyses of combination chemotherapy trials. (Unpublished data, 1977.)

22. Einhorn, L. H., and Donohue, J.: Cis-diamminedichloroplatinum, vinblastine and bleomycin combination chemotherapy in disseminated testicular cancer. *Ann Intern Med 87: 293–298, 1977.*

23. Fisher, B., Ravdin, R. G., and Ausman, R. K.: Surgical adjuvant chemotherapy of the breast: Results of a decade of cooperative investigation. *Ann Surg 168: 337–356, 1968.*

24. Frei, E., III, Freireich, E. J., Gehan, E., Pinkel, D., Holland, J. F., Selawry, O., Haurani, F., Spurr, C. L., Hayes, D. M., James, G. W., Rothberg, H., Sodee, D. B., Rundles, R. W., Schroeder, L. R., Hoogstraten, B., Wolman, I. J., Traggis, D. G., Cooper, T., Gendel, B. R., Ebaugh, F., and Taylor, F. (Acute Leukemia Cooperative Group B): Studies of sequential and combination antimetabolite therapy in acute leukemia—6-mercaptopurine and methotrexate. *Blood 18: 431–454, 1961.*

25. Goldenberg, I. S., Sedransk, N., Volk, H., Segaloff, A., Kelley, R. M., and Haines, C. R.: Combined androgen

and antimetabolite therapy of advanced female breast cancer. *Cancer 36: 308–310, 1975.*

26. Goldin, A., Greenspan, E. M., and Schoenbach, E. B.: Studies on the mechanism of action of chemotherapeutic agents in cancer: VI. Synergistic (additive) action of drugs on a transplantable leukemia in mice. *Cancer 5: 153–160, 1952.*

27. Gordon, I., and McArthur, J.: Thio-TEPA and cyclophosphamide in the treatment of advanced mammary cancer. *Scot Med J 10: 27–33, 1965.*

28. Greenspan, E.: Combination cytotoxic chemotherapy in advanced disseminated breast cancer. *J Mt Sinai Hosp NY 33: 1–27, 1966.*

29. Greenspan, E. M., Fieber, M., Lesnick, G., and Edelman, S.: Response of advanced breast carcinoma to the combination of the antimetabolite, methotrexate, and the alkylating agent, thio-TEPA. *J Mt Sinai Hosp NY 30: 246–267, 1963.*

30. Gutterman, J. U., Cardenas, J. O., Blumenschein, G. R., Hortobagyi, G., Burgess, M. A., Livingston, R. B., Mavligit, G. M., Freireich, E. J., Gottlieb, J. A., and Hersh, E. M.: Chemoimmunotherapy of advanced breast cancer: Prolongation of remission and survival with BCG. *Br Med J 2: 1222–1225, 1976.*

31. Heuson, J. C.: Current overview of EORTC clinical trials with tamoxifen. *Cancer Treat Rep 60: 1463–1466, 1976.*

32. Hoge, A. F., Bottomly, R. H., Shaw, M. T., and Assal, N. R.: Adrenalectomy and oophorectomy plus limited-term chemotherapy in the treatment of breast cancer. *Cancer Treat Rep 60: 857–865, 1976.*

33. Hoogstraten, B., George, S. L., Samal, B., Rivikin, S. E., Costanzi, J. J., Bonnet, J. D., Thigpen, T., and Braine, H.: Combination chemotherapy and adriamycin in patients with advanced breast cancer: A Southwest Oncology Group study. *Cancer 38: 13–20, 1976.*

34. Ingle, J. N., Tormey, D. C., Bull, J. M., and Simon, R. M.: Bone marrow involvement in breast cancer: Effect on response and tolerance to combination chemotherapy. *Cancer 39: 104–111, 1977.*

35. Jones, S. E., Durie, B. G. M., and Salmon, S. E.: Combination chemotherapy with adriamycin and cyclophosphamide for advanced breast cancer. *Cancer 36: 90–97, 1975.*

36. Keiser, L. W., Capizzi, R. L.: Principles of combination chemotherapy, in *Cancer, Vol. 5*, Becker, Ed. Plenum Press, New York and London, 1977, pp. 163–190.

37. Kennedy, B. J.: Hormonal therapies in breast cancer. *Semin Oncol 1: 119–130, 1974.*

38. Kennedy, B. J., and Kiang, D. T.: The effects of short-term cyclophosphamide on estrogen therapy in metastatic breast cancer. *Med Pediatr Oncol 1: 265–270, 1975.*

39. Legha, S. S., Davis, H. L., Jr., and Muggia, F. M.: Hormonal therapy of breast cancer: New approaches and concepts. *Ann Intern Med 88: 69–77, 1978.*

40. Lewison, E. F.: Castration in the treatment of advanced breast cancer. *Cancer 18: 1558–1562, 1965.*

41. Li, M. C., Whitmore, W. F., Jr., Golbey, R., and Grabstald, H.: Effects of combined drug therapy on metastatic cancer of the testis. *JAMA 174: 1291–1299, 1960.*

42. Lloyd, R. E., Salmon, S. E., Jones, S. E., and Jackson, R. A.: Randomized trial of low-dose adriamycin and cyclophosphamide ± calusterone for advanced breast cancer (Abstract). *Proc AACR ASCO 17: 126, 1976.*

43. Moore, F. D., Van Devanter, S. B., Boyden, C. M., Lokich, J., and Wilson, E.: Adrenalectomy with chemotherapy in the treatment of advanced breast cancer: Objective and subjective response rates; duration and quality of life. *Surgery 76: 376–388, 1974.*

44. Nemoto, T., Horton, J., Cunningham, T., Sponzo, R., Rosner, D., Diaz, R., and Dao, T. L.: Update report: A comparison of combination chemotherapy (FCP) vs. adriamycin (ADM) vs. adrenalectomy (ADX) in breast cancer (Abstract). *Proc AACR ASCO 16: 46, 1975.*

45. Ramirez, G., Klotz, J., Strawitz, J. G., Wilson, W. L., Cornell, G. N., Madden, R. E., and Minton, J. P. (Central Oncology Group): Combination chemotherapy in breast cancer: A randomized study of 4 versus 5 drugs. *Oncology 32: 101–108, 1975.*

46. Simone, J. V., Aur, R. J. A., Hustu, H. O., Verzosa, M., Pinkel, D.: Combined modality therapy of acute lymphocytic leukemia. *Cancer 35: 25–53, 1975.*

47. Skipper, H. E., Chapman, J. B., and Bell, M.: The antileukemia action of combinations of certain known antileukemic agents. *Cancer Res 11: 103–112, 1951.*

48. Smalley, R. V., Carpenter, J., Bartolucci, A., Vogel, C., and Krauss, S.: A comparison of cyclophosphamide, adriamycin, 5-fluorouracil (CAF) and cyclophosphamide, methotrexate, 5-fluorouracil, vincristine, prednisone (CMFVP) in patients with metastatic breast cancer: A Southeastern Cancer Study Group project. *Cancer 40: 625–632, 1977.*

49. Stott, P. B., Zelkowitz, L., and Tucker, W. G.: Combination chemo-hormonal therapy for disseminated breast carcinoma. *Cancer Chemother Rep 57: 106, 1973.*

50. Talley, R. W., Vaitkevicius, V. K., and Leighton, G. A.: Comparison of cyclophosphamide and 5-fluorouracil in the treatment of patients with metastatic breast cancer. *Clin Pharmacol Ther 6: 740–748, 1965.*

51. Taylor, S. G., III, Pocock, S. J., Shnider, B. I., Colsky, J., and Hall, T. C.: Clinical studies of 5-fluorouracil + premarin in the treatment of breast cancer. *Med Ped Oncol 1: 113–121, 1975.*

52. Tormey, D. C.: Combined chemotherapy and surgery in breast cancer: A review. *Cancer 36: 881–892, 1975.*

53. Tormey, D. C.: Adriamycin in breast cancer: An overview of studies. *Cancer Chemother Rep 6: 319–327, 1975.*

54. Tormey, D. C., Falkson, H., Falkson, G., and Davis, T. E.: Evaluation of chemotherapy ± tamoxifen in breast cancer (Abstract). *Proc AACR ASCO 19: 34, 1978.*

55. Tormey, D. C., Simon, R., Falkson, G., Bull, J., Bank, P., Perlin, E., and Blom, J.: Evaluation of adriamycin and dibromodulcitol in metastatic breast carcinoma. *Cancer Res 37: 529–534, 1977.*

56. Van Dyk, J. J., Falkson, G.: Extended survival and remission rates in metastatic breast cancer. *Cancer 27: 300–303, 1971.*

Hormonotherapy of breast cancer

20

Pablo Viladiu, M.D.

Introduction

Endocrine therapy is an old therapeutic weapon in advanced breast cancer. In 1896 Beatson[1] demonstrated the effects of bilateral ovariectomy in the treatment of several premenopausal breast cancer patients.

After these experiments, which were forgotten for a period of time, the relationship between hormonal manipulation and the regression of certain human tumors was identified. The phenomenon has been called hormone dependency.

Since then, adrenalectomy and hyphophysectomy have been introduced, and it has been clearly established that certain breast cancer patients obtain striking remissions from endocrine ablation. These ablative procedures presumably remove sources of circulating hormones which are related to maintenance and growth of breast tumor tissues. Alternatively, breast cancer regression can be achieved by administering pharmacological doses of estrogen, androgen, progestin, or glucorticoid. However, fewer than half of the treated patients benefit from these empirical approaches in years of collected experience.

The choice of endocrine therapy for an individual patient has been largely based on a number of clinical observations which can provide the physician with valuable information in selecting those patients who are most likely to benefit from endocrine treatment.

These factors are principally:

a) Age and menopausal status: Premenopausal women respond to ovophorectomy in approximately one third of the cases. The response rates to adrenalectomy and hypophysectomy are reported between 30% and 45%. Older patients have a higher probability of response; the longer interval since naturally occurring menopause, the better response rate.

b) Free interval: Patients with a prolonged free interval from first treatment to relapse have a better probability of responding to endocrine treatment.

c) The response to previous hormonal treatments.

d) The localization of metastases. As a general rule, patients with soft tissues metastases have a better chance of responding to endocrine treatment than ones with osseous involvement; visceral metastases, especially to the liver or to the brain, respond most poorly, while nodular pulmonary lesions respond moderately well.

More recently, determination of estrogen receptors has correctly identified patients with hormonally responsive tumors. Very few responses occur if the estrogen receptor protein is absent. We shall review various endocrine treatments bearing in mind that most results predated introduction of estrogen receptors.

Ablative therapy

Starting with the classic reports in 1952 on the use of adrenalectomy by Huggins and Bergenstal[2] and in 1958 on hypophysectomy by Luft, et al.[3] and Ray and Pearson,[4] no substantial alterations in these original reports have been made. Simplified procedures for doing hypophysectomies have been described but many are subject to either incomplete ablation or unusual complications.

Adrenalectomy obtains 30–45% responses with an average duration of 12–15 months. Similar results have been regularly reported hypophysectomy.

In premenopausal women, castration applied therapeutically either by radiotherapy or surgery induces 25–35% of responses with an average duration of 10–14 months.

"Medical adrenalectomies" have been subsequently introduced. Pharmacological doses of glucocorticoid has been used with limited success. Griffiths, et al.[5] used aminoglutethimide, a potent steroidogenesis inhibitor, plus physiological amounts of dexamethasone, and they observed partial tumor regression.

Because of a drug interaction between aminoglutethimide and dexamethasone, which caused accelerated catabolism of the latter, a new regimen using hydrocortisone has been developed.[6] Hormone monitoring tests have established that daily administration of 1000 mg of aminoglutethimide and 40 mg of hydrocortisone suppresses the blood levels of estrogen precursors. The overall rate of objective response in 50 valuable patients was 38%. These results together with those of Gale and Newsome[7,8] indicate that the response rates obtained may be similar to those obtained by surgical ablative procedures.

Additive hormonotherapy

This treatment had a purely empirical basis. Estrogens and androgens have been commonly used with a remission rate not exceding 30% in large series of patients. The Council on Drugs[9] in 1960 carried out a study to determine the effectiveness of estrogen and androgen. The results are presented in Table 1. These results have not changed substantially in subsequent studies. As a result, estrogens have been preferred in menopausal patients, and androgens in premenopausal, although they can also be used in postmenopause. With estrogens the responsiveness was higher in soft tissue (40.7%) than in viscera (32%) and bones (32.4%). Significant side effects are produced by both estrogens and androgens.

In order to minimize the androgenic side effects of testerone propionate other compounds have been investigated, such as fluoxymesterone, dromostanolone, and calusterone, with similar efficacy, and perhaps a slightly different spectrum of toxicity. Testolactone was also shown to have some efficacy, although totally lacking androgenic effects.

Progestational agents have been much less investigated. Some remission rates as high as 20–25% have been reported, but also some negative studies exist. High doses of medroxyprogesterone acetate are also being investigated. Corticoids have also been employed in breast cancer treatment, as indicated under "medical adrenalectomy." A 10–15% response rate has been noted.

Important drugs under investigation are the antiestrogens. Three compounds have been used in advanced breast cancer: Clomiphene Citrate, Nafoxidine, and Tamoxifen. One of the firsts reports was published by Bloom[10] on 52 postmenopausal breast cancer patients treated with Nafoxidine. The rate of objective remission was 37% with a median remission time of 9 months.

In EORTC[11] studies with Nafoxidin, a 28% rate of remissions was obtained in 108 breast cancer patients. Nafoxidine had, however, undesirable toxic effects on the skin. Tamoxifen, therefore, has become the antiestrogen of choice for the treatment of advanced breast cancer. Tamoxifen is a molecule derived from tri-phenil-ethilene and chemically related to clomiphene.

The first clinical evidence of effectiveness of Tamoxifen was presented by Cole, et al.[12] in 1971. They obtained a 23% remission rate in 96 postmenopausal patients, using daily dosages of 10 or 20 mg of Tamoxifen.

The drug was also effective in a group of 145 patients premenopausal women with breast cancer, otherwise untreated for 3 months before treatment with Tamoxifen.[13] Some degree of tumor response was observed in 104 (72%) of those receiving Tamoxifen (dose of 20 mg twice a day). A series of reports[14–18] using standard criteria of response is presented in Table 2. The table includes only patients who were postmenopausal and received Tamoxifen, 20 mg twice a day.

For these results we conclude that antiestrogens are at least as active as previous endocrine treatments and are less toxic and much better tolerated. It is likely that antiestrogens will substitute for the more agressive ablative procedures.

Hormone receptors

One might inquire: why do tumors respond to hormone deprivation or excess hormones? Studies of intracellular macromolecules with affinity for various steroid hormones have revealed the existence of specific protein receptors in hormone target tissues. It was considered that if we could isolate those tumors which contain steroid receptors,

TABLE 1

Percent Responses to Hormonal Treatment According to Interval from Menopause

Postmenopause	Androgens	Estrogens
<8 years	16.3%	27%
>9 years	27.7%	37.7%

TABLE 2

Tamoxifen: Summary of Results in Postmenopausal Women

Author	No. of Cases	CR	PR	CR + PR Total (%)	Mean Duration (Months)
Lerner[14]	44	3	16	43	7.5
Morgan[15]	72	7	17	33	9.5
Manni[16]	39	—	19	48.7	11
Viladiu[17]	31	4	12	51.6	13.9
Kiang[18]	59	7	12	32	9

we would have the datum which would enable us to select those patients with a certain probability of response to hormonal treatment.

Determination of estrogen receptors (ER) is best known and most commonly studied technique.[19,20]

Table 3 shows a detailed quantification of ER in breast cancer tissues of 155 patients. About 70% of human breast tumors contain detectable quantities of receptors in primary or metastatic tissues. The wide range in ER content could be explainable from different cell populations within a tumor.

Relationship of age with ER is shown in Table 4. There is a higher percentage of positive receptor tumors in patients over 50 years of age when compared to the group under 50.

Encouraging results have been forthcoming concerning the practical application of the estrogen receptors assay, to aid in the selection of patients for endocrine therapies.

Data compiled from a symposium in Bethesda[21] grouping 436 cases with various forms of endocrine treatment showed that when estrogen receptors are negative less than 8% will respond to any hormal treatment. When the estrogen receptors are positive, about 57% will respond to hormonal treatment.

In an effort to improve on the predictiveness of positive tests, several additional parameters have

been tested. The actual quantity of ER may be important.

McGuire has presented data on a group of patients with both estrogen and progesterone receptors, determinations correlated with response to hormonal treatment.[22] When both receptors are positive, the response rate was 84%, and it was 25% when only the ER was positive. Similarly, androgen and estrogen receptors have also been studied and correlated in order to assess the selectivity of both tests combined. Engelsman's data[23] indicates that when both receptors are positive, a 67% response rate is achieved, but the rate drops when one or both are negative.

The presence of receptors may have prognostic implications in the absence of therapy. Recently Walt, et al.[24] indicated that a shorter survival rate and a greater likelihood of visceral metastases was associated with a negative estrogen-receptor.

The interval to recurrence was found by De Sombre, et al.[25] to be shorter for patients with low levels of ER in the lesions. Median time to recurrence for 17 positive ER breast cancer patients was 23 months while that of 38 patients with negative ER was 9 months.

Knight, et al.[26,27] have studied the correlations between ER levels, recurrence rates, and survival on a group of 145 breast cancer patients followed for a 20-month period after mastectomy. Recur-

TABLE 3

Quantification of Estrogen Receptors in Breast Cancer Tissues

ER; fm/mg	No. of Cases	%
<3	51	32.9
3–5	6	3.9
6–20	31	20.0
21–100	30	19.4
>100	37	23.9

TABLE 4

Age and Estrogen Receptors in Breast Cancer

Age (Years)	Negative[a] ER/ No. of Cases	%
<50	25/53	47.2
>50	78/100	78
Total	103/153	67.3

$p < 0.01$.
[a] ER > 3 fm/mg.

TABLE 5

Free Interval (Mean) According to Estrogen Receptor and Lymph Node Status at Mastectomy

	ER+ (Months)	ER− (Months)	
LN (−)	78.3	24.2	52
	(9)[a]	(8)[a]	
LN (+)	28.5	18.3	23
	(15)[a]	(13)[a]	
	53.5	21.5	

[a] ( ) Number of cases.

rence rates for the negative ER group was 37% vs. 15% for the positive one. Survival was also significantly longer for positive ER patients when compared with the negative group (death rates at 20 months were 6% vs. 20%). ER status was a prognostic factor for survival within each group of patients. Death rates for premenopausal women were 22% for ER− and 4% for ER+. Postmenopausal rates were 23% for ER− and 5% for ER+.

Kinne, et al.[28] studied ER in a group of 173 patients: 96 were ER positive, 64 negative, and 13 borderline. Recurrence rates at 30 months postmastectomy were 43.7% in ER negative patients and 28.1% in ER positive patients. The favorable prognosis of ER positive patients applies also for subgroups of positive or negative lymph nodes.

Therefore, ER is a useful predictor of recurrence especially in patients with negative nodes. Conversely, the absence of ER in primary breast specimen is a major prognostic indicator for early recurrence and worse survival, independent of other known prognostic factors such as axillary lymph node involvement, tumor size, and menopausal status.

We conducted a similar retrospective study on 45 metastasic breast cancer patients relating the length of the free interval from mastectomy to relapse, the status of lymph nodes at mastectomy, and the levels of ER in the metastatic deposits. Table 5 indicates the mean length of the intervals related to both these factors and their predictive values appear to be independent from each other. These findings will probably be employed in future trials of adjuvant therapy.

Hormones and chemotherapy

The last point that I want to touch upon is the possibility of increasing the therapeutic efficiency of hormonotherapy and chemotherapy by combining both. Hormones and cytotoxic agents may act on different tumoral cell lines which are present in variable proportions from one tumor to another. Hormonal effects on endocrine sensitive cells could leave a smaller tumor volume for chemotherapy and thus increase its effectiveness. On the otherhand, if proliferation is slowed by hormonal effects, chemotherapeutic efficacy might be interfered with.

As early as 1966, Greenspan[29] found a higher remission rate when he combined prednisone and testosterone with polychemotherapy.

Hoge, et al.[30] in a nonrandomized study combining adrenalectomy with chemotherapy in 25 patients observed a remission rate of 80% with 10 complete remissions.

Brunner, et al.[31] in a randomized study showed a higher remission rate but did not find any significant difference when a combination of hormone and polychemothreapy was compared with polychemotherapy alone.

Heuson[32] in a EORTIC study combined Tamoxifen with Adriamycin and Vincristine cyclicly and alternating with CMF, obtaining 73% of responses.

According to these results, we carried out a small preliminary study using Tamoxifen 20 mg twice daily combined with Adryamycin (60–75 mg/m^2 9 3w) in 16 postmenopausal patients. Thirteen out of 16 patients responded with objective remission.[33] Similarly, using a combination of CMF and Tamoxifen in 55 postmenopausal patients we obtained a remission rate of 59%.

We hope that by selecting patients according to estrogen receptor levels, these new combination treatment approaches might yield increasing remission rates in advanced breast cancer patients.

References

1. Beatson, G. T.: On the treatment of inoperable cases of carcinoma of the mamma: Suggestions for a new method of treatment with illustrative cases. *Lancet 2: 104–107, 1896.*

2. Huggins, C., and Bergenstal, D. M.: Inhibition of human mammary and prostatic cancer by adrenalectomy. *Cancer Res. 12: 134–141, 1952.*

3. Luft, R., Olivercrona, H., Ikkos, D., Nilsson, L. B., and Mossberg, H.: Hypophysectomy in the management of metastatic carcinoma of the breast. In *Endocrine Aspects of Breast Cancer*, A. R. Currie, Ed. Edinburgh, Livingston, 1958, pp. 27–35.

4. Ray, B. S., and Pearson, O. H.: Surgical hypophysectomy in the treatment of advanced cancer of the breast. In *Endocrine Aspects of Breast cancer*, A. R. Currie, Ed. Edinburgh, Livingston, 1958, pp. 36–45.

5. Griffiths, C. T., Hall, T. C., Saba, Z., Barlow, J. J., and Nevinny, H. B.: Preliminary trial of aminoglutethimide in breast cancer. *Cancer 32: 31–37, 1973.*

6. Santen, R. J., Samojlik, E., Lipton, A., Harvey, H., Ruby, E. B., Wells, S. A., and Kendall, J.: Kinetic, hormonal and clinical studies with aminoglutethimide in breast cancer. *Cancer 39: 2948–2958, 1977.*

7. Gale, K. E., Sheehe, P. R., Gould, L. V., and Rohner, R.: Treatment of advanced breast cancer with aminoglutethimide (abstr). *Clin Res 24: 376A, 1976.*

8. Newsone, H. J., Jr., Brown, P., Terz, O., and Lawrence, W. O.: Plasma steroids and clinical response with medical adrenalectomy for advanced breast carcinoma (abstr.). *Clin Res 24: 379A, 1976.*

9. Council on Drugs: Androgens and estrogens in the treatment of disseminated mammary carcinoma. *JAMA 172: 1271–1283, 1960.*

10. Bloom, H. J. G., and Boesen, E.: Antiestrogens in treatment of breast cancer: Value of nafoxidin in 52 advanced cases. *Br Med J 2: 7–10, 1974.*

11. Tagnon, H. J.: Antiestrogens in treatment of breast cancer. *Cancer (Suppl) 39: 2959–2964, 1977.*

12. Cole, M. P., Jones, C. T. A., and Todd, I. D. H.: The treatment of advanced carcinoma of the breast with the antiestrogenic agent Tamoxifen (ICI 46,474). A series of 96 patients. *Adv Antimicr Antineoplastic Chemother 2: 529–531, 1972.*

13. Ward, H. W. C., Arthur, K., Banks, A. J., Bond, W. H., Brown, I., Freeman, W. E., Holme, G. M., Jones, W. G., Newsholme, G. A., and Ostrowski, M. J.: Antiestrogen therapy for breast cancer—a report on 300 patients treated with Tamoxifen. *Clin Oncol 4(1): 11–17, 1978.*

14. Lerner, H. J., Band, P. R., Israel, L., and Leung, B. S.: Phase II Study of Tamoxifen: Report of 74 patients with stage IV breast cancer. *Cancer Treat Rep 60: 1431, 1976.*

15. Morgan, L. R., Schein, P. S., Wooley, P. V., Hoth, D., MacDonald, J., Lippman, M., Posey, L. E., and Beazley, R. W.: Therapeutic use of Tamoxifen in advanced breast cancer correlation with biochemical parameters. *Cancer Treat Rep 60: 1437, 1976.*

16. Manni, A., Trujillo, J., Marshall, J. S., and Pearson, O. H.: Antiestrogen induced remissions in stage IV breast cancer. *Cancer Treat Rep 60: 1445, 1976.*

17. Viladiu, P., Bosch, F. X., Benito, E., and Alonso, M. C.: Antiestrogen Tamoxifen in the treatment of advanced breast cancer: A series of 32 patients. *Cancer Treat Rep 61: 899, 1977.*

18. Kiang, D. T., and Kennedy, B. J.: Tamoxifen (antiestrogen) therapy in advanced breast cancer. *Ann Intern Med 87(6): 687–690, 1977.*

19. Jensen, E. V., De Sombre, E. R., and Jumblut, P. W.: Estrogen receptors in hormone responsive tissues and tumors. In *Endogenons Factors Influencing Host-Tumor Balance*, R. W. Wissler, T. L. Dao, and S.

Wood, Jr., Eds. Chicago, University of Chicago Press, 1967, pp. 15–30.

20. McGuire, W. L., Horwitz, K. B., Pearson, O. H., and Segaloff, A. Current status of estrogen and progesterone receptors in breast cancer. *Cancer (Suppl) 39: 2934–2947, 1977.*

21. McGuire, W. L., Carbone, P. P., Sears, M. E., and Escher, G. C. Estrogen receptors in human breast cancer: An overview. In *Estrogen Receptors in Human Breast Cancer*, W. L. McGuire, P. P. Carbone, and E. P. Vollmer, Eds. Raven Press, New York, 1975, pp. 1–7.

22. McGuire, W. L., and Horwitz, B. K.: Progesterone receptors in breast cancer. In *Hormones, Receptors and Breast Cancer*, W. L. McGuire, Ed. Raven Press, New York, 1978, pp. 31–42.

23. Engelsman, E., Persijn, J. P., and Korsten, C. B.: Experience with estrogen and androgen receptors in breast cancer: correlation with clinical data. *Proc Int Symposium, Lyon, June 1977.*

24. Walt, A. J., Sighakawinta, A., Brooks, S. C., and Cortez, A.: The surgical implications of estrophile estimations in carcinoma in the breast. *Surgery 80: 506–512, 1976.*

25. De Sombre, E. R., Greene, G. L., and Jensen, E. V.: Estropilin and endocrine responsiveness of breast cancer. In *Hormones, Receptors and Breast Cancer*, W. L. McGuire, Ed. Raven Press, New York, 1978, pp. 1–14.

26. Knight, W. A., Livingston, R. B., Gregory, E. J., and McGuire, W. L.: *Cancer Res 37: 4669–4671, 1977.*

27. Knight, W. L., Livingston, R. B., Gregory, E. J., Walder, A. I., McGuire, W. L., and Coltman, C. A., Jr.: Absent estrogen receptor and decreased survival in human breast cancer. Communication to the XIIth International Congress of Cancer, Buenos Aires, October 1978.

28. Kinne, D. W., Menendez-Botet, C., Rosen, P. P., Wang, Y. Y., Schwarts, M., Fracchia, A. A., and Ashikari, R.: Estrogen Receptor protein values of primary breast cancer as a predictor of recurrence. Communication to the XIIth International Congress of Cancer, Buenos Aires, October 1978.

29. Greenspan, E.: Combination cytotoxic chemotherapy in advanced disseminated breast cancer. *J Mt Sinai Hosp 33: 1–27, 1966.*

30. Hoge, A. F., Bottomley, H., and Shaw, M. T.: Adrenalectomy with adjuvant chemotherapy in advanced breast cancer. *Proc Am Soc Clin Oncol 16: 248, 1975.*

31. Brunner, K. W., Sonntag, R. V., Alberto, P., Senn, H. J., Martz, G., Obrecht, P., and Maurice, P.: Combined chemotherapy and hormonal therapy in advanced breast cancer. *Cancer 39: 2923–2933, 1977.*

32. Heuson, J. C.: Current overview of EORTC Clinicals trials with Tamoxifen. *Cancer Treat Rep 60: 1463, 1976.*

33. Bosch, F. X., Alonso, M. C., Ojeda, B., and Viladiu, P.: Asociación de Tamoxifen y Adriamicina en el tratamiento del carcinoma avanzado de mama. *Oncología 80(3): 111, 1977.*

21

The role of radiotherapy in breast cancer

Ignacio Petschen, M.D.*

Carlos Prats, M.D.†

Radiotherapy in breast cancer is a very controversial form of therapy. The reason for this is based on the fact that the percentage of cures has not clearly increased since it was first introduced. The actual problem lies in determining which line of therapy—which usually includes surgery, radiotherapy, chemical therapy, and hormone therapy—can result in a higher survival with minimum morbidity.

The present tendency to limit aggressive surgery is obvious; the classic radical mastectomy is being replaced by more conservative techniques. Chemotherapy is broadening its field of action to include earlier stages. Today, hormone therapy may be guided by determining hormonal receptors. Hormone antagonist substances may be utilized in this therapeutic field. As far as radiotherapy is concerned, the indications tend to be more accurate, depending on the stage of the disease and the associated therapies. The latter aspect is the one we wish to analyze in the light of the latest publications and our limited personal experience.

Stage I

The spectrum of lines of therapy followed in this stage ranges from radical mastectomy (Halsted technique) through radiotherapy to partial mastectomy alone. In spite of this, the results published do not appear to reveal significant statistical differences.[9,14,20,31,56,57,106] Let us analyze the therapeutic possibilities from greater to lesser aggressiveness.

We will not discuss classical radical mastectomy on its own,[93,102] or followed by radiotherapy,[58] because it seems excessively aggressive in this stage. We think that modified radical mastectomy is sufficiently "radical" and has a lower morbidity rate.[106,107] This technique, according to Patey, is the one followed in the majority of our patients. Postoperative radiotherapy has been applied in cases of axillary lymph node invasion or in those others where the primary tumor lay in medial quadrants or in the central mammary area. Our results are shown in Table 1. The tendency to substitute radical mastectomy by modified radical mastectomy (conservation of the pectorals) can be inferred from the work of Albert,[1] which gives the frequency of the different types of mastectomy done in Detroit between 1973 and 1976, in 6132 patients diagnosed of cancer of the breast; for Stage I radical mastectomy is reduced from 32.4% (1973) to 16.4% (1976), whereas the modified radical mastectomy increased from 37.9% (1973) to 53.1% (1976). A variant of modified radical mastectomy would be total mastectomy with axillary lymph node dissection, a technique described by Rosen.[90]

Another line of therapy followed is simple mastectomy and postoperative radiotherapy; its pioneer was McWirther[62] in Edinburgh, and some schools still follow this line today, based on the results obtained, which proved to be similar to those of radical surgical techniques.[46,50,52,60]

Another therapeutic alternative would be to perform only a simple mastectomy, with additional postoperative radiotherapy being administered in those cases where signs of lymph node involvement would be apparent.[9,20,47,67] The study done by the Cancer Research Campaign, which compares simple mastectomy followed by radiotherapy with simple mastectomy alone would not appear to show

*Chief of the Departments of Radiotherapy, La Fe Medical Center and Institute of Oncology, Valencia, Spain.

† Associate chief of the Departments of Radiotherapy, La Fe Medical Center and Institute of Oncology, Valencia, Spain.

TABLE 1

Five-Year Survival Rates for the Different Stages of Breast Cancer Treated Between 1971 and 1973 (1971-1974*), 334 Cases, "La Fe" Medical Center, Valencia

Stage	No. Patients	Patients Alive	Survival (%)
I	59	43	73
II	51	31	61
III*	173	69	40
IV	51	3	6

any difference in results when comparing both groups.

Another approach to treatment many radiotherapists prefer is that which combines conservative surgery (tumorectomy or variants of the same: "lumpectomy," segmentectomy, etc.) with subsequent radiotherapy on the remaining mammary parenchyme and lymphatic drainage systems. A greater number of long-term relapses and carcinogenetic effects from irradiation of the breast have been put up as arguments against this method.[82,90,93,102,107] However, the excellent results obtained by numerous workers (see Table 2), comparable to those of radical surgery, and taking into account the great aesthetic advantages, make this procedure one of the most attractive.[6,17,28,38,42,55,58,63,68,76,79,81,82,86,87,109,111] We consider it completely valid for those patients who have small peripheral tumors (T_1), without associated mammary pathology (fibrocystic mastopathy, hints of multifocal disease), and in those cases where the loss of the gland would imply a severe

TABLE 2

Results of Conservative Treatment (Tumorectomy plus Radiotherapy) in Stage I Breast Cancer According to Different Authors

Author	Survival (%) 5 years	10 years
Peters (1967)—Stages I and II	76	45
Wise (1971)	95	62
Mustakallio (1972)	79	61
Atkins (1972)	78	—
Rissanan (1969/74)	79	73 (T_1)
		49 (T_2)
Amalric (1976)	86	—
Pierquin (1977)	89 (T_1)	—
	84 (T_2)	—
Durand (1977)	85	72

psychic trauma. We have a limited but very positive personal experience in this respect; the seven patients treated in this way between 1972 and 1974 are still alive and relapse-free.

A technical variant of the mentioned therapeutic approach consists of completing external radiotherapy with interstitial curietherapy (Ir-192) at the level of the primary tumoral bed or of the tumor itself, if this has not been removed, or has been incompletely excised.[79,82,109]

Finally there exists an ultraconservative line of thought which believes in partial mastectomy—in the above conditions of small tumor, not central, etc.—without subsequent radiotherapy, this being reserved for those cases of local or regional failure. The defender of this idea, Crile, reports success figures in every way comparable to those obtained with more drastic procedures.[21,22]

All mentioned therapeutic approaches are still in use, as neither of them show a clear advantage over the others. But what is striking to us are the results of the trials done by the Cancer Research Campaign[20] and by Crile.[21,22] How could one explain that these results are no worse in the group of patients in which the axillary lymph nodes are not treated initially, knowing that in stage I there exists a frequency of tumoral axillary lymph node involvement of 15–40%?[32,90,107] And all the more so when we know that systematic axillary radiotherapy or surgery would eradicate the axillary tumoral disease.

The theory which could justify these findings would be based on two facts[9,20,22,32]:

1. Long-term failures are conditioned by early spreading of the disease, before the diagnosis.

2. The loco-regional treatment (surgery or radiotherapy) of these tumors allows control of loco-regional disease quite easily, without having to be aggressive from the beginning.

If this is so, we would be forced to think that the only valid treatment in this phase or stage of evolution is the local one. The regional therapeutic approach would not make any sense except when the mass of the tumoral lymphatic nodes would produce clinically detectable deformation (treatment on demand). The only way to improve the results would be, according to this argument, the setting up of a systemic treatment from the start.

We consider that this hypothesis is excessively simplistic, although it seems to be the only one which could justify the results of the studies men-

TABLE 3

Influence of Type of Lymph Node Involvement (Macro- or Micrometastases) and Level of Axillary Invasion in 8-Year Survivals from Patients with Breast Cancer (Huvos[51])

	Micrometa (%)	Macrometa (%)	Total (%)
N(−)	—	—	82
N(+) Level I	94	62	71
N(+) Level III	59	29	55

tioned above. In fact, this must be much more complex; let us consider the following in order to try to explain these facts.

a) There has been some controversy over the reliability of the results of random studies carried out up to date.[13,32,46,56,57,84] We will not go into them, but let us remember the works of Levitt and Fisher who seriously cast doubts on the conclusions of the majority of these studies.

b) According to specific papers,[10,51,88,92] one of the most important being that of Huvos, the prognosis gets progressively and notably worse according to two sets of circumstances, namely the level at which the axillary lymph nodes are affected and the size of the lymph-node metastases. As we see in Table 3, the prognosis is better if only the lower lymphnode level is affected (level I), than when the invasion reaches the high level or the axillary apex (level III). In the same way micrometastases imply a better prognosis than macrometastases. According to this, how could the prognosis of stage I breast cancer with micrometastases at the lymph node level I—these being eradicated by means of an effective therapy—be the same as when they are allowed to develop till they reach higher levels and are transformed into (palpable) macrometastases?.

c) We cannot forget the immunity status of the host and its possible alterations. If we accept that in certain circumstances the host's immunocompetence may be able to eradicate the neoplasm, especially at the lymph-node level, we should admit that either surgical or radiotherapeutic management on the regional lymphnodes could have adverse effects.[3,30]

Nevertheless, although we know that radiotherapy produces peripheral lymphopenia, it is not clear that it has immunosupressive effects.[29,43,61,94]

Stjernswärd's thesis[96–98] based mainly on the depletion of T. lymphocytes (considered to be the chief responsible cells for cellular immunity) has not been confirmed by other authors.[12,77] These, on the contrary, observe basically a decrease in B. lymphocytes. The immunity depletion could be due more to the tumor growth than to the therapeutic methods.[72,73]

d) Finally the technique of irradiation and administered dose plays an important role. In some, statistical studies treatment is done with conventional radiotherapy; in others, the doses are insufficient. The volumes of treatment also vary from some schools to others. Therefore, it is not surprising that some authors have high rates of relapses administrating doses of 2000–4000 rad,[5,15,87] whereas others who use a more precise technique and give doses of up to 5000 rad, obtain better results.[38,50,58]

Because of the above reasons—and also becasue of the logical tumoral progression which occurs in the majority of neoplasias—it is difficult for us to believe that in any initial phase (T_{1-2} N_0 M_0) the success or failure of the treatment ia predetermined by the existence or nonexistence, at the moment of diagnosis, of widespread blood-born metastases. It is also difficult for us to believe that the degree of lymph-node neoplastic involvement does not entail a potential risk of dissemination, thereby justifying not to act therapeutically on early ganglionar metastases and to wait till these become detectable by palpation. In that case what explanation could be given to the results of the Cancer Research Campaign and Crile studies?. Let us try to explain this.

A stage I may or not have axillary lymph-node involvement. When there is no involvement, the therapeutic lymph-node treatment—be it surgical or radiotherapeutic—would not make any sense, as it does no good; and it could even have negative effects because of the resultant immunitary depression. A local hypothetical relapse would meet with a changed immunocompetence in the treated lymphnode area, bringing with it greater risk of dissemination. On the other hand, in other cases of stage I where there might exist subclinical lymphnode invasion, it is reasonable to think that the host's immunitary capacity alone would not manage to eradicate the tumor; in such cases regional treatment (surgery or radiotherapy) would be beneficial.

Continuing on this hypothetical level, surgical intervention and/or lymph-node radiotherapy, in the first group of stage I given, could make the results worse, and in the second group it would improve them; however, analyzing stage I as a whole, there might be a balance between the two groups without significant statistical differences being detected in the survival rates.

What parameters can we establish to determine in which cases surgery and/or radiotherapy would be suitable in clinical stage I? Without any kind of previous lymph-node surgery, we could only evaluate the more or less aggressive features of the primary tumor (degree of histological differenciation, invasion in the mammary lymph channels, extension to soft tissues, etc.[11,69] and the general state of immunity of the patient (cutaneous test, lymphocyte count, etc). Hormonal receptors could also be a prognostic and therapeutic indicator. This is why we think, as others, that limited lymphnode surgery (with more diagnostic than therapeutic purposes) could be very useful.[17,38,39,55,63,67,80,82,105] The resection of the inferior and central axillary groups, considered as the first step in the breast's lymphatic drainage, should give us additional data. We would then be able to determine not only if the nodes are involved but also other parameters, as for example, the degree of tumoral invasion (macro- or micrometastases) and histologic signs of the immunitary competence of the host. These parameters, which will allow us to decide if radiotherapy is needed, will be more thoroughly analyzed when we discuss stage II.

To conclude stage I, we should like to approach the question of tumoral dissemination. It is possible to think, as we have already said, that if the failures are only due to the fact that there is dissemmination at the time of diagnosis, then the only way to eliminate them would be the routine setting up of a systemic treatment (chemotherapy or hormone therapy). On the other hand, we must think that chemotherapy is not harmless, since it also produces—and to a certain, even greater extent then surgery and radiotherapy—immunitary depression. The present trend is to administer it in those cases where there exists important axillary lymphnode invasion; because it is thought that in these circumstances the possibilities of spreading would be greater.[9,104] This could be one more reason, according to some workers, to prescribe axillary lymph-node dissection, however limited, in addition to the tumorectomy or total mastectomy in stage I.[17,28,38,55]

Stage II

Given the fact that palpable axillary adenopathy exists in this stage, the histological confirmation of the presumed tumoral invasion strikes us as obvious. The usual therapy, however, in these cases is modified radical mastectomy. Although some authors propose conservative attitudes similar to those analyzed in stage I,[17,79,82] we consider that here they are less justified. We do not think that mammary surgery alone is acceptable, waiting for the evolution of the nodes in order to decide whether these progress or diminish spontaneously.[20-22] We think that a greater risk than that of stage I is being run by waiting for the immunocompetence of the host to be capable of eliminating very important (palpable) neoplastic masses. On the other hand, the eradication of these without histological confirmation does not seem advisable either.

We think correct, at present, in these stages, a total surgery of the mammary gland (a tumorectomy could only be considered on very small peripheral tumors), and a dissection of the axillary nodes, that is, any one of the so-called modified radical mastectomies.[22,106,107] Our opinion is that, in the case where the removed axillary nodes are negative for tumor, (N−), further radiotherapy would not be necessary, provided that the primary tumor is located in the medial quadrants or in the central mammary area. If there is tumor in the axillary nodes (N+), the controversy arises again with reference to associate radiotherapy.

Some authors claim to obtain better results using postoperative radiotherapy.[36,49,50] Others, however, obtain worse results.[67,97,98] What is certain is that, in the majority of the studies carried out, there has been no modification of statistically significant figures.[14,31,32,56,57,84] In order to explain this, we must use arguments similar to those given when referring to stage I.

Subgroups within stage II must exist where radiotherapeutic treatment after surgery would be effective, not only obtaining a notable decrease in the loco-regional relapses[14,36,38,40,56,57,58,106]— which has been clearly proved—but also obtaining greater survival rates. On the other hand, radiotherapy could be, if not harmful, at least totally useless in a different subgroup. Therefore, the

TABLE 4

Relation between Lymph Node Immuno-Histologic Pattern and Survival Rates in Patients with Breast Cancer (Tsakraklides[101])

Histologic	Survival (%)	
Pattern	5 Years	10 Years
Lymphocyte Predominance	84	75
Germinal Center Predominance	72	54
Unstimulated	63	39
Lymphocyte Depletion	36	33

matter is to determine which is the first above-mentioned subgroup that would justify irradiation and which is the second subgroup that would not need it.

These two subgroups have been formed in relation to the number of affected axillary nodes; that is, less than four nodes = low risk = no postoperative radiotherapy; more than four nodes = high risk = postoperative radiotherapy.[98] Perhaps this limit is not suitable enough and other parameters in addition to the number of nodes will have to be established. These parameters could indicate the lymph-node group or level involved, the micro- or macroinvasion of the node and the histological factors indicative of the immunitary response. In this respect Tsakraklides, as we show in Table 4, gives an excellent prognosis when examination of the nodes indicates lymphocitic predominance; the prognosis is fair when there is germinal center predomiance or lack of stimulation, while lymphocitic depletion presupposes the worst prognosis. In addition to this we must bear in mind factors dependent on the primary tumors which have already been given in stage I, that is, lymphatic tumoral invasion, the existence of lymphoid perivenous infiltration, the existence of estrogen receptors, etc.

Another question to analyze, noted by some authors, is that of knowing whether chemotherapy could completely substitute radiotherapy in this stage II.[98] We think not. Radiotherapy is an excellent method of loco-regional neoplastic control, better in this respect than chemotherapy. Let us not forget that both therapeutic methods show a parallelism of action as far as radiosensitivity and chemosensitivity are concerned and that ionizing radiations because they can be directed locally, preserving the healthy, remaining organism achieve greater intensity of locoregional action.

With the further associated use of chemotherapy, the possibilities of loco-regional control must increase. They are then additive or even potentiating therapeutics, but not mutually excluding methods. This reasoning is what leads our therapeutic guidelines on any type of chemo- and radiosensitive tumor, for example lymphomas, Wilms' tumor, Ewing's sarcoma, etc; the notable effectiveness of chemotherapy has not eliminated radiotherapy, this being applied almost systematically at a loco-regional level.

It is also reasonable to think that when chemotherapy recovers those cases with worst prognosis because of the existence of generalization at the time of diagnosis—which are those cases which fundamentally condition the long term failures rates—the benefits obtained from a definitive loco-regional control by ionizing radiations could be made more outstanding.

Stage III

We have divided stage III into two subgroups, taking into account the different therapeutic modality usually applied by most workers. We will call these subgroups "early" and "advanced."

Early stage III, includes groups $T_3 N_0 M_0$, and $T_3 N_2 M_0$. In these cases therapeutic considerations will be similar to those seen in stage II. Modified radical mastectomy continues to be the initial treatment most often used in our cases, and we consider it suitable, except in some N_2 cases where the large size of the axillary nodes might require preoperative radiotherapy. Under no circumstances would a tumorectomy be justified. In stage T_{3b} a radical mastectomy could be considered because of the possible infiltration of the pectoral muscle. Postoperative radiotherapy is systematically administered; only in specified cases of node negativity $(N-)$ and primary tumor in the outer quadrants of a voluminous gland, without skin fixation or to muscle planes, could radiotherapy be disregarded.

As we are referring to a subgroup of stage III, it is not easy to find studies related to rates of survival with or without postoperative radiotherapy. Whatever the case may be, a similar reasoning to that of stage II could be made.

Advanced stage III, includes $T_4 M_0$ (any N) and $N_3 M_0$ (any T) and this is what we consider true advanced loco-regional cancer. In this case almost no author doubts the necessity of radiotherapy. However, what is not completely unified is the way in which irradiation must be interwoven into the therapeutic strategy. In some of our cases, an initial mastectomy, usually radical, has been performed, and the patient treated with postoperative radiotherapy. However, in most cases, treatment with ionizing radiations has been the first initiated, an approach which seems to us the most appropriate, since post-irradiation mastectomy brings with it greater guarnatees of radicality.

Let us remember that radiotherapy is capable of obtaining loco-regional control of the tumor in the majority of cases.[6,7,35,44,53,75,99,103,113] Zucali, for example, reports 50% complete remission, 40% partial remission, and only 10% without response. In any case, as these controls are not definitive and local or lymph-node relapses often occur at a later date, we think that surgery is indicated after irradiation, either simple or radical mastectomy, according to the circumstances.[16,23,35,45,85,91,95,113] Some authors think that an interstitial curie therapy can facilitate the control of the disease.[2,109] The histological findings in our 10 cases where radical radiotherapy was followed by mastectomy support the criterion of radiosurgical association, since seven of those (70%) still had tumor. This finding is similar to that of other authors.[13]

Exceptionally, the special anatomy of a pendulous breast, with the subsequent technical difficulties for suitable radiotherapy, could lead us to perform a mastectomy from the start.[65]

One special form of advanced breast cancer is the inflammatory variety (the French PEV), which presupposes the existence of tumoral infiltration of the dermic lymph channels, which produces cutaneous edema and capillary congestion. Everyone knows the seriousness and bad prognosis of this clinical form, and the prevention of an initial surgical attitude.[8,59,89,100,108] Our therapeutic proposal in the PEV stage, without distant metastases, is that of immediate loco-regional irradiation associated with chemotherapy. In this form we are more careful to prescribe further surgery; we only advise it in those cases where the inflammatory signs have disappeared with a palpable tumor still remaining.

Although we have discussed loco-regional treatment with almost exclusive reference to radiotherapy and surgery, we cannot forget that chemotherapy and hormone therapy—which in these stages play as important a role as systemic therapy, since there is an increased possibility of hidden distant metastases—also offer loco-regional effect which will enhance the rates of local neoplastic control, increasing the relapse-free periods.[25,26,33,98] The polychemotherapy in stage III has been established even by some important schools (M. D. Anderson Hospital in Houston and the National Institute of Tumors in Milan) as the only initial therapy; after three or four cycles of chemotherapy they go on to irradiation, to establish hereafter, in some cases, surgery.[25,26,65] We believe that immediate chemotherapy does not justify a delay in the irradiation. Radiotherapy and polychemotherapy can be applied simultaneously, bearing in mind that the structures to be irradiated do not, to any great extent, compromise the medular reserves, being therefore well tolerated. In this way a quicker and more effective loco-regional recovery doubtlessly takes place, together with a systemic concomitant effect. From 4–6 weeks after irradiation, surgical treatment may be undertaken with polychemotherapy thereafter.

Stage IV

When distant metastases exist, radiotherapy plays a secondary role; it is restricted at attaining palliative effects. We still do not have enough experience to determine to what extent TBI (total body irradiation) or half TBI might have measurable systemic effect.[34,98] In a patient with only one metastasis, which is theoretically controllable, we could consider an aggressive loco-regional approach such as that described in stage III; in any case systemic therapy (chemotherapy and hormone therapy) play a major role.

Osseous metastases are those which are most often irradiated, especially those which cause pain or threaten to fracture.[24,41,53] Pathological fractures of long bones, especially the femur and the humerus, should be irradiated preferably after the internal osseous fixation. Epidural lesions which cause medular compression can also regress with radiotherapy[53]; an alternative is laminectomy. Radiotherapy can in itself be effective in the palliation of the symptoms produced by cerebral metastases and by metastases in the choroid or retina.[27]

A frequent indication for radiotherapy are recurrences in the chest wall which appear after a mastectomy. If only surgical intervention was performed, therapy with ionizing radiations combined with chemotherapy controls the tumor in more than 50% of the cases.[18,110,112] If, on the other hand, they appear after a mastectomy plus radiotherapy of the chest wall, a new course with ionizing radiations is most problematic. However some authors like Laramore[54] irradiate again at the recurrence site using electrons and reaching 4000 rad; this author controls 62% of his cases. As we have said before, this must be done in connection with chemotherapy which, in addition to its systemic effects, increases local control rates when added to radiotherapy. In this respect Olson[70] obtained 60% control rates with radiotherapy alone and 79% with radiotherapy and actinomycin D.

Summary

This work tries to update the indications of radiotherapy on breast cancer, based on the analysis of world bibliography and the personal experience of the authors.

Lately the need for radiotherapy, especially in the initial stages in the treatment of breast cancer, has been questioned. And this is based on statistical studies where radiotherapy does not seem to bring an increase in the survival rates. On the other hand, mention has also been made of the possible dangers of radiotherapy on account of the immunitary depression of the host. This is why we have analyzed the indications of radiotherapy in breast cancer, according to clinical stages, reaching the following conclusions:

1) We defend the idea of considering completely valid the alternative of radiotherapy after conservative surgery, as opposed to radical surgery in certain cases of Stage I. It seems advisable to associate a partial axillary lymph-node dissection with the tumorectomy in order to determine the state of the lymph nodes.

2) In stage II, we do not recommend systematic postoperative irradiation but rather establishing a series of parameters, fundamentally histologic, which allow us to determine in which cases radiotherapy can be beneficial. The "wait-and-see" attitude towards the lymph-node axillary areas when nodes are already palpable is not justified in our view.

3) In stage III, radiotherapy plays an important role in the loco-regional control of the disease. This is why radiation treatment in the so-called stage III "advanced" must precede surgical methods. We should also use associated chemotherapy.

4) In stage IV, systemic treatments relegate radiotherapy to a merely symptomatic palliative level. Radiotherapy of distant metastases especially osseous is, however, particularly effective.

5) As drugs are becoming more and more effective some have replaced radiotherapy. However, both therapies tend to be complementary.

6) We must not forget the importance of a suitable radiotherapeutic technique in order to allow the homogeneous irradiation of the tumor volume, with sufficient doses to meet the degree of neoplastic involvement, which should produce minimum morbidity.

7) We emphasize the need to continue with random studies to solve the points not yet sufficiently clear.

References

1. Albert, S., et al.: Recent trends in the treatment of primary breast cancer. *Cancer 41: 2399-2404, 1978.*

2. Alderman, S. J.: Combination teletherapy and iridium implantation in the treatment of locally advanced breast cancer. *Cancer 38: 1936-1938 1976.*

3. Alexander, P., and Hall, J.: The role of inmunoblasts in host resistance and immunotherapy of primary Sarcomata. *Adv. Cancer Res 13: 37, 1970.*

4. Amalric, R., et al.: Radiotherapie curative a esperance conservatrice des cancers du sein operables. 403 cas de 5 ans. *Bull Cancer 63(2): 239-248, 1976.*

5. Atkins, H., et al.: Treatment of early breast cancer. A report after ten years of a clinical trial. *Br Med J 2: 423-429, 1972.*

6. Bacless, F.: Five year results in 431 breast cancer treated solely by roentgen rays. *Ann Surg 161: 103-104, 1965*

7. Bacless, F., et al.: Cancer du sein. Association de cobaltotherapie a hautes—chirurgie. Confrontation des resultats histologiques, cliniques et evolutifs; a propos de 105 cas. *Eur J Cancer 5: 219-229, 1969.*

8. Barker, J. L., et al.: Inflamatory carcinoma of the breast. *Radiology 121: 173-176, 1976.*

9. Baum, M., and Coyle, P. J.: Simple mastectomy for early breast cancer and the behaviour of the untreated axillary nodes. *Bull Cancer 64(4): 603-610, 1977.*

10. Berg, J. W.: The significance of axillary mode levels in the study of breast carcinoma. *Cancer 8: 776, 1955.*

11. Black, M. M., et al.: Prognosis in breast cancer utilizing histologic characteristics of the primary tumor. *Cancer 36: 2048-2055, 1975.*

12. Blomgren, H., et al.: Effect of radiotherapy on blood lymphocyte population in mammary carcinoma. *Int. J. Radiation Oncol Biol Phys 1: 177–188, 1976.*

13. Bouchard, J.: Advanced cancer of the breast treated primarily with irradiation. *Radiology 84: 823–841 1963.*

14. Brady, L. W., et al.: Cancer of the breast. The role of radiation therapy after mastectomy. *Cancer 39: 2868–2874, 1977.*

15. Bruce, J.: Enigma of breast cancer. *Cancer 24: 1314–1318, 1969.*

16. Bucalossi, P., et al.: Risultati della radioterapia pre-operatoria nel carcinoma mammario T3. *Tumori 58: 203–211, 1972.*

17. Calle, R., et al.: Place et limites des therapeutiques a visee conservatrice des epitheliomas mammaries. Resultats a 10 ans. *Bull Cancer 64(4): 633–648, 1977.*

18. Chu, F. C. H., et al.: Locally recurrent carcinoma of the breast. Results of radiation therapy. *Cancer 37: 2677–2681, 1976.*

19. Clement, J. A., and Kramer, S.: Immunocompetence in patients, with solid tumors undergoing cobalt 60 irradiation. *Cancer 34: 193–196, 1974.*

20. Report (Cancer Research Campaign): Management of early cancer of the breast. *Br Med J 1: 1035–1038, 1976.*

21. Crile, G., Jr., et al.: Partial mastectomy for carcinoma of the breast. *Surg Gynecol Obstet 136: 929–933, 1973.*

22. Crile, G.: Management of breast cancer. Limited mastectomy. *JAMA 230(1): 95–98, 1974.*

23. Delarue, N. C., et al.: Preoperative irradiation of locally advanced breast cancer. *Arch Surg 91: 136–153, 1965.*

24. Delclos, L. and Johnson, G.C.: Palliative irradiation in breast cancer. *Radiology 83: 272, 1974.*

25. De Lena, M., et al.: Controlled study with adriamycin plus Vincristine followed by radiotherapy in T3b-T4 breast cancer. Proc. 11th Int. Cancer Congress. Florence (1974). Abstract 2017.

26. De Lena M., et al.: Combined chemotherapy and radiotherapy in inoperable (T3/T4) breast cancer. *Proc Am. Assoc. Cancer Res 16: 273, 1975.*

27. Deutsch, M., et al.: Radiotherapy for intracranial metastases. *Cancer 34: 1607–1611, 1974.*

28. Durand, J. C., and Pilleron, J. P.: Cancers du sein: Exérèse limité suivie d'irradiation. *Bull Cancer 64(4): 611–618, 1977.*

29. Einhorn, N. and Einhorn, J.: Effect of radiotherapy and surgery on immune reactivity to target tissue. *Radiation Ther Oncol 7: 120–126, 1972.*

30. Ellis, R. J., et al.: Immunologic competence of regional lymph nodes in patients with breast cancer. *Cancer 35: 655–659, 1975.*

31. Fisher, B., et al.: Postoperative radiotherapy in the treatment of breast cancer. Results of NSABP Clinical Trial. *Ann Surg 172: 711, 1970.*

32. Fisher, B., et al.: Comparison of radical mastectomy with alternative treatments for primary breast cancer. *Cancer 39: 2827–2839, 1977.*

33. Fisher, B., et al.: L-Phenylalanine mustard (L-PAM) in the management of primary breast cancer. *Cancer 39: 2883–2903, 1977.*

34. Fitzpatrick, P. J. and Rider, W. D.: Half body radiotherapy. *Int J Radiat Oncol Biol Phys 1: 197–207, 1976.*

35. Fletcher, J., et al.: Radical irradiation of advanced breast cancer. *Am J Roentgenol 93: 573–583, 1965.*

36. Fletcher, G. H., and Montague, E. D.: Does adequate irradiation of the internal mammary chain and supraclavicular nodes improve survival rates? *Int J Radiat Oncol Biol Phys 4 (5/6): 481–492, 1978.*

37. Fletcher, G. H.: *Text Book of Radiotherapy.* Lea and Febiger, Philadelphia, 1973, pp. 457–497.

38. Fletcher, G. H., et al.: Combination of conservative surgery and irradiation for cancer of the breast. *Am J Roentgenol 126(2): 216–222, 1976.*

39. Forrest, A. P. M., et al.: Simple mastectomy and pectoral node biopsy. *Br J Surg 63: 569, 1976.*

40. Forrest, A. P. M.: Conservative local treatment of breast cancer. *Cancer 39: 2813–2821, 1977.*

41. Garmatis, C. J., and Chu, F. C. H.: The effectiveness of radiation therapy in the treatment of bone metastases from breast cancer. *Radiology 126(1): 235–237, 1978.*

42. Ghossein, N. A., et al.: Local control of breast cancer with tumorectomy plus radiotherapy or radiotherapy alone. *Radiology 121(2): 455–459, 1976.*

43. Glas, U., and Wasserman, J.: Effect of radiation treatment on cell-mediated immune response in carcinoma of the breast. *Acta Radiol (Ther) 13: 83–94, 1974.*

44. Guttmann, R.: Radiotherapy in locally advanced cancer of the breast. *Cancer 20: 1046–1050, 1967.*

45. Haagensen, C. D., et al.: Metastasis of carcinoma of breast to periphery of regional lymph node filter. *Ann Surg 169: 174–190, 1969.*

46. Halnan, K. E.: Postoperative radiotherapy and breast cancer. *Lancet: 1401, 1976.*

47. Hayward, J.: The conservative treatment of early breast cancer. *Cancer 33(2): 593–599, 19xx.*

48. Hendrickson, F. R., et al.: Radiation therapy for osseous metastases. *Int J Rad Oncol Biol Phys 1: 275–281, 1976.*

49. Host, H.: Postoperative radiotherapy in breast cancer (European Radiology Conference, Edinburgh). Cited by Halnan, K. E.: *Lancet: 1401, 1976.*

50. Host, H., and Brennhoud, I. O.: The effect of postoperative radiotherapy in breast cancer. *Int J Radiat Oncol Biol Phys 2: 1061–1067, 1977.*

51. Huvos, A. G., et al.: Significance of axillary macrometastases and micrometastases in mammary cancer. *Ann Surg 173(1): 44–46, 1971.*

52. Kaae, S., and Johansen, H.: Simple mastectomy plus postoperative irradiation by the method of McWirther for mammary carcinoma. *Ann Surg 179: 895, 1969.*

53. Keys, H. M., and Rubin, P.: The changing role of radiation therapy in breast cancer. In *Breast Cancer. Advances in Research and Treatment,* W. McGuire, Ed. Churchill, Livingstone, 1977.

54. Laramore, G. E., et al.: The use of electron beams in treating local recurrence of breast cancer in previously irradiated fields. *Cancer 41: 991–995, 1978.*

55. Levene, M. B., et al.: Treatment of carcinoma of the breast by radiation therapy. *Cancer 39: 2840–2845, 1977.*

56. Levitt, S. H., et al.: Radiotherapy in the postoperative treatment of operable cancer of the breast. Part I. *Cancer 39: 924–932, 1977.*

57. Levitt, S. H., et al.: Radiotherapy in the postoperative treatment of operable cancer of the breast. Part II. *Cancer 39: 933–940, 1977.*

58. Loeffler, R. K.: A technique for the local and regional control of carcinoma of the breast using 25-MeV × radiation. *Cancer 36: 1496–1505, 1975.*

59. Lucas, F. V., and Perez-Mesa, C.: Inflammatory carcinoma of the breast. *Cancer 41: 1595–1605, 1978.*

60. Lythgoe, J. P., et al.: Manchester Reg. Breast Study. Preliminary results. *Lancet 1(8067): 744–747, 1978.*

61. McCredie, J. A., et al.: Effect of postoperative radiotherapy on peripheral blood lymphocytes in patients with carcinoma of the breast. *Cancer 29: 349–356, 1972.*

62. McWirther, R.: The value of simple mastectomy and radiotherapy in the treatment of cancer of the breast. *Br J Radiol 21: 599, 1948.*

63. Million, R. R.: Segmental mastectomy plus radiation therapy for stage 1 cancer of the breast. *Am J Clin Pathol 64: 767–773, 1975.*

64. Montague, E. D.: Physical and clinical parameters in the management of advanced breast cancer with radiation therapy alone. *Am J Roentgenol 99: 995–1001, 1967.*

65. Montague, E. D.: Radiation management of advanced breast cancer. *Int J Radiation Oncol Biol Phys 4: 305–307, 1978.*

66. Montague, E. D.: Radiation management of advanced breast cancer. *Int J Radiation Oncol Biol Phys 4: 305–307, 1978.*

67. Murray, J. G., et al.: Cancer reserach campaign Study of the management of early breast cancer. *Eng World J Surg 1(3): 317–319, 1977.*

68. Mustakallio, S.: Conservative treatment of breast cancer. Review of 25 years followup. *Clin Radiol 23: 110–116, 1972.*

69. Nime, F. A., et al.: Prognostic significance of tumor emboli in intramammary lymphatics in patients with mammary carcinoma. *Ann J Surg Pathol: 1–6, 1977.*

70. Olson, C. E., et al.: Review of local soft tissue recurrence of breast cancer irradiated with and without Actinomycin-D. *Cancer 39(5): 1981–1983, 1977.*

71. Orton, C. G., and Ellis, F.: A simplification in the use of the NSD concept in practical radiotherapy *Br J Radiol 46: 529–537, 1973.*

72. Papatestas, A. E. and Kark, A. E.: Peripheral lymphocyte counts in breast carcinoma. An index of immune competence. *Cancer 34: 2014–2017, 1974.*

73. Papatestas, A. E., et al.: The prognostic significance of peripheral Lymphocyte counts in patients with breast carcinoma. *Cancer 37: 164–168, 1976.*

74. Paterson, R., and Rusell, M. H.: Clinical trials in malignant disease. Part II—Breast cancer: evaluation of postoperative radiotherapy. *J Fac Radiol 10: 175, 1959.*

75. Pearlman, N. W., et al.: Primary inoperable cancer of the breast. *Surg Gynecol Obstet 143: 909–913, 1976.*

76. Peters, M. V.: Wedge resection and irradiation. An effective treatment in early breast cancer. *JAMA 200(2): 144–145, 1967.*

77. Petrini, B., et al.: Blood lymphocyte subpopulations in breast cancer patients following radiotherapy. *Clin Exp Immunol 29: 36–42, 1977.*

78. Petschen, I., et al.: Dosimetría de la radioterapia del cancer de mama. *Radiologic 20: 247–256, 1978.*

79. Pierquin, B., et al.: Radiotherapie radicale des cancers du sein. Experience de Creteil. *Bull Cancer 64(4): 649–658, 1977.*

80. Priesching, A.: Therapeutische taktik beim Mammakarzinom. In *Krebsbehandlung als interdisziplinäre Aufgabe* K. H. Kärcher, Ed. Springer-Verlag, Berlin, 1975.

81. Prosnitz, L. R., and Goldenberg, I. S.: Radiation therapy as primary treatment for early stage carcinoma of the breast. *Cancer 35: 1587–1596, 1975.*

82. Prosnitz, L. R., et al.: Radiation therapy as initial treatment for early stage cancer of the breast without mastectomy. *Cancer 39: 917–923, 1977.*

83. Raventos, A.: Post-operative radiation therapy. *Cancer 28: 1651–1653, 1971.*

84. Raventos, A.: Clinical trials of adjuvant radiotherapy for breast cancer. *Cancer 39: 941–944, 1977.*

85. Reeves, G. I., et al.: Prognostic factors in breast carcinoma. *Int J Radiat Oncol Biol Phys 4, Suppl 2: 176–177, 1978.*

86. Rissanen, P. M.: A comparison of conservative and radical surgery combined with radiotherapy in the treatment of stage I carcinoma of the breast. *Br J Radiol 42: 423–426, 1969.*

87. Rissanen, P. M., and Holsti, P.: Vergleich zwischen konservativer und radikaler chirurgie, kombiniert mit strahlentherapie, bei der Behandlung des Brustkrebses in Stadium I. *Strahlentherapie (Sonderb) 147(4): 370–374, 1974.*

88. Robbins, G. F.: Long-term survivals among primary operable breast cancer patients with metastatic axillary lymph nodes at level III. *Acta Un Int Cancer 18: 864, 1962.*

89. Robbins, G. F., et al.: Inflammatory carcinoma of the breast. *Surg Clin North Am 54: 801–810, 1974.*

90. Rosen, P. P., et al.: "Residual" mammary carcinoma following simulated partial mastectomy. *Cancer 35: 739–747, 1975.*

91. Rubens, R. D., et al.: Prognosis in inoperable stage III carcinoma of the breast. *Eur J Cancer 13: 805–811, 1977.*

92. Say, C. C., and Donegan, W. L.: Invasive carcinoma of the breast: prognostic significance of tumor size

and involved axillary lymph nodes. *Cancer 34: 468–471, 1974.*

93. Schottenfeld, D., et al.: Ten-year results of the treatment of primary operable breast carcinoma. *Cancer 38: 1001–1007, 1976.*

94. Slater, J. M.: Effect of therapeutic irradiation on the immune responses. *Am J Roentgenol 126(2): 313–320, 1976.*

95. Spratt, J. S.: Locally recurrent cancer after radical mastectomy. *Cancer 20: 1051, 1967.*

96. Stjernswärd, J., et al.: Lymphopenia and change in distribution of human B and T lymphocytes in peripheral blood induced by irradiation for mammary carcinoma. *Lancet 1: 1352–1356, 1972.*

97. Stjernswärd, J.: Decreased survival related to irradiation postoperatively in early operable breast cancer. *Lancet 2: 1285–1286, 1974.*

98. Stjernswärd, J.: Adjuvant radiotherapy trials in breast cancer. *Cancer 39: 2846–2867, 1977.*

99. Stoker, T. A. M., and Ellis, H.: Post-irradiation toilet mastectomy in the management of locally advanced carcinoma of the breast. *Br J Radiol 48: 851–, 1972.*

100. Stocks, L. H., and Patterson, F. M. S.: Inflammatory carcinoma of the breast. *Surg Gynecol Obstet 143(6) 885–889, 1976.*

101. Tsakraklides, V., et al.: Prognostic significance of the regional lymph node histology in cancer of the breast. *Cancer 34: 1259–1267, 1974.*

102. Urban, J. A.: Changing patterns of breast cancer. *Cancer 37: 111–117 1976.*

103. Vaeth, J. M., et al.: Radiotherapeutic management of locally advanced carcinoma of the breast. *Cancer 30: 107–112, 1972.*

104. Valagussa, P.: Patterns of relapse and survival following radical mastectomy. Analysis of 716 consecutive patients. *Cancer 41: 1170–1178, 1978.*

105. Veronesi, U., et al.: Traitement conservatif du cancer du sein. *Bull Cancer 64(4): 619–626, 1977.*

106. Wallgren, et al.: L'essai de Stockholm de Radiotherapie pre-operatoire dan le cancer du sein operable. *Bull Cancer 64(4): 627–631, 1977.*

107. Wanebo, H. J., et al.: Treatment of minimal breast cancer. *Cancer 33: 349–357, 1974.*

108. Wang, C. G.: Management of inflamatory carcinoma of the breast. *JAMA 201: 123, 1967.*

109. Weber and Hellman, S.: Radiation as Primary Treatment for local control of breast carcinoma. *JAMA 234(6) 608–611, 1975.*

110. Weichselbaum, R. R., et al.: The role of postoperative irradiation in carcinoma of the breast. *Cancer 37: 2682–2690, 1976.*

111. Wise, L., et al.: Local excision and irradiation—An alternative method for the treatment of early mammary cancer. *Ann Surg 174: 392–401, 1971.*

112. Zimmerman, K. W., et al.: Frequences, anatomical distribution and management of local recurrences after definitive therapy for breast cancer. *Cancer 19: 67–74, 1966.*

113. Zucali, R., et al.: Natural history and survival of inoperable breast cancer treated with radiotherapy and radiotherapy followed by radical mastectomy. *Cancer 37: 1422–1431, 1976.*

22

Critical summation of current status of breast cancer chemotherapy

Ezra M. Greenspan, M.D.

Since the author first introduced combination chemotherapy for breast cancer in the early 1960s, various two-, three-, and four-drug combinations have yielded progressive increases in regression rates and survival. Intensive polychemotherapy with five to seven different cytotoxic agents should be expected to inhibit 65–85% of previously untreated "fresh" metastatic recurrent or inoperable breast cancers, as observed by myself,[2] Cooper,[1] and others. Although such high response rates are equal to that seen in Hodgkin's disease and the lymphomas, the breast cancer patient's survival declines rapidly after 2 years and falls below 50% after 3 years despite long-term polychemotherapy, including drug sequences and crossovers given up to 2 years in duration.[3] Why does the median survival of patients after these combinations fail to exceed 3 years, despite the increasing efficiency of multiple drug combinations in advanced and recurrent breast cancer?

Detailed and critical analysis of certain relatively neglected factors specially related to the clinical aspects of breast cancer might help in elucidating these disappointing results. Fateful delays, suboptimum treatment schedules in the surgical adjuvant setting, and inadequate stratification and adjustment to metastatic patterns in the advanced patients seem paramount.

In an attempt to avoid tumor resistance various crossovers of combinations in sequence have been developed. These result in the substitution of one drug couplet or triplet for another. Yet, this approach leads to a potentially harmful deletion of certain agents which could be avoided by replacing the sequence concept with an accretion (piling on)

program of six to nine agents. Optimal temporal interdigitation also has not been developed with agents which have a better action when used in specific sequence. Methotrexate is usually not given preceding fluorouracil, but rather simultaneously with it, contrary to current evidence that this is not optimal therapeutically. Synchronization with agents such as adriamycin and vincristine prior to the use of the alkylating agents and the schedule-dependent cell cycle agents has also not been assessed in breast cancers.

Absence of priming or loading doses of cell-cycle specific agents (FU or MTX), is a feature of most cooperative group protocols. This results in inadequate doses of several agents within many combinations. In the CMF (Bonadonna) regimen the M & F dosage is often hit or miss since many patients never become toxic on MTX or FU throughout their management. We fail to modify and alter the individual drug emphasis within polychemotherapy schedules in accordance with the predominant presenting metastatic pattern. Thus, optimum treatment of the cohort with metastatic hepatomegaly may require different drugs compared to patients with pulmonary lymphangitic carcinomatosis or inflammatory cancer or CNS metastases. No studies have been done to determine which schedules are more effective against which metastatic patterns.

Too many delays occur due to the deliberate use of non-life-saving radiotherapy. The effect of radiotherapy on survival is either negligible or nonexistent in many heterogeneous series of patients, and is certainly under the 5% recognizable limits in clinical studies world wide. The very poor survival reported by Cooper when adjuvant polychemotherapy was delayed until day 57, to allow completion of radiotherapy, instead of beginning

Mount Sinai School of Medicine, New York, New York.

on day 23, is most provocative and cannot be overemphasized. Postoperatively, surgeons and others often delay the decision-making process for several weeks due to lack of candor. In the high-risk patient immediately after operation, a few weeks delay may well be the most important single cause for the failure of breast cancer chemotherapy in the long run, as the recent controlled Scandinavian study[4] has shown that treatment begun 3 days after operation with only one drug (cyclophosphamide for 1 week), is far more likely to save lives 10 years later, than treatment begun 23 days after operation.

In experimental models of surgical adjuvant therapy, treatment beginning 2 or 4 days postop makes a major difference in results. Current American surgical adjuvant programs begin 2–4 weeks after operation.

Delays also occur in cooperative group case acquisition due to the data requirements before acceptance of patients within many studies. If several weeks delay reduces the regression rate and remission interval in the postsurgical patient, it most likely plays a significant role also in the advanced patient. Rigid predetermined dose regimens intrinsic to protocol studies do not invariably represent the best treatment for the individual patient, although the regimens represent necessary "convenience packages" for the group. In protocols, most drugs are not individually and consistently pushed to the limits of tolerable toxicity despite some dose adjustment allowances. Thus, a fraction, perhaps 10% of the good-risk patients, may be undertreated, and, conversely, a fraction of the poor-risk patients may be routinely overtreated (10%). In the use of methotrexate today all too often patients never show methotrexate toxicity throughout their entire clinical course, although they are considered to have become resistant or to have failed after adequate use of methotrexate.

All of these factors could account for the 50–65% response rates in studies of five and six drug regimens by many cooperative groups. Higher response rates within private group practice have been attributed to overenthusiasm, case selective, vague criteria for response, and other pejorative factors intrinsic to private practice, but the possibility that a more prompt intensive individual custom-tailored polychemotherapy has been employed has not been considered.

The 8–12 week delay involved in evaluating solo hormone therapy on the basis of estrogen titers is certainly unwarranted, except perhaps in elderly females with indolent chest wall recurrent cancers. Of therapeutic importance is the fact that 20–25% of patients who have developed end-stage polychemotherapy-resistance are nevertheless capable of developing a regression by the addition of nolvadex (tamoxifen).[5] This observation reinforces the concept that hormonal therapy and polychemotherapy can and should be promptly employed *simultaneously* in many women with breast cancer.

Current search for the best surgical adjuvant program indicates the need for a prompt precise adoption of the Cooper's five-drug regimen which differs in certain important details from so-called "Cooper-type" regimen of ECOG and CALGB. The prospects for cure of breast cancer are certainly enhanced by Cooper's current long-term follow-up recently analyzed by Holland.[6] This now shows that, in women with four or more nodes positive, even though treatment was begun postoperatively on day 23, there are from 40–70% of patients remaining "free of disease," 5–8 years after treatment. What would have been the results if treatment had been begun in the first week rather than the fourth week after operation? When will Cooper's precise regimen be tested in prospective randomized studies? Clinical cure seems to be in reach today in breast cancer, just as it is in lymphomas. But, this can only be proved by studies based on the concept of intensive prompt, precise, and holistic therapy adjusted to an individually-induced tolerable toxicity.

References

1. Cooper, R. G.: Combination chemotherapy in hormone resistant breast cancer. (Abstr. #57 AACR). *Cancer Res 1969.*

2. Greenspan, E. M.: Chemotherapy of breast cancer. Hahnemann Symposium, "Cancer Chemotherapy III," 1978.

3. Burchenal, J. H.: Adjuvant therapy-theory, practice and potential. *Cancer 37: 46–57, 1976.*

4. Nissen-Meyer, R., Kjullgren, K., Malmio, K., Mansson, B., and Norin, Torseen: Surgical adjuvant chemotherapy. Results with one short course with cyclophosphamide after mastectomy for breast cancer. *Cancer 41: 2088–2098, 1978.*

5. Glick, J. H.: Tamoxifen studies; Proc. American Soc. Clinical Oncology. *Cancer 19: 354, 1978.*

6. Holland, J.: Therapy of primary breast cancer. *Israeli J Med Sci 13: 8, 1977.*

23

Hodgkin's disease: Introduction

Constantino Herranz, M.D.

The investigations on the Hodgkin's disease have reached an enormous interest in the last years. The teamwork of numerous investigators have changed radically the prognosis of this process, which has turned into a curable disease in a great proportion of the cases.

The story began in 1833, when Thomas Hodgkin read to the Medical-Chirurgical Society his historic paper "On same morbid appearances of the absorbent glands and spleen."[1] Samuel Wilks, in 1865, described another ten cases and suggested the apellation "Hodgkin's disease."[2] At this time Virchow already used the term "lymphoma" to describe a group of diseases of lymphoid involvement,[3] and Billroth suggested the term "malignant lymphoma" to include a series of diseases of lymphoreticular system. The next century accumulated knowledge concerning Hodgkin's disease, at first very slowly, in a parallel way to the development of oncology and, in the last 10–15 years, very fast, reaching the current encouraging status. At the turn of the century, Sternberg[4] and Reed[5] described the pathological patterns of this illness, and, in particular, the peculiar cells, which retain their name.

In 1902, Pusey[6] first initiated his tests of palliative radiotherapy applied to Hodgkin's disease, which showed radio-sensitivity and served as the basis for subsequent progress, in the hands of Renè Gilbert,[7] Vera Peters[8] and other investigators. Current methods were defined by Henry Kaplan and his school of Stanford, which established through studies the evolution of curative radiotherapy.[9]

The classification of Gall and Mallory in 1942 first clarified confusing relationships in malignant lymphomas.[10] Two years later Jackson and Parker spoke about Hodgkin's paragranulomas, granulomas, and sarcomas,[11] and finally, in 1965, the Symposium held in Rye (New York) adopted the classification which has reached our days[12] and also has been the key of all current work, which was fundamental to the progress in the treatment of the disease.

Another important step in the struggle against Hodgkin's disease was the demonstration of the clear relationship between the extension of the disease and its evolution. This induced Vera Peters and other radiotherapists to recommend the necessity for clear studies on disease spread. A series of clinical classifications were established, which led to that adopted in Ann Arbor (Michigan) in 1971.[13] In these years, there was a parallel change in the concept of the disease, evolving from a systemic and generalized process to consideration of it as a unicentric process with regional dissemination. This led to efforts in improving the means of determining the exact localization of the zones affected (staging). Thus, the appearance of protocols including a series of physical, byochemical, radiological, isotopic, and other types of studies. The important steps in this aspect were, first of all, the introduction of lymphography which enabled one to visualize the abdominal nodal areas, inaccessible to other physical procedures, and later, the introduction of laparotomy and splenectomy at Stanford.[14] The diagnostic importance of this surgical maneuver has been demonstrated in numerous works. The infectious processes described, especially in children,[15] have been a factor in prompting reevaluation of the indications of this procedure.

Finally, the chemotherapy of Hodgkin's disease has been also evolving. After an amount of experience and identification of active agents with monochemotherapy,[16] the field was revolutionized with polichemotherapeutic combinations, which have been very successful, the original Mopp being the classical scheme.[17] New active drugs have further extended the possibilities of chemotherapy,[18,19] mainly upon recurrence.

The success in the therapy of Hodgkin's disease is today the result of the collaboration of radiotherapists, internists, surgeons, and many other specialists in relation with this process.

Servicio de Oncología Médica, C.S., La Fe, Valencia.

In short, Hodgkin's disease is one of the most stimulating themes in oncology today. There are many aspects to be clarified, such as the etiology of the disease, with the possible role of viruses, the influence of genetic, immunological, and environmental factors and other questions, which are the subject of work being done by investigators now and which we hope to see solved in the next few years.

References

1. Hodgkin, T.: On some morbid appearances of the absorbent glands and spleen. *Med Chir Trans 17: 68–114, 1832.*

2. Wilks, S.: Cases of enlargement of the lymphatic glands and spleen (or Hodgkin's disease), with remarks. *Guys Hosp Rep 11: 56–67, 1865.*

3. Virchow, R.: Weisses Blut. *Neue Notizen Geb Natur Heilk 36: 151–156, 1845.*

4. Sternberg, C.: Über eine eigenartige unter dem Bilde der Pseudoleukämie verlaufende Tuberculose des lymphatischen Apparates. *Z. Heilk 19: 21–90, 1898.*

5. Reed, D. M.: On the pathological changes in Hodgkin's disease, with special reference to its relation to tubercluosis. *Johns Hopkins Hosp Rep 10: 133–196, 1902.*

6. Pusey, W. A.: Cases of sarcoma and of Hodgkin's disease treated by exposures to X-rays: a preliminary report. *JAMA 38: 166–169, 1902.*

7. Gilbert, R.: Radiotherapy in Hodgkin's disease. *Am J Roentgen 41: 198–241, 1939.*

8. Peters, M. V., and Middlemiss, K. C. H.: A study of Hodgkin's disease treated by irradiation. *Am J Roentgen 79: 115–121, 1958.*

9. Kaplan, H. S.: Role of intensive radiotherapy in the management of Hodgkin's disease. *Cancer 19: 356–367, 1966.*

10. Gall, E. A., and Mallory, T. B.: Malignant lymphoma. A clinical-pathologic survey of 618 cases. *Am J Pathol 18: 381–429, 1942.*

11. Jackson, H., and Parker, F.: Hodgkin's disease. II. Pathology. *N Engl J Med 231: 35–44, 1944.*

12. Lukes, R. J., Craver, L. F., Hall, T. C., Rappaport, H., and Rubin, P.: Report of the nomenclature committee. *Cancer Res 26: 1311, 1966.*

13. Carbona, P. P., Kaplan, H. S., Musshoff, K., Smithers, D. W., and Tubiana, M.: Report of the committee on Hodgkin's disease staging classification. *Cancer Res 31: 1860–1861, 1971.*

14. Glatstein, E., Guernsey, J. M., and Rosenberg, S. A.: The value of laparotomy and splenectomy in the staging of Hodgkin's disease. *Cancer 24: 709–718, 1969.*

15. Chilcote, R. R., and Baehner, R. L.: The incidence of overwhelming infections in children staged for Hodgkin's disease. *Proc Am Assoc Cancer Res 16: 224, 1975.*

16. Carter, S. K., and Livingston, R. B.: Single-agent therapy for Hodgkin's disease. *Arch Intern Med 131: 377–387, 1973.*

17. De Vita, V. T., Serpick, A. A., and Carbone, P. P.: Combination chemotherapy in the treatment of advanced Hodgkin's disease. *Ann Intern Med 73: 881–895, 1970.*

18. Bonadonna, G., Uslenghi, C., and Zucali, R.: Recent trends in the medical treatment of Hodgkin's disease. *Eur J Cancer 11: 251–266, 1975.*

19. Rozencweig, M., Von Hoff, D. D., Davis, H. L., Jacobs, E. M., Muggia, F. M., and De Vita, V. T.: Hodgkin's disease. In *Randomized Trials in Cancer: A Critical Review by Sites,* M. J. Staquet, Ed. Raven Press, New York, 1978, pp. 103–130.

24

Prognostic factors and chemotherapy of Hodgkin's disease

J. Vicente

Introduction

Drug therapy of Hodgkin's disease is as old as cancer chemotherapy itself. Aside from the use of potassium arsenite in the form of Fowler's solution, no significant advance was made before the 1940s when the modern era of cancer chemotherapy was ushered in by the introduction of polyfunctional alkylating agents.

The first major landmark in this field was the report by Gilman and Philips,[42] soon followed by those by Goodman, et al.[45] and Jacobson, et al.,[51] of significant clinical responses in patients with Hodgkin's disease and other lymphomas treated with methyl-bis-β-chloroethylamine hydrochloride (HN2, nitrogen mustard) and the closely related compound tris-β-chloroethylamine hydrochloride.

The development of new alkylating agents and other major drugs like antimetabolites and corticosteroids, all of which were tested in Hodgkin's lymphoma, made additional contributions. An important step was the identification in the early 1960s of two new classes of drugs, the *vinca* alkaloids[7,40,53] and Procarbazine, the first almost specific compound for Hodgkin's disease.[62,63,86] Both agents showed no cross-resistance with each other and with alkylating agents, presumably due to their completely different mechanism of action.

The second landmark was the introduction of combination chemotherapy. Stemming from the success of intensive cyclic quadruple combination chemotherapy (VAMP) in acute lymphocytic leukemia of childhood,[39] two early attempts, at combination included the use of Chlorambucil and Vinblastine investigated by Lacher and Durant[56] and the quadruple combination of Cyclophosphamide, Vincristine, Methotrexate and Prednisone (MOMP) of DeVita, Moxley et al.,[27] achieved remarkable results in comparison with previous single agent chemotherapy. This led the latter investigators shortly afterwards to develop the MOPP regimen,[28] exploiting the full potential of the then most active drugs against this lymphoma. This regimen eventually became established as the first drug treatment capable of achieving cures of Hodgkin's disease.

Since that time additional drugs have appeared which show efficacy. Almost each new group of drugs entering trial has shown some activity, but, in particular, the nitrosoureas,[57,76,78] DTIC,[38] and the antitumor antibiotics, bleomycin[6] and adriamycin.[5] These new agents, lacking cross-resistance among them and with the conventional drugs outlined above, were soon incorporated into combination regimens in several on-going studies, rather than being used alone, as single agents. This led soon to "salvage" chemotherapy, which began with the design and report by Bonadonna, et al.[10] of the ABVD regimen, lacking cross-resistance with MOPP; this made possible the recovery of patients refractory to standard chemotherapy and prompted the development of other similar combinations.

In the following paragraphs the actual facts and significance of these findings will be briefly reviewed at the light of present knowledge.

Single agent chemotherapy

The results obtained with conventional single agents have been extensively reviewed.[15,36] As with

Oncology Department, Fundación Jiminez Diaz, Madrid, Spain.

x-ray therapy and other systems, the dose-response curve was steep with respect to toxicity and both frequency and magnitude of disease regression, so that maximum tolerated dose was necessary to achieve optimal therapeutic effect.[36]

Response rates with alkylating agents ranged from 54 to 65%, the lower figure being for Cyclophosphamide and the higher for Mechlorethamine or nitrogen mustard, with complete remissions in 12–16% of the treated cases.

Vinca alkaloids showed similar overall response rates between 58 and 68% but a more impressive complete remission rate of 30–36% is attributed to Vincristine. Patients with prior treatment with radiotherapy or other chemotherapy showed a lower response rate, particularly in terms of the complete remission rate.[14] This was not the case with Procarbazine; this agent showed the same response frequency and quality in patients with or without previous treatments. Overall response rate was similar to that achieved with the other agents, 69%, but the average complete remission rate of 38% was the highest known at that date, some series reaching more than 50% of complete remissions.[82]

Glucocorticoids, particularly prednisone and prednisolone at medium or high dosage, also showed some activity, about 60% of overall responses, but with no complete remissions reported.

The median duration of response was shorter in unmaintained remissions achieved with these drugs. They ranged between 2 and 4 months. Scott[77] reported, however, that continued treatment after complete remission prolonged the median duration of this remission, and this become common practice. Notwithstanding this, remissions rarely exceeded 1 year. With Procarbazine, the average duration of complete remissions was 13.5 months.[82] It was traditional to give the agents sequentially, changing treatment when the disease no longer responded; therapy generally started with an alkylating agent followed by Vinblastine and then by Procarbazine; finally, upon relapse corticosteroids or new agents were used. Overall median survival from onset of chemotherapy was about 2 years[81] and was longer in patients responding to more than one drug in the sequence (40–42 months) than in those responding to only one or not at all (9–18 months).[1]

The experience with new drugs is quite compa-rable, although based on limited data. None appears superior to Procarbazine, but they again are not cross-resistant with each other or with conventional drugs,[5,6,38,57,76,78] so that their use in combinations can be fully exploited.

Combination chemotherapy—The MOPP regimen

As mentioned in the introductory paragraphs, the first approach to combination chemotherapy for Hodgkin's disease was the report of Lacher and Durant in 1965,[56] using Chlorambucil plus Vinblastine.

DeVita, Moxley, et al.[27] reported in abstract form and later extended[66] the preliminary results of a pilot study in 14 patients of a four-drug combination (MOMP, NCI-I) plus radiotherapy to the involved areas. The agents used were Cyclophosphamide, Vincristine, Methotrexate, and Prednisone administered together at nearly full dosage in 2-week-a-month courses, repeated thrice in a cyclic fashion. Radiotherapy was employed between the first and second or second and third courses of chemotherapy and was not used in five advanced patients. The overall response rate was 90% in stage II-B up patients, 80% being complete remissions; with two exceptions, the complete remission was achieved during or immediately following the first course of chemotherapy and preceded radiotherapy, so that the regressions may be properly ascribed to the combination chemotherapy.[56] With the exception of three earlier relapses (two in partial responders), the remissions persisted without maintenance therapy for 30+ months. Radiotherapy may have played an important role, especially in the duration of response, since the remissions were sustained in eight of nine patients who received radiotherapy, but in one out of five treated with chemotherapy alone. Toxicity was comparable to that observed after the usual therapeutic doses of the individual drugs, proving the feasibility and safety of combination chemotherapy.

These promising results prompted the NCI group of investigators to undertake new approaches to devise an optimum combination. Procarbazine was substituted for Methotrexate, which was the least active in the original combination; Nitrogen Mustard, Mechlorethamine, replaced Cyclophosphamide as the best representative of the alkylating agents; duration of treatment was extended to a minimum of 6 months or six cycles as remission induction and no radiotherapy was employed. This was the MOPP program, which actually opened the way to cure for advanced Hodgkin's disease and has by now already passed the test of time.[24-26,28,29]

The overall response rate in previously untreated cases was 95%, with 81% complete remissions, slightly lower in the most advanced stages (77% for stage IV-B) and symptomatic patients, all "A" cases achieving complete remission. The complete remission rate was also decreased by prior treatment, especially if the patient had received chemotherapy or a combination of radiotherapy and chemotherapy and less so, or not at all, with prior radiotherapy alone. Patients younger than 16 appeared to respond poorer than the adults. No major influence was noted for other host factors, including immunologic depression.

Ten-year follow-up results are now available. The actuarial median disease-free survival has not yet been reached: 66% of patients achieving complete remission remain relapse-free at 5 and 10 years after all treatment was discontinued. The relapse rate was highest during the first 18 months and no relapses were noted after 42 months. The duration of response was influenced by age, histology, and "B" symptoms: patients under 16 years or nodular sclerosing histology had shorter complete remissions; no "A" but 40% of "B" patients have relapsed at 5 years. The 5- and 10-year survival for the whole series (n = 194) was 65% and 58%, whereas for the 155 patients who achieved complete remissions the figures were 82% and 72%, respectively. Survival was adversely affected by age under 16 (median 36 months) and "B" symptoms, but no influence was noted of histology or type of organ involvement. Thirteen patients have died

while in complete remission, and ten were autopsied and found free of disease.

The above facts soon stimulated efforts to duplicate this experience and determine the MOPP efficacy in other series of patients.[13,37,44,49,52,64,68,79,85] Our own, recently reported in abstract form[85] included 66 evaluable patients treated between 1970 and 1976. At present, more than 60% of the patients have been followed up longer than 5 years after completion of six cycles of induction treatment; usually two more cycles were administered as consolidation and no patient with a follow-up of less than 2 years is included. Most patients, in fact 90%, were symptomatic and 85% Ann Arbor Performance Status (PS) IV; 14% were of lymphocytic predominance (most of them of the epithelioid variant), 32% nodular sclerosis, 33% mixed cellularity and 15% lymphocytic depletion; 34 cases had received prior treatment (eight single drug chemotherapy, nine radiotherapy, and 17 both), and 32 had none.

Overall response rate was 91% (Table 1). Previous therapy influenced response, particularly in terms of the complete remission rate; 53% of the whole series achieved a complete remission and 38% a partial remission; among those without prior treatment, the figures were 69% complete and 25% partial remissions; patients with prior radiotherapy behaved like previously untreated patients; complete remissions decreased somewhat in patients with prior single agent chemotherapy, 63%, but fell to a mere 13% in the group of cases who received both. No difference was observed in response according to histology, 57%, 54%, and 60% complete remissions for nodular sclerosis, mixed cellularity, and lymphocytic depletion, respectively, except for the singular epithelioid variant, which lessened the

TABLE 1

MOPP Results in 66 Consecutive Patients of Advanced Hodgkin's Disease (F.J.D. Series)

	All Patients No. (%)	No Prior Treatment, No. (%)	Prior Treatment			
			Radiotherapy No. (%)	Chemotherapy No. (%)	RT + CT No. (%)	All Cases No. (%)
Total cases	66 (100%)	32 (100%)	9 (100%)	8 (100%)	17 (100%)	34 (100%)
CR + PR	60 (91%)	30 (94%)	9 (100%)	7 (88%)	14 (83%)	30 (88%)
CR	35 (53%)	22 (69%)	6 (67%)	5 (63%)	2 (12%)	13 (38%)

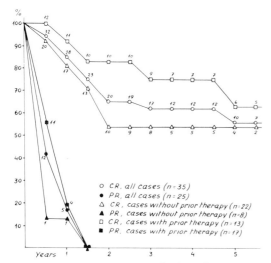

FIGURE 1. F.J.D. series. Actuarial relapse-free survival after six cycles of MOPP treatment according to the existence or not of prior treatment.

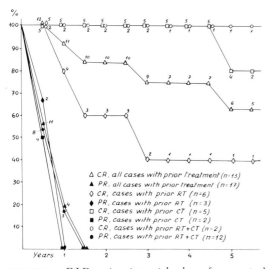

FIGURE 2. F.J.D. series. Actuarial relapse-free survival after six cycles of MOPP treatment according to the prior therapy.

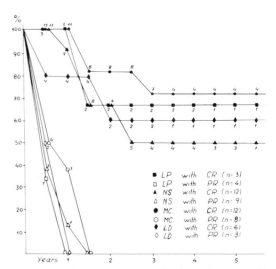

FIGURE 3. F.J.D. series. Actuarial relapse-free survival after six cycles of MOPP treatment according to histology.

complete remission rate of the lymphocytic predominance cases, in which group it is included to only 33%.

Actuarial median disease-free survival (Fig. 1) for the whole series has not been yet reached in complete responders; 56% of these patients remain relapse-free at 5 years; all partial responses progressed soon so that the median interval to progression was mostly shorter than 12 months. The duration of the complete remissions was little influenced by prior treatment and, curiously, it was even better in the cases with prior therapy; a no-

table exception was the small number of patients previously treated with radiotherapy alone, who showed an actuarial median relapse-free survival of only 30 months, in contrast to the figure of more than 80% of the other groups remaining free of disease at 5 years (Fig. 2). Duration of the complete remissions was also affected by histology (Fig. 3): nodular sclerosis patients had shorter complete remissions than those with lymphocytic predominance and mixed cellularity ($p = 0.03$), even shorter than lymphocytic depletion patients, and these had shorter complete remissions than mixed cellularity cases ($p < 0.05$).

Actuarial median survival is shown in Figure 4: 62% of all treated patients and 70% of responders are alive at 5 years. Only 40% of partial responders remain alive at 5 years, with a median survival of 20 months. In contrast, the 5-year survival for complete responders is 90%. For nonresponders the survival is less than 6 months (median 4 months). Partial responders who had prior treatment seemed to survive longer than those without it, but there is no difference in survival for complete responders with or without prior therapies. Survival was also influenced by histology (Fig. 5): it was longer, 75% at five years ($p < 0.05$) for patients with nodular sclerosis than for those with other histologies, including lymphocytic predominance, which had about the same than lymphocytic depletion and mixed cellularity, about 60% at 5 years; after separation of the cases with the particular epithelioid

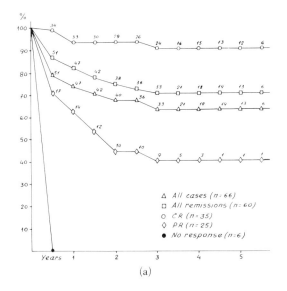

(a)

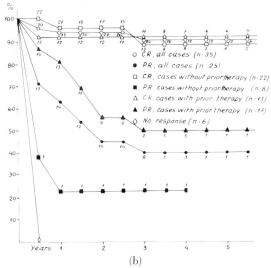

(b)

FIGURE 4. F.J.D. series. Actuarial survival after six cycles of MOPP treatment according to remission (a) and to prior therapy (b).

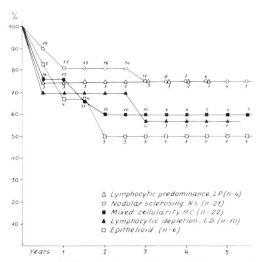

FIGURE 5. F.J.D. series. Actuarial survival after six cycles of MOPP treatment according to histology.

variant of histology, however, it became clear that true lymphocytic predominance patients behaved like those with nodular sclerosis, whereas 5-year survival fell to 50%, 56%, and 60% for epithelioid, lymphocytic depletion, and mixed cellularity respectively.

The very high response rate and, especially, the amazing complete remission rate and long duration have been consistently reported for patients with advanced Hodgkin's disease treated with MOPP, although generally not at the levels originally observed by the NCI workers.[13,37,44,49,52,64,68,79] They were always significantly better than previous results with single-drug therapy, when historically compared. However, at least three randomized, controlled studies[13,49,79] confirmed that this was indeed the case, when compared against repeated high-dose nitrogen mustard or against similar drugs and doses as used in MOPP but in a sequential manner. The complete response rate ranged from 48% up to 91%, with an average rate of 60%.[44] The median duration of the complete responses has also been reported with ample variations but always exceeding 15 months. These variations undoubtedly are accounted in large part by inclusion of patients with inadequate prior treatment, and departures from the original protocol design. Reports in fact confirm the adverse affect on both complete remission rate and duration of prior therapy, specially chemotherapy with or without added radiotherapy.[37,68,79] We have found no influence of radiotherapy when used alone as previous treatment and little effect of single-agent chemotherapy, but an ample effect of the prior usage of both chemotherapy plus radiotherapy on the complete remission rate, with little or no effect at all on the overall response rate. On the other hand, prior treatment in our series has not impaired the duration of response. These groups are, however, handicapped with regards to achieving complete remission.

Our cases were mostly PS-IV and symptomatic "B" patients, so that we could not examine the effect of this parameter on response and survival.

Frei, et al.[37] found significant differences between their cases with III-A, B, IV-A stages and those with stage IV-B in complete remission rates but not in the duration of the relapse-free survival. Stutzman and Glidewell[79] reported no differences in the complete remission rate and very slight in the duration of response for stages III and IV; systemic symptoms adversely affect the duration but not the rate of the complete remissions, and this fact has been also noted by others,[64] whereas Nixon and Aisenberg[68] have found significant impairment of both complete remission rate and duration in symptomatic patients. Some adverse influence of older age[52,64,68] and bone marrow involvement[64] has been reported on the duration of the relapse-free survival.

In our series we have also confirmed the findings of DeVita, et al.[24] concerning the response of nodular sclerosing variety. The patients with this histology relapse more frequently than those with other histologies, but live longer; in addition, we have found that lymphocytic depletion also shows a decreased duration of the complete remissions as compared with lymphocytic predominance and mixed cell histologies. Epithelioid types respond less to MOPP, and was the only histologic feature affecting response rate, a finding contrary to what has been reported by others.[69]

After confirmation that MOPP chemotherapy represented a major breakthrough in the treatment of Hodgkin's disease, clinical trials explored several means of preventing relapse and increasing survival. We shall review in sequence the question of maintenance treatments, MOPP varients, non-cross-resistant combinations or "salvage" regimens, and combined modality approaches; including radiotherapy.

The question of maintenance

The original NCI study provided for no maintenance therapy[26] partly based on experience on previous lymphoma studies.[14] This proved to be scientifically useful, permitting the evaluation of the actual need for a maintenance treatment.

The Southwestern Oncology Group studied the need for maintenance after MOPP. They undertook in 1968 a controlled study to determine the effect of the duration of MOPP treatment on the duration of the remission in advanced Hodgkin's disease.[37] The results in 178 evaluable patients were reported: the complete remission rate was 66% after six courses of MOPP treatment. Patients in complete remission were then randomly allocated either to continued MOPP treatment every 2 months for a total of 18 months (maintained remissions) or to no further treatment (unmaintained remissions). The relapse rate was significantly less in patients with maintained remissions, 75% of whom remained in remission, versus only 46% of the unmaintained patients 3 years after the start of the study and seemed to support the advantages of maintenance treatment. Subsequently, no difference emerged in overall survival. Evidently, patients who received only six cycles of MOPP treatment and subsequently relapsed had an excellent chance of reentering complete remission on retreatment with MOPP (13 out of 17 or 77%), whereas patients who were treated during 24 months and relapsed on treatment were no longer responsive to this therapy.

At about the same time, the NCI workers[89] started a clinical trial with 86 patients, 64 of whom (74%) entered complete remission after MOPP given for a minimum of six cycles. Fifty-seven of these could be used for the study and were randomized to one of three regimens: no additional therapy, two cycles of MOPP every 3 months for 15 months or treatment with BCNU for the same period. No significant differences were found at 4 years, but complications and infections were more frequent in the patients receiving maintenance therapy.

Some variations between both studies here could also be responsible for the conflicting results[26,89]: In the NCI series all patients received at least six cycles of MOPP, but, if evidence of continued response to therapy short of a complete remission occurred at six cycles, then therapy was continued until complete remission was attained and supplemented with the additional cycles. Approximately one-quarter of the patients received more than the proposed six cycles of therapy before complete remission was achieved, while, in the SWOG study, treatment in the unmaintained arm was stopped at six cycles. This approach could result in a fraction of patients with relatively incomplete remissions being falsely considered as complete. This fact has been also reported for some MOPP variants,[31] and stresses once more the relevance of achieving a complete remission. An additional small difference between both studies was the slightly larger fraction of nodular sclerosing histology patients randomized by the SWOG to the unmaintained arm, which as we now know, may have adversely affected the duration of the complete remission.[26] An updated report of the original SWOG series at 7.2 years revealed[22] that, although the median duration of the maintained remissions had not been yet reached by that time and the curve remained continuously above that of unmaintained remissions, the median of which was reached at 35 months, the difference was no longer statistically significant ($p = 0.10$). On the other hand, the survival estimates showed that 58% of unmaintained versus 48% of maintained remissions were alive at that period, again without statistically significant difference.

These facts cast some doubt on the value of maintenance MOPP treatment. The median time to complete remission is about 3 months.[25,29] The implication of very late complete remissions is unknown. So far, no maintenance treatment has proven advantageous with MOPP variants either,[31,33,65] and some more studies are in due course. A no maintenance arm unfortunately was not included in some studies. The overall 4- or 5-year survival does not seem to substantially differ from unmaintained series.[46,52,67]

In view of these facts and the risks involved[2,67,75,89] in prolonged treatment, maintenance should only be undertaken in the context of prospective controlled studies, and not as a clinical routine. Very slow responders might best be treated with alternative regimens rather than unduly prolong induction therapies to which possibly they are refractory.

MOPP variants

Many investigators have attempted to devise a more effective and less toxic drug combination than MOPP. Some trials have directly compared MOPP to other combinations, but most studies have not, rendering small differences difficult to interpret. Moreover, many lack sufficient follow-up so that their actual comparability is uncertain. So far a clear superiority of any regimen over MOPP has not emerged.

Three-drug combinations are clearly inferior to MOPP. The very first one to be studied was COP,[61] which used Cyclophosphamide, Vincristine, and Prednisone administered in 5-day cycles every 2

weeks for at least six courses. The original report included 107 patients. Those achieving complete remission were continued on treatment for four more cycles and then randomized to no treatment or to maintenance with the same regimen at 4-week intervals. The unmaintained treatment, a minimum of 10 courses being administered, was roughly equivalent in drugs and dosage to MOPP regimen but without Procarbazine. The complete remission rate was only 36% with a median duration of 5 months, unmaintained, or 10 months, maintained. Survival was not reported beyond 80 weeks.

The Acute Leukaemia Group 5 compared[79] MOPP to a schedule, consisting of six 2-week treatment periods alternating Vincristine plus Procarbazine and Vinblastine plus chlorambucil plus Prednisone. The patients thus received roughly half the Procarbazine and alkylating agent and about the same amount of Prednisone and Vinca alkaloid than in six cycles of MOPP therapy. Median time to complete response was 60 days, as against 5 weeks with MOPP, and the complete remission rates were the same, 61%. Remission duration, however, was 27+ months for MOPP and only 9 months for the sequential regimen, considering all patients treated.

This same group has reported a study comparing four-drug and three-drug combinations, all MOPP derivates, in a randomized trial in 537 patients.[67] The 4-drug combinations were MOPP and the latter BOPP, derived by substitution of BCNU for Nitrogen Mustard in the MOPP regimen, and the two 3-drug were derived by removing in the former the Procarbazine (BOP) or the Nitrosourea (OPP). At six cycles of treatment, the former combinations gave significantly higher frequency of complete remissions (BOPP 67%, MOPP 63%) than the 3-drug regimens (BOP 40%, OPP 42%). After remission, all complete and partial responders were subjected to maintenance treatment with Vinblastine or with Chlorambucil or with Chlorambucil plus monthly Vincristine plus Prednisone for 24 months, after which they were again randomized to no therapy or to reinforcement treatment consisting of three courses of the therapy employed in their initial induction, following which the maintenance program was resumed for another 9 months. No significant difference in relapse rate was demonstrated with any of these procedures of maintenance or late reinforcement. When all responders are considered together, the two four-drug regimens led to significantly longer remissions than the two 3-drug ones ($p = 0.002$). Median survival for the patients on four-drug combinations was about 5 years in contrast with only 2 years for the two three-drug regimens. Use of half-dose Vincristine in the four-drug combinations gave no significant differences in complete remission rate or duration.

The British National Lymphoma Investigation[12] has examined the value of Prednisone in the MOPP regimen in stage IV Hodgkin's disease, by comparing it with MOP, that is, the same without Prednisone. It found only half as many complete remissions with the later (MOPP 80%, MOP 44%). Although this study used Prednisone in each cycle as against only in the first and fourth cycles employed in the original schedule, this cannot fully account for the contrasting report of Jacobs et al.,[50] who found no difference between both regimens. This discrepancy may in part be related to retrospective nature of the latter study, motivated by the reported problems arising with corticosteroid administration and rapid withdrawal in patients previously subjected to lung or heart irradiation.[18]

From the above facts, therefore, it seems that the presence of alkylating agent and Procarbazine are essential for the complete remission rate in the MOPP regimen. Procarbazine may also be essential for the duration of the remission, whereas a lower dosage of Vincristine does not appear to have much effect. Improvement of MOPP therapy may call for substitutions, or additions to the four components, rather than a reduction in the number.[67]

The substitution of Vinblastine for Vincristine of MOPP regimen with reinforcement of Prednisone administration, which was given in all the six cycles, as the MVPP combination, was endeavored by the London investigators of the St. Bartholomew's Hospital, whose report was updated in 1973.[46] Although no direct comparison with MOPP was made, the results do not significantly differ in terms of remission rate, duration, survival and prognostic factors involved. This is true in spite of the fact that a 4-week gap, as against a 2-week one in MOPP. Neurotoxicity was lower but marrow toxicity was greater with MVPP than with MOPP.

DeVita et al.[29] treated a small group of patients without prior therapy by a modified MOPP regi-

men in which Cyclophosphamide was substituted for Nitrogen Mustard (COPP, C-MOPP) and obtained 64% complete remissions. The high incidence of alopecia observed led this combination to be abandoned. Morgenfeld et al.[65] have reported the results with COPP in a series of 138 patients; overall complete remission rate was 66% but increased to 77% in patients who received six cycles of induction treatment and decreased to 45% in those having only three to five courses; prior chemotherapy adversely affected the complete remission rate. Patients achieving complete remission were then allocated by Institutions, either to no therapy or to maintenance treatment with one cycle of COPP every 3 months, biweekly Vinblastine or the later plus one cycle of COPP every 6 months. The median duration of complete remissions was longer for patients who completed six cycles of treatment, 30 months, as against 10 months for those with less treatment courses. Four-year survival of complete responders was 65%. No statistically significant differences were noted between the patients distributed to maintenance or to no treatment. All "A" patients (100%) achieved a complete remission and were alive at 48 months as against only 75% and 52% respectively for symptomatic "B" patients. The poorest survival was accounted for by the IV-B patients who represented more than half the whole population treated. These results are comparable but somewhat inferior to those achieved with MOPP and the same is true for CVPP (Cyclophosphamide and Vinblastine substituted for Nitrogen Mustard and Vincristine respectively in the MOPP regimen) as reported by Høst and Abrahamsen.[48]

Two other regimens using Cyclophosphamide and Vinblastine plus Procarbazine and Prednisone have been reported, but, again, none of these studies has directly compared them with MOPP. Bloomfield, et al.[4] used a combination stemming from the original St. Bartholomew's Hospital schedule, but substituted Cyclophosphamide, at half equivalent dosage, for Nitrogen Mustard; three weekly doses of Vinblastine were employed in each cycle, Prednisone being administered as in MOPP regimen only in the first and fourth cycles. The gap between courses was 4 weeks, and treatment lasted a minimum of six cycles; maintenance with the same combination was used at 2–3-month intervals. The complete remission rate was 74%; nodular sclerosis patients had lower complete remission rate,

74%, than mixed cellularity, 100%. The median duration of complete remissions at the time of the report is 27+ months, so that the results seem very comparable to the original MOPP report.

Diggs, et al.,[31] on the other hand, have used an entirely different regimen, with only one large dose of Cyclophosphamide, two doses of Vinblastine and 7-day courses of Procarbazine and Prednisone, with 2-week gaps between courses. Responding patients received a minimum of six cycles; those achieving complete remission received three more courses, but those who did not, continued treatment until maximal response. Complete responders were then randomized either to no further therapy or to maintenance treatment with alternating monthly doses of CCNU and Vinblastine for one more year. The complete remission rate was 62%; prior chemotherapy, in addition to irradiation, significantly decreased the chance of obtaining complete remission: 37.5% as compared to 79% in the previously irradiated only group ($p < 0.05$). Median time to complete remission was 3 months. Median duration was about 35 months with no statistically significant difference found between maintained versus unmaintained remissions.

A five-drug combination has been used by Prosnitz, et al.[73] sequentially combined with low-dose radiotherapy to the sites of bulk disease. They used Nitrogen Mustard, Procarbazine, and Prednisone and both Vincristine and Vinblastine administered in three 6-week cycles with 2-week gaps between courses to previously untreated patients with III-B or IV disease or patients previously irradiated in relapse, stages II, III, and IV. Radiotherapy followed, and two additional cycles of chemotherapy were given. The results after the first three cycles, before radiotherapy, were 75% of complete remissions, which are comparable to those achieved with MOPP.

Cooper, et al.[23] have reported preliminary results of a more recent cancer and acute leukemia Group B study which randomized patients into four four-drug combinations MOPP, MVPP, and the same two combinations with CCNU substituting for Nitrogen Mustard. So far, of 438 patients entered, 327 were evaluated at the time of the report. The complete remission rate ranged from 59% to 66%, and no statistically significant difference was noted between the four regimens in the whole series. Differences were observed in the patients with prior treatment favoring CCNU-containing combinations. All remissions were maintained with either periodic reinductions or Vinblastine. Remission duration was also longer with CCNU-containing regimens, with 33% less relapses on C(CCNU)OPP and 68% less relapses on C(CCNU)VPP ($p < 0.05$), which also was the less toxic of all four combinations. No survival data have been yet analyzed so that the actual merit of these combinations must await the test of time.

Durant, et al.[32] reported a study by the SECSG testing three four-drug combinations containing BCNU and Procarbazine and either Cyclophosphamide plus Vincristine (BCOP), Cyclophosphamide plus Vinblastine (BCVP), or Vincristine plus Vinblastine (BOVP) in 61 patients, most of them with extensive prior therapy, including radiation and multiple-drug treatments. The last regimen, combining both Vinca alcaloids was used in only eight patients, but it was dropped because of severe and prolonged neuromyalgic toxicity. BCOP, administered to 31 patients, gave nine (29%) complete remissions and, similarly, BCVP achieved nine complete remissions in 22 patients (41%). These studies were the forerunners of the five-drug combination BCVPP, which was extensively studied by the group and also by the Eastern Cooperative Oncology Group (ECOG). ECOG compared BCVPP versus standard MOPP, as an induction treatment for 6 months, and also investigated the ability of BCVPP or BCG vaccine to maintain remission. The SECSG has undertaken the task of comparing the effect of the combination at six cycles in patients stratified according to amount of prior therapy and that of continuation treatment either with BCVPP or MOPP or no treatment. The study was activated in 1971 and accesion of patients was completed on December, 1975.

So far, only preliminary results in 220 patients have been reported in the ECOG study, in abstract form.[3] The induction treatment yielded the same results in terms of complete remission rate with both regimens: MOPP 69%, BCVPP 70%. Maintenance with both combinations or BCG or no maintenance at all yielded identical results. Other findings were that BCVPP could induce remissions in patients resistant to MOPP, and that gastrointestinal toxicity and neurotoxicity were somewhat milder with BCVPP, but hematologic toxicities were similar to MOPP.

The SECSG study has been recently reported in

detail in their study of 324 patients at 4 years of observation.[33] The complete remission rates were not significantly different for patients with no prior treatment (68%) and patients with prior radiotherapy only (73%), but were significantly lower in patients with major prior chemotherapy (28%, $p < 0.01$). There were no evident differences in the duration of remission or survival among patients included in the prior treatment groups, or between the curves of survival and disease-free survival originally have suggested that maintenance therapy significantly prolonged a complete remission or survival in previously untreated patients. However, multivariate analysis did not demonstrate maintenance therapy to be a significant prognostic factor; rather, favorable prognostic indicators were shown to be related to host factors. For all patient groups, female sex and an initial lymphocyte count of >1372 were favorable factors; for those with little or no prior therapy, age below 40, Caucasian race and having lymphocytic predominance or nodular sclerosis histology favorably influenced the outcome as well. Although platelet and neurologic toxicities were less with BCVPP, pulmonary fibrosis has been reported with a fatal outcome in five cases out of the six.

Bleomycin has also been studied as an addition to MOPP. This investigation was undertaken by the SWOG in order to determine whether this antibiotic drug could improve the results obtained with MOPP alone.[21] These have been recently updated.[20] Between 1971 and 1974, 253 patients entered the study; they were randomized to receive MOPP alone or MOPP plus one of two different dose levels of Bleomycin (low dose: ldB, 2 units/m²; high dose: hdB, 10 units/m²) on days 1 and 8 of the first six cycles of MOPP. Complete responses were maintained for 18 months with any one of two MOPP schedules or with these plus radiotherapy. Patients with significant compromise of pulmonary function were excluded from the randomization and treated with MOPP alone. The complete remission rate for MOPP alone was 70%, MOPP + ldB, 84%, MOPP + hdB, 76%, and MOPP alone in the special group of compromised pulmonary function, 64%. The high-dose Eleomycin arm was closed early because of three episodes of irreversible myelosuppression, and MOPP alone was closed at about the same time because it confirmed previous SWOG studies on 384 patients with a complete remission rate of 64%. Complete response was sig-

nificantly adversely affected by marrow involvement, poor performance status, and 10% weight loss in the prior six months. Overall response rate favored MOPP + ldB (96%) when compared to MOPP alone (84%, $p = 0.03$), but, there were no significant differences between the complete remission rates ($p = 0.076$), duration ($p = 0.26$), or survival ($p = 0.06$).

Bonadonna, et al.[8] devised another five-drug combination by substituting Adriamycin and Bleomycin for Procarbazine in the MOPP regimen. This combination, called MABOP, yielded induction results, after six monthly cycles, comparable to MOPP in stages III and IV. Median duration of complete remissions in stage IV patients was 13 months. Although the study was not controlled, it is clear that this combination is inferior to MOPP and points out again the important role of Procarbazine in the chemotherapy of Hodgkin's disease.

Thus, so far, MOPP-derived three-drug regimens are evidently inferior, and no four-drug or five-drug regimen has been conclusively proven to be better than MOPP.

Combinations non-cross-resistant with MOPP and "salvage" chemotherapy

About 40% of Hodgkin's disease patients achieving complete remissions with any of the above reviewed combinations will relapse and require additional treatment. Late relapses may respond again with prolonged disease-free survival to retreatment with MOPP,[35,37] but the more prevalent early relapses exhibit a poorer response with the same or slightly different reinduction regimen.[32,33] Relapses occurring during the first 6 months of follow-up after MOPP therapy usually do not respond to a new induction with the same combination.[64] Thus 25% of the patients treated, and 20–30% of patients, initially shown refractory to induction treatment, will require other therapies.

Bonadonna, et al.[10] developed the first combination with four drugs not previously used in the MOPP regimen. The new combination included two antibiotics, Adriamycin and Bleomycin, a Vinca alkaloid, Vinblastine and the imidazole-carboxamide derivate dimethyltriazene or DTIC, being the Vinca alkaloid, the only near similarity with the MOPP regimen or its variants. It was named by its acronym ABVD and administered in six monthly cycles, as standard therapies. In an updated report[11] on 56 patients not having prior chemotherapy, the results obtained with MOPP in half of them are compared to those of the ABVD regimen in the other half, after six cycles of induction treatment. Overall response rate, as well as complete remission rate, showed no statistical differences (complete remission rate, MOPP 62%, ABVD 70%) and was adversely affected by the presence of symptoms but not by histology, in both regimens. After primary treatment failure or relapse, crossover treatment was given to a total of 10 patients and continued until further relapse or progression was evident; only one out of five patients crossed-over to MOPP showed a partial response; ABVD induced two complete remissions in five treated patients. In another series which is not part of the above study, six cycles of ABVD produced complete remission in seven of ten patients resistant to MOPP, for a duration ranging from 3 to 24+ months; thus, a total of nine out of 15 patients (60%) achieved a complete remission.

We have reported preliminary results in 18 patients treated with ABVD after MOPP failure and followed up for at least 1 year after completion of six cycles of therapy[83,84]; usually two more cycles were given after complete remission documented at the end of the six-cycles induction treatment. Overall response rate was 83% with a complete remission rate of 61%. Nine cases had had MOPP within 6 months prior to ABVD; one case had not responded to MOPP and did not respond to ABVD either; the remaining eight patients had achieved seven partial and one complete remissions with MOPP and all responded to ABVD (two partial and six complete remissions). Three cases received ABVD 10–12 months after MOPP to which they had responded (one partial and two complete remissions) and responded again to the alternate regimen, all three with complete remissions. Another six cases had received MOPP 13 and 58 months (median 26.8 months) earlier and had been in complete remission; after ABVD, however, two did not respond and there were two complete and two partial remissions. At the time of this report, median actuarial interval to progression in patients achieving partial remissions only was 5 months, whereas the median duration of complete remissions was 16 months (Fig. 6). The regimen was well tolerated, considering that all patients had received

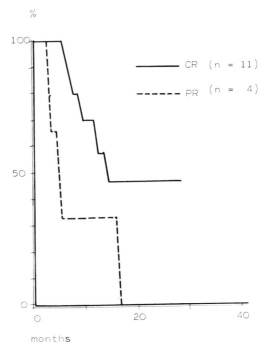

FIGURE 6. F.J.D. series. Actuarial relapse-free survival after six cycles of ABVD according to remission.

prior combination chemotherapy at least; alopecia was mild, myelosuppression moderate, and cardiopulmonary toxicity was not observed; more than 80% of the projected dose of each drug was in fact administered. This small series thus confirmed the lack of cross resistance with MOPP regimen, and the valuable remission index seemed promising. However, the duration of complete remission was shorter than commonly observed after primary treatments.

Case, et al.[16] have reported their results with minor modifications of this regimen in 24 patients previously treated with MOPP and radiotherapy, after either progression of the disease while receiving MOPP or recurrence within 2 months following discontinuance of this regimen. Fifteen (63%) achieved significant objective response, although only one reached a complete remission status, with a median duration of 6.5+ months.

Clamon and Corder have reported[19] their results in nine stage IV patients, who had failed either while receiving MOPP or shortly following remission, treated with the original ABVD. Seven patients progressed in spite of the new treatment, receiving only 1–3½ cycles. Two patients were able to receive at least six cycles of ABVD: one progressed and the other achieved a partial response which lasted 4 months. This group was particularly unfavorable since the median interval from MOPP to ABVD was 3 months; six patients had bone marrow or bone involvement, and the other three patients had extensive lung involvement.[11]

Other combinations have been reported such as one developed by Lokich, et al.,[60] which consists of Bleomycin, DTIC, Vincristine, Prednisone, and Adriamycin (acronym B-DOPA) administered in 6-day cycles every three weeks, for six to eight courses. Of 15 evaluable patients, who were induction failures or relapses after MOPP. Twelve patients achieved response (80%) and nine were complete (60%), with a median duration at the time of the report of 14+ months (range, 2 to 21+).

Vinciguerra, et al.[87] designed another combination, the BVDS regimen, consisting of at least 12 monthly cycles of Bleomycin, Vinblastine, Doxorubicin (Adriamycin), and Streptozotocin, and treated 10 patients who had failed standard MOPP or C(CCNU)OPP variant chemotherapy. Five patients (50%) achieved objective response, and three of them (30%) a complete remission, after two to three cycles of therapy, one remaining in remission without further treatment.

Loh, et al.[59] have treated 22 patients with a combination of Adriamycin, Bleomycin, and DTIC (ABDIC) and achieved five complete remissions (23%) with 68% overall objective responses. Goldman and Dawson[43] reported a cooperative study of British Hospitals of a combination of CCNU, Vinblastine, and Bleomycin (CVB), which was administered for a minimum of six monthly cycles and continued thereafter with monthly courses of the same without Bleomycin. All but one of the 39 patients treated had responded to a previous chemotherapy (MOPP or MVPP) but then had subsequently progressed or recurred shortly (3–6 months) after treatment. Overall response rate to CVB was 85%, and complete remission rate was 26%. The duration of the remissions was not reported.

Kurnick, et al.[55] have informed on their results with a similar combination without Vinblastine; CCNU was administered at 6-week intervals, but Bleomycin was given twice a week for 5 weeks and weekly thereafter. They have reported 18 patients with 72% overall response rate; two patients (11%) achieved complete remission lasting 20 and 36+ months respectively. Williams et al., on the other

hand, have reported[88] preliminary results in 10 patients with a combination of Adriamycin and CCNU; eight patients achieved objective remission, and five (50%), a complete remission status.

Another four-drug combination has been studied by Osieka, et al.[71] consisting of Adriamycin, Bleomycin, CCNU, and DTIC. They treated 15 patients, who had previously responded to C-MOPP before becoming refractory to it. This yielded two complete remissions and 11 partial responses.

The SCAB regimen, a combination of Streptozotocin, CCNU, Adriamycin and Bleomycin has been investigated by Levi, et al.[58] They have administered monthly cycles of this regimen to 17 evaluable patients with prior treatment and achieved an overall response rate of 60% with complete remissions in 33%. A study of the combination in a small group of 10 previously untreated patients yielded eight complete remissions, including six who were symptomatic[30]; duration of the responses at the time of the report is from 2+ to 23+ months (unmaintained), and one relapse has occurred at 6 months following completion of chemotherapy. Thus, so far, the regimen is very comparable to MOPP and lacks cross resistance with it, although toxicity seems to be greater.

A similar regimen BCAVe has been evaluated by Porzig, et al.[72] It consists of Bleomycin, CCNU, Adriamycin, and Vinblastine and is administered in 6-week cycles up to maximum tolerated adriamycin dose (7–10 cycles). This regimen yielded 77% objective responses and 50% complete remissions in a group of 22 patients who developed disease progression during or after MOPP therapy. The median actuarial survival for the whole series was 16.4 months and that of complete responders 24 months; median relapse-free survival has not been yet reached for complete remissions (35+ months).

We must conclude that many of these results seem promising for the rescue of patients who have failed to achieve or continue on complete remission after MOPP. More data are urgently needed on the quality of the new remissions and on the characteristics of the patients who respond. Previously unresponsive patients seem to do worse, implying either an inherent refractoriness to known chemotherapy or an easily acquired resistance to the combinations of available drugs.[33] In addition to that, two other trends may help in answering the dilemma: If these refractory patients are identifiable, use of more than one regimen for remission induction may be considered or the combined usage of chemotherapy plus radiotherapy. These will be briefly reviewed in the following paragraphs.

Supraintensive combination chemotherapy

The studies of ECOG and SECSG with MOPP and BCVPP[3,33] showed that the latter regimen could induce remissions in patients who failed or became resistant to MOPP, but it was incapable of improving the quality of the complete remissions achieved with the first treatment. Both combinations were at least partially cross resistant, the only different drugs being only two, BCNU and the Vinca alkaloid; and the treatment was done after six cycles of induction with the other regimen. Therefore, this trial does not address itself well to the question of initial use of non-cross-resistant combinations.

Bonadonna, et al. have reported the preliminary results[9] of an eight-drug, two-regimen combination in a group of 39 patients with proved extranodal extensions. These were randomly allocated to receive either 12 cycles of MOPP (17 cases) or six cycles of MOPP monthly alternating with six cycles of ABVD (22 cases). All patients were previously thoroughly stratified. After a minimum of six cycles, overall response rate was higher for the two-regimen arm (91%) than for the MOPP alone arm (65%), but the complete remission rate was comparable in both armas (55% versus 53%). All complete responders of the MOPP plus ABVD arm remain alive and relapse free at 2 years of follow-up, whereas there are 90% surviving and 65% relapse free in the MOPP alone arm at that time. Considerably more prolonged follow-up is necessary, but these preliminary results seem encouraging.

The only other study so far announced, not including radiotherapy, is the comparison by Cancer and Leukemia Group B of 12 cycles of the BVDS regimen, 12 cycles of the MOPP variant with CCNU instead of Nitrogen Mustard, and alternating sequential monthly cycles of both regimens.[87] A report of the results is not presently available.

The combined modality (chemotherapy plus radiotherapy) approach

Several studies have investigated the value of moderate or low-dose radiotherapy in addition to full induction or split-course combination chemotherapy.

Such a strategy was initially employed by the NCI workers prior to MOPP.[27,66] That investigation was uncontrolled so that the value of radiotherapy could only be inferred: complete remission persisted 30+ months in eight of nine patients who received radiotherapy to involved areas in addition to chemotherapy, but only in one out of five who were treated with chemotherapy alone. Jacquillat, et al.[52] found significant differences in remission duration and survival in stage III patients who received irradiation after remission induction with MOPP and Vinblastine maintenance. Here again, the use of radiotherapy was not randomized, and the results are not different than achieved with MOPP alone. Gamble, et al.[41] employed MOPP plus radiotherapy (3000–4000 rad) in stage III-A and B patients, but overall results are not better than those which can be achieved with MOPP alone (68% overall 5-year survival).

Similar considerations apply to work of the Yale group reported by Prosnitz, et al.[73] A split course 5-drug combination chemotherapy plus low-dose radiotherapy to the sites of bulk disease, nodal or parenchymal, yielded 75% complete remissions in a series of 80 patients. All but one of the remissions were achieved during the 6-month chemotherapy period, prior to radiotherapy, so that the latter was only intended to enhance the duration. However, 5-year survival rates are not very different from those obtained with MOPP alone (overall 68%; complete remissions 92%). Other uncontrolled studies have not yet reported prolonged enough follow-up for proper evaluation of the results.

Bonadonna, et al.,[11] in the study outlined in a previous paragraph, have also attempted to increase response and survival by adding moderate dose (2000–25 000 rad) radiotherapy to all nodal and extranodal areas of pre-existing disease, except bone marrow, after complete remission or good partial response (>75%) achieved with chemotherapy (MOPP or ABVD, randomized). Unfortunately, they have not randomized patients to chemotherapy alone. At the time of the report, 30 months of observation only, the results for survival and for duration of response are similar to their MOPP plus ABVD study without radiotherapy. Although results appear somewhat better than those for MOPP alone,[9] the time of follow-up is still too short to warrant any interpretation.

A most aggressive approach has been reported by Case, et al.[17] but again with preliminary results and nonrandomized. The protocol alternates monthly courses of MOPP and ABDV with 200-rad radiotherapy, given in the fifth month to areas of originally bulky disease without chemotherapy. The chemotheraply is continued thereafter monthly up to 8 months, and then bimonthly up to 2 years. Complete remission has been achieved in 13 out of 14 previously untreated patients, four out of six with prior radiotherapy, and all four with prior chemotherapy for a rate of 87.5%. The results in patients with prior chemotherapy may be valuable; however, more extensive experience is needed before any conclusion can be drawn.

Kun, et al.,[54] on the other hand, have reported a poor outcome in 28 previously untreated patients who received wide field irradiation after complete MOPP treatment for stages II-B and III-B disease. There was considerable morbidity associated with the treatment contrarily to other reports,[47,70,74] and the combined true and marginal recurrence rate was 14% with a disease-free survival of only 61%, which is inferior to MOPP alone.

The only controlled study so far reported is that of Rosenberg et al.[74] on 33 patients with PS-IV disease (excepting those with liver involvement, who were treated on a separate protocol). The patients were randomized to receive either six cycles of MOPP chemotherapy alone or split-course MOPP chemotherapy combined with total nodal irradiation. No difference has been observed in survival or relapse-free survival after a follow-up of 7 years. This study casts doubt on the value of adjuvant radiotherapy implied in the preceding studies.

Studies on the opposite strategy: namely, the use of chemotherapy as an adjuvant to radiation therapy in early stages have also been carried out. Tubiana[80] has reported an analysis at 5 years of the cooperative trial by the EORTC group on clinical stages I and II, in which 296 patients were randomized to receive or not a 2-year treatment with weekly injections of Vinblastine after extended field radiotherapy (mantle field for supradiafragmatic regions and an inverted Y field for infradi-

afragmatic lesions). Recurrences in irradiated regions were low (4%) and similar in both groups as well as were extranodal or widespread recurrences (about 20%), the only significant difference being in the recurrences in the nonirradiated areas (30% versus 15%). The difference in relapse-free survival was significant, but this did not carry over to overall survival for the whole group. Unfavorable histologic forms and patients older than 30 years of age, did demonstrate differences in survival favoring the combined approach.

O'Connell, et al.[70] reported preliminary results of a prospective randomized trial on stages I-A, II-A and -B, III-B with megavoltage extended field radiation therapy alone or megavoltage radiotherapy limited to the involved lymph node sites followed by MOPP. At 3 years of follow-up, 10 out of 41 patients in the extended field group had relapsed, but only one out of 31 in the group of limited radiotherapy plus chemotherapy, the difference being significant ($p < 0.03$) and the results encouraging. Hellman, et al.[47] also found promising results in a group of stage III-B patients treated with split-course MOPP chemotherapy plus mantle and para-aortic nodal or total nodal irradiation versus irradiation alone. The study was uncontrolled and the patients with added chemotherapy were presumably selected for more advanced disease. However, only three out of 21 in this group suffered relapse as against four out of seven in the irradiation alone group. The comparison of both kinds of treatment in stage II-B patients failed to demonstrate such differences.

The Stanford controlled trials, recently updated,[74] have shown that although adjuvant MOPP chemotherapy significantly improves the initial relapse-free survival in I, II, and III stage patients (with the exception of I-B and II-B), improvement in survival is not significant at 3–9 years of follow-up. On favorable cases, stages I-A and II-A, including II_E-A with favorable histology, the results so far point out that chemotherapy may permit the use of more limited radiotherapy, with comparable results to extended field radiotherapy alone, and under this light there should be seen the result sof O'Connell, et al.[70] reviewed above. The results of the Stanford group in stage III-B patients with the combined treatment are not better than those reported with MOPP alone, indicating that these patients should be treated mainly with combination chemotherapy, although the relapse-free survival seem to be better for the combined treatment as it was the case with the cases reported by Hellman et al.[47] Studies by the SWOG in process also show similar trends. Comparative trials with careful stratification of known prognostic factors[33] are needed to explore the role of these therapies alone and in combination. However, a major deterrent to extending studies on aggressiveness of treatment is the problem of secondary malignancies, namely acute leukemia, which develop with increasing frequency with the combined approach. Moreover, as combination chemotherapy becomes applied in an optimal manner (i.e., with its proper intensity and in patients in better condition), results are likely to improve. Nevertheless, a resistant group of patients does exist, for which proper identification of host factors and exploration of therapies through comparative may be quite valuable.

References

1. Aisenberg, A. C., and Goldman, J. M.: Prolongation of survival in Hodgkin's disease. *Cancer 27: 802–805, 1971.*

2. Arseneau, J. C., Sponzo, R. W., Levin, D. L., Schnipper, L. E., Bonner, H., Young, R. C., Canellos G. P., Johnson, R. E., and DeVita, V. T., Jr.: Nonlymphomatous malignant tumours complicating Hodgkin's disease. Possible association with intensive therapy. *N Engl J Med 287: 1119–1122, 1972.*

3. Bakemeier, R. F., DeVita, V. T., and Horton, J.: Chemotherapy and immunotherapy of Hodgkin's disease. *Proc Am Assoc Cancer Res and ASCO 17: 293, 1976.*

4. Bloomfield, C. D., Weiss, R. B., Fortuny, I., Vosika, G., and Kennedy, B. J.: Combined chemotherapy with cyclophosphamide, vinblastine, procarbazine and prednisone (CVPP) for patients with advanced Hodgkin's disease. An alternative program to MOPP. *Cancer 38: 42–28, 1976.*

5. Blum, R. H., and Carter, S. K.: Review of adriamycin, a new anticancer drug with significant clinical activity. *Ann Intern Med 80: 249–259, 1974.*

6. Blum, R. H., Carter, S. K., and Agre, K.: A Clinical review of bleomycin, a new antinoplastic agent. *Cancer 31: 903–913, 1973.*

7. Bohannon, R. A., Miller, D. G., and Diamond, H. D.: Vincristine in the treatment of lymphomas and leukaemias. *Cancer Res 23: 613–617, 1963.*

8. Bonadonna, G., De Lena, M., Monfardini, S., Rossi, A., Branbilla, C., Uslenchi, C., and Zucali, R.: Combination usage of Adriamycin (NSC 123127) in malignant lymphomas. *Cancer Chemother Rep (Part 3) 6: 381–388, 1975.*

9. Bonadonna, G., Fossati, V., and De Lena, M.: MOPP versus MOPP plus ABVD in Stage IV Hodgkin's disease. *Proc Amer Assoc Cancer Res and ASCO 19: 363, 1978.*

10. Bonadonna, G., Zucali, R., Monfardini, S., De Lena, M., and Uslenghi, C.: Combination chemotherapy of Hodgkin's disease with adriamycin, bleomycin, vinblastine and imidazole carboxamide versus MOPP. *Cancer 36: 252–259, 1975.*

11. Bonadonna, G., Zucali, R., De Lena, M., and Valagussa, P.: Combined chemotherapy (MOPP or ABVD) Radiotherapy approach in advanced Hodgkin's disease.

12. British National Lymphoma Investigation: Value of prednisone in combination chemotherapy of stage IV Hodgkin's disease. *Br Med J 3: 413–414, 1975.*

13. Brook, J., and Gocka, C.: Combination of single agent with combination therapy in Hodgkin's disease. *Proc Am Assoc Cancer Res 12: 12, 1971.*

14. Carbone, P. P., Spurr, C., Schneiderman, M., Scoto, J., Holland, J. F., and Schneider, B.: Management of patients with malignant lymphoma. A comparative study of cyclophosphamide and Vinca alkaloids. *Cancer Res 28: 811–822, 1968.*

15. Carter, S. and Livingston, R.: Single agent therapy of Hodgkin's disease. *Arch Intern Med 131: 377–387, 1973.*

16. Case, D. C., Jr., Young, C. W., and Lee, B. J., III: Combination chemotherapy of MOPP-resistant Hodgkin's disease with adriamycin, bleomycin, dacarbazine and vinblastine (ABDV). *Cancer 39: 1382–1386, 1977.*

17. Case, D. C., Young, C. W., Nisce, L., Lee, B. A. J. and Clarkson, B. D.: Eight-drug combination chemotherapy (MOPP-ABDV) and local radiotherapy for advanced Hodgkin's disease. *Cancer Treat Rep 60: 1217–1223, 1976.*

18. Castellino, R. A., Glatstein, E., Turbon, M. M., Rosenberg, S., and Kaplan, H. S.: Latent radiation injury of lung or heart activated by steroid withdrawal. *Ann Intern Med 80: 593–599, 1974.*

19. Clamon, G. H., and Corder, M. P.: ABVD treatment of MOPP failures in Hodgkin's disease: A re-examination of goals of salvage therapy. *Cancer Treat Rep 62: 363–367, 1978.*

20. Coltman, C. A., Jr.: MOPP plus low dose Bleomycin for advanced Hodgkin's disease. A five year follow-up. (Abstract, pp. 15–16, Session I). Symposium on Recent Development on Bleomycin Treatment, XII Int. Cancer Congress, Buenos Aires, October 1978.

21. Coltman, C. A., Jr. and Delaney, F. C.: Five drug combination chemotherapy for advanced Hodgkin's disease. *Clin Res 21: 876, 1973.*

22. Coltman, C. A., Jr., Hall, W., Frei, E., III, and Moon, T. E.: MOPP maintenance versus unmaintained remission for MOPP-induced complete remissions of advanced Hodgkin's disease: 7.2 year follow-up. *Proc Am Assoc Cancer Res and ASCO 17: 289, 1976.*

23. Cooper, M. R., Spurr, C. L., Glidewell, O., and Holland, J. F.: The superiority of a nitrosourea (CCNU) containing four-drug combination over MOPP in the treatment of stage III and IV Hodgkin's disease. *Proc Am Assoc Cancer Res and ASCO 16: 111, 1975.*

24. DeVita, V., Canellos, G., Hubbard, S., Chabner, B., and Young, R.: Chemotherapy of Hodgkin's disease with MOPP: a ten-year progress report. *Proc Am Assoc Cancer Res and ASCO 17: 269, 1976.*

25. DeVita, V. T., Canellos, G. P., and Moxley, J. H., III.: A decade of combination chemotherapy of advanced Hodgkin's disease. *Cancer 30: 1495–1504, 1972.*

26. DeVita, V. T., Jr., Lewis, B. J., Rozencweig, M., and Muggia, F. M.: The chemotherapy of Hodgkin's disease. Past experiences and future directions. *Cancer 42: 979–990, 1978.*

27. DeVita, V. T., Moxley, J. H., III, Brace, K., and Frei, E., III: Intensive combination chemotherapy and x-irradiation in the treatment of Hodgkin's disease. *Proc Am Assoc Cancer Res 6: 15, 1965.*

28. DeVita, V. T., and Serpick, A. A.: Combination chemotherapy in the treatment of advanced Hodgkin's disease. *Proc Am Assoc Cancer Res 8: 13, 1967.*

29. DeVita, V. T., Serpick, A. A., and Carbone, P. P.: Combination chemotherapy in the treatment of advanced Hodgkin's disease. *Ann Intern Med 73: 881–895, 1970.*

30. Diggs, C. H., Wiernik, P. H., and Aisner, J.: SCAB (Streptozotocin, CCNU, Adriamycin, Bleomycin) for advanced untreated Hodgkin's disease. *Proc Am Assoc Cancer Res and ASCO 19: 370, 1978.*

31. Diggs, C. H., Wiernik, P. H., Levi, J. A., and Kvols, L. K.: Cyclophosphamide, vinblastine, procarbazine and prednisone with CCNU and vinblastine maintenance for advanced Hodgkin's disease. *Cancer 39: 1949–1954, 1977.*

32. Durant, J. R., Bartolucci, A., Gams, R. A., Dorfman, R. F., and Velez-Garcia, E.: Southeastern Cancer Study Group trials with nitrosoureas in Hodgkin's disease. *Cancer Treat Rep 60: 781–787, 1976.*

33. Durant, J. R., Gams, R. A., Velez-Garcia, E., Bartolucci, A., Wirtschafter, D., and Dorfman, R.: BCNU, velban, cyclophosphamide, procarbazine and prednisone (BVCPP) in advanced Hodgkin's disease. *Cancer 42: 2101–2110, 1978.*

34. Durant, J. R., and Lessner, H. E.: Development of four-drug BCNU combination chemotherapy regimens. *Cancer 32: 277–285, 1973.*

35. Fisher, R. I., DeVita, V. T., Hubbard, S. M., and Young, R. C.: Prolonged disease-free survival in Hodgkin's disease following reinduction with MOPP. *Proc Am Assoc Cancer Res and ASCO 18: 318, 1977.*

36. Frei, E., III, and Gamble, J. F.: Progress in the chemotherapy of Hodgkin's disease. *Cancer 19: 378–384, 1966.*

37. Frei, E., III, Luce, J. K., Gamble, J. F., Coltman, C. A., Jr., Constanzi, J. J., Tally, R. W., Monto, R. W., Wilson, H. E., Hewlett, J. S., Delaney, F. C., and Gehan, E. A.: Combination chemotherapy in advanced Hodgkin's disease: Induction and maintenance of remission. *Ann Intern Med 79: 376–382, 1973.*

38. Frei, E., III, Luce, J. K., Talley, R. W., Vaitkivicious, V. K., and Wilson, H. E.: 5-(3,3-Dimethyl-1-triazeno) imidazole-4-carboxamide (NSC-45388) in the treatment of lymphoma. *Cancer Chemother Rep 56: 667–670, 1972.*

39. Freireich, E. J., Karon, M., and Frei, E., III: Quadruple combination therapy (VAMP) for acute lymphocytic leukaemia of childhood. *Proc Am Assoc Cancer Res 5: 20, 1964.*

40. Frost, J. W., Goldwein, M. I., and Bryan, J. A.: Clinical experience with vincaleukoblastine in far advanced Hodgkin's disease and various malignant states. *Ann Intern Med 58: 854–859, 1962.*

41. Gamble, J. F., Fuller, L. M., Ibrahim, E., Butler, J. J., and Schullenberger, C. C.: Combined chemotherapy-radiotherapy management of stage III Hodgkin's disease. *Arch Intern Med 131: 435–441, 1973.*

42. Gilman, A., and Philips, F. S.: The biological actions and therapeutic applications of the β-chloroethylamines and sulfides. *Science 103: 409–415, 1946.*

43. Goldman, J. M., and Dawson, A. A.: Combination therapy for advanced resistant Hodgkin's disease. *Lancet 2: 1224–1227, 1975.*

44. Goldsmith, M. A., and Carter, S. K.: Combination chemotherapy of advanced Hodgkin's disease. *Cancer 33: 1–8, 1974.*

45. Goodman, L. S., Wintrobe, M. M., Damesherk, W., Goodman, W. J., Gilman, A., and McLennan, M. T.: Nitrogen mustard therapy. Use of methyl-bis (beta-chloroethyl) amine hydrochloride and tris (beta-chloroethyl) amine hydrochloride for Hodgkin's disease, lymphosarcomas, leukemia and certain allied and miscellaneous disorders. *JAMA 132: 126–132, 1946.*

46. Hamilton, Fairley G., and McElwain, T. J.: Chemotherapy In *Hodgkin's Disease*, D. Smithers, Ed. Churchill-Livingstone, London, 1973, pp. 221–228.

47. Hellman, S., Mauch, P., Goodman, R. L., Rosenthal, D. S., and Moloney, W. C.: The place of radiation therapy in the treatment of Hodgkin's disease. *Cancer 42: 971–978, 1978.*

48. Høst, H., and Abrahamsen, A. F.: Combination chemotherapy with cyclophosphamide, vinblastine, procarbazine and prednisone in the treatment of malignant lymphomas. *Scand J Haematol 10: 170–176, 1973.*

49. Huguley, C. M., Jr., Durant, J. R., Moores, R. R., Chan, Y. K., Dorfman, R. F., and Johnson, L.: A comparison of nitrogen mustard, vincristine, procarbazine and prednisone (MOPP) versus nitrogen mustard in advanced Hodgkin's disease. *Cancer 36: 1227–1240, 1975.*

50. Jacobs, C., Portlock, C. S., and Rosenberg, S. A.: Prednisone in MOPP chemotherapy for Hodgkin's disease. *Br Med J 2: 1469–1471, 1976.*

51. Jacobson, L. O., Spurr, C. L., Guzman Barron, E. S., Smith, T., Lushbaugh, C., and Dick, G. F.: Nitrogen mustard therapy. *JAMA 132: 263–271, 1946.*

52. Jacquillat, C., Weil, M., Auclerc, G., Desprez-Curely, J. P., Chelloul, N., Goguel, A., Dana, M., Weisgerber, C., Teillet, F., Izrael, V., Chastang, C., Heaulme, M., Boiron, M., and Bernard, J.: Traitement initial de la maladie de Hodgkin par la polychimiotherapie. *Nouv Presse Med 3: 2073–2078, 1974.*

53. Johnson, J. S., Armstrong, J. G., Gorman, M., and Burnett, J. P.: The vinca alkaloids: a new class of oncolytic agents. *Cancer Res 23: 1390–1398, 1963.*

54. Kun, L. E., Devita, V. T., Young, R. C., and Johnson, R. E.: Treatment of Hodgkin's disease using intensive chemotherapy followed by irradiation. *Int J Radiat Oncol Biol Phys 1: 619-626, 1976.*

55. Kurnick, J. E., White, M., Ware, D. E., and Robinson, W. A.: Bleomycin (NSC-125066) and CCNU (NSC-79037) in the combination chemotherapy of MOPP-resistant Hodgkin's dsiease. *Cancer Chemother Rep 59: 1147-1150, 1975.*

56. Lacher, M. J., and Durant, J. R.: Combined vinblastine and chlorambucil therapy of Hodgkin's disease. *Ann Intern Med 62: 468-476, 1965.*

57. Lessner, H.: BCNU (1,3,bis (2-chloroethyl)-1-nitrosourea) effects on advanced Hodgkin's disease and other neoplasia. *Cancer 22: 451-456, 1968.*

58. Levi, J. A., Wiernik, P. H., and Diggs, C. H.: Combination chemotherapy of advanced, previously treated Hodgkin's disease with streptozotocin, CCNU, adriamycin and bleomycin. *Med Pediatr Oncol 3: 33-40, 1977.*

59. Loh, K. K., Gamble, J. F., Shullenberger, C. C., and Fuller, L. M.: Combination chemotherapy in MOPP resistant Hodgkin's disease. *Proc Am Assoc Cancer Res and ASCO 18: 267, 1977.*

60. Lokich, J. J., Frei, E., III, Jaffe, N., and Tullis, J.: New multiple-agent chemotherapy (B-DOPA) for advanced Hodgkin's disease. *Cancer 38: 667-671, 1976.*

61. Luce, J. K., Gamble, J. F., Wilson, H. E., Monto, R. W., Isaac, B. L., Palmer, R. L., Coltman, C. A., Hewlett, J. S., Gehan, E. A. and Frei, E., III.: Combined cyclophosphamide, vincristine and prednisone therapy of malignant lymphoma. *Cancer 28: 306-317, 1971.*

62. Martz, G., d'Alessandri, A., Keel, H. J., and Bollag, W.: Preliminary clinical results with a new antitumor agent RO 4-6467 (NSC-77213). Cancer Chemother Rep 33: 5-14, 1963.

63. Mathe, G., Schweisguth, O., Schneider, M., Amiel, J. L., Berumen, L., Brule, G., Cattan, A., and Schwarzenberg, L.: Methylhydrazine in the treatment of Hodgkin's disease. *Lancet 2: 1077-1083, 1963.*

64. Moore, M. R., Jones, S. E., Bull, J. M., William, L. A., and Rosenberg, S. A.: MOPP chemotherapy for advanced Hodgkin's disease. Prognostic factors in 81 patients. *Cancer 32: 52-60, 1973.*

65. Morgenfeld, M. C., Pavlovsky, A., Suarez, A., Somoza, N., Pavlosky, S., Palau, M'., and Barros, C. A.: Combined Cyclophosphamide, Vincristine, Procarbazine and Prednisone (COPP) therapy of malignant lymphoma. *Cancer 36: 1241-1249, 1975.*

66. Moxley, J., DeVita, V., Bruce, K., and Frei, E.: Intensive combination chemotherapy and X-irradiation in Hodgkin's disease. *Cancer Res 27: 1258-1263, 1967.*

67. Nissen, N. I., Pajak, T. F., Glidewell, O., Pedersen-Bjergaard, J., Stutzman, L., Falkson, G., Cuttner, J., Blom, J., Leone, L., Sawitsky, A., Coleman, M., Haurant, F., Spurr, C. L., Harley, J. B., Seligman, B., Cornell, C., Henry, P., Senn, H., Brunner, K., Martz, G., Maurice, P., Bank, A., Shapiro, L., James, G. W., and Holland, K. F.: A comparative study of a BCNU containing 4-drug program versus MOPP versus 3-drug combinations in advanced Hodgkin's disease (A Cooperative Study by the Cancer and Leukaemia Group B). *Cancer 43: 31-40, 1979.*

68. Nixon, D. W., and Aisenberg, A. C.: Combination chemotherapy of Hodgkin's disease. *Cancer 33: 1499-1504, 1974.*

69. O'Connell, J. M., Schimpff, S. C., Kirschner, R. H., Abt, A. B., and Wiernik, P. H.: Epitheloid granulomas in Hodgkin's disease. A favorable prognostic sign? *JAMA 233: 886-889, 1975.*

70. O'Connell, M. J., Wiernik, P. H., Brace, K. C., Byhardt, R. W., and Greene, W. H.: A combined modality approach to the treatment of Hodgkin's disease; preliminary results of a prospectively randomized clinical trial. *Cancer 35: 1055-1064, 1975.*

71. Osieka, R., Bruntsch, U., Gallmeier, W. N., Seeber, S., and Schmidt, C. G.: Post-MOPP-Chemotherapie des Morbus Hodgkin. *Dtsch Med Wochenschr 101: 1177-1184, 1976.*

72. Porzig, K. J., Portlock, C. S., Robertson, A., and Rosenberg, S. A.: Treatment of advanced Hodgkin's disease with B-CAVe following MOPP failure. *Cancer 41: 1670-1675, 1978.*

73. Prosnitz, L. R., Farber, L. R., Fischer, J. J., Bertino, J. R., and Fischer, D. B.: Long term remissions with combined modality therapy for advanced Hodgkin's disease. *Cancer 37: 2826-2833, 1976.*

74. Rosenberg, S. A., Kaplan, H. S., Glatstein, E. J., and Portlock, C. S.: Combined modality therapy of Hodgkin's disease. A report on the Stanford trials. *Cancer 42: 991-1000, 1978.*

75. Rosner, F., and Grunwald, H.: Hodgkin's disease and acute leukaemia, report of eight cases and review of the literature. *Am J Med 58: 339-353, 1975.*

76. Schein, P., O'Connell, M., Blom, J., Hubbard, S., Magrath, I., Bergevin, P., Wiernik, P., and DeVita, V.: Clinical antitumor activity and toxicity of streptozotocin. *Proc Am Assoc Cancer Res and ASCO 15: 168, 1974.*

77. Scott, J. L.: The effect of nitrogen mustard and maintenance chlorambucil in the treatment of advanced Hodgkin's disease. *Cancer Chemother Rep 27: 27, 1963.*

78. Selawry, O., and Hansen, H.: Superiority of CCNU over BCNU in the treatment of advanced Hodgkin's disease. *Proc Am Assoc Cancer Res and ASCO 13: 46, 1972.*

79. Stutzman, L., and Glidewell, O.: Multiple chemotherapeutic agents for Hodgkin's disease. Comparison of three routines: A cooperative study by Acute Leukaemia Group B. *JAMA 225: 1202-1212, 1973.*

80. Tubiana, M.: The place of radiotherapy in the treatment of malignant lymphoma. *Clin Haematol 3: 161-193, 1974.*

81. Vincente, J.: Enfermedad de Hodgkin: clínica, diagnóstico y evaluación. *Bol Fund Jiminez Diaz 6: 535-558, 1974.*

82. Vincente, J.: Aspectos actuales de la quimioterapia del Cáncer. *Rev Clin Esp (Europa Medica) 119: 501-516, 1970.*

83. Vicente, J., and Cortes-Funes, H.: ABVD for the

treatment of advanced resistant lymphomas. *Proc Am Assoc Cancer Res and ASCO 17: 189, 1976.*

84. Vicente, J., Cortes-Funes, H., and Murias, A.: ABVD regimen in MOPP resistant Hodgkin's disease. XIIth International Cancer Congress, Buenos Aires, 1978, Abstract No. 11, Vol. 3, Nos. 44–46, p. 218.

85. Vicente, J., Cortes-Funes, H., Murias, A., and Holgado, J.: MOPP chemotherapy of advanced Hodgkin's disease with prolonged follow-up. XIIth International Cancer Congress, Buenos Aires, 1978, Abstract No. 12, Vol. 3, Nos. 44–46, pp. 218–219.

86. Vicente, J., Torres, J. A., and Serrano, F.: Experiencia clínica con Natulan (Ro-4-6467). *Arch Cancerol 5:* 37–45, 1966.

87. Vinciguerra, V., Coleman, M., Jarowski, C. I., Degnan, T. J., and Silver, R. T.: A new combination chemotherapy for resistant Hodgkin's disease. *JAMA 237:* 33–35, 1977.

88. Williams, S., Einhorn, L., and Rohn, R.: Combination chemotherapy of refractory Hodgkin's disease (HD) with Adriamycin (ADR) and CCNU. *Proc Am Assoc Cancer Res and ASCO 18: 269, 1977.*

89. Young, R. C., Canellos, G. P., Chabner, B. A., Schein, P. S., and DeVita, V. T.: Maintenance chemotherapy for advanced Hodgkin's disease in remission. *Lancet 1: 1339–1343, 1973.*

25

Present state of radiotherapy of Hodgkin's disease

J. Albert Solis

From a historical point of view, radiotherapy in the treatment of Hodgkin's disease can be divided into three fundamental phases,each of them represented by a figure, distinguished for his contribution to this therapy.

The first one was René Gilbert, in the year 1920, who for the first time applied radiation with wide fields, instead of exclusively treating the affected regions, using low-dose and low-voltage therapy. The application of this technique succeeded in doubling the survival of patients affected by this disease.

The most relevant figure of the second phase is Dr. Vera Peters of Toronto, who followed the course established by Gilbert, introducing an acceptable classification by stages, increasing the dose and studying the influences on age, survival, sex, duration of disease before treatment, presence of systemic symptoms, irradiation of proximal lymph-node regions, and the radiotherapy with adjuvant chemotherapy, thus obtaining long periods of survival.

The third phase began in 1950 when the kilovoltage radiotherapy was substituted by supervoltage. The most relevant figure of this stage was Dr. Henry Kaplan, who advocated the mantle, demonstrating the effectiveness of wide fields with high dose to reduce the number of relapses.

Although the above-mentioned are the most outstanding figures in this field, it would also be advisable to add the names of other personalities to whom patients affected by this disease have been greatly indebted for their contribution and dedication. These include names such as Fuller, Easson, Russel, Tubiana, Smithers, et al.

Meetings held in Paris, Rye, London, and Ann Arbor, have also contributed to the knowledge and treatment of Hodgkin's disease. In the course of these meetings, important conclusions have been attained as to histological classification, clinical stage, with essential contributions of clinical methods. Among these we should like to point out lymphography, biopsy of the bone marrow and laparotomy and, lastly, delineation of the therapeutic methods, radio- and chemotherapy..

The utilization of the present techniques of radiotherapy are justified by the comparison of the results obtained before and after their application, with a clear advantage of the latter.

Regarding the dose administrated, after the works performed by Kaplan and his Stanford group, it has been concluded that the ideal dose is 4000 rad, in 4 weeks of treatment. With this dose relapses are at a minimum.[7]

Irradiation technique

The principal idea is to admistrate the above-mentioned dose to the lymph-node regions, and to protect the neighboring organs. The main fields employed are the following:

1. *Mantle:* Includes the medistinum, bilateral hilar nodes, and the bilateral lymph-node cervical, axillary, supra- and infraclavicular previously protecting the lungs, larynx, cervical spinal cord, posterior cerebral fossa, buccal cavity, and humeral heads, by blocks of lead.

2. *Inverted-Y:* Includes the spleen or the splenic pedicle, if laparotomy has been applied, and the para-aortic, iliac, inguinal and bilateral femoral, nodes with protection of the rectum, bladder, and iliac, and upper femoral bone marrow.

Gap is left in the union with the mantle to avoid myelitis.

3. *Spade:* Includes the spleen, splenic pedicle, and the lymph-node para-aortic and common iliac

Servicio de Radioterapia, Fundacion Jimenez Diaz, Madrid

chains with double protection for the gonads and pelvic structures.

4. Para-aortic/hepatic: Encompasses the splenic hilar nodes, the para-aortic nodes, and the right hepatic lobe.

5. Pelvic field: Includes the external iliac lymph-nodes, inguinal and femoral, with protection of the rectum, bladder and iliac, and upper femoral bone marrow.

6. Waldeyer ring: Encompasses the pre-auricular lymph nodes and the lymphatic tissues of the Waldeyer ring. Employed when these tissues are affected or whenever high cervical lymph nodes are noted.

There are special techniques existing which are not always applied. Among them, we shall describe the principal ones.

1. Split cycle of treatment whenever large mediastinic masses exist. Normal dose administrated is from 1500 to 2000 rad, in 2 weeks, with a 1- or 2-week interruption to allow regression of the adenopathies and perform a staging laparotomy. Lastly the mantle is resumed with a smaller mediastinic field.

2. Usage of thinner protection blocks (30% of transmission on one or both pulmonary fields, whenever there is an existence of hilar nodes, with the purpose of administrating 1600 rad to the entire lung in a period of 4 weeks, exceeding the maximum tolerated dose of this organ.

3. Minimantle. It is similar to the mantle but protecting the mediastinum and the hilar nodes.

An important point is the junction of the mantle and the infradiaphragmatic fields, which must be calculated individually for each particular patient with the purpose of preserving the spinal cord from overdosage and providing a suitable irradiation of the lymph node.

A 4-week recess is normally recommended between the supra- and infradiaphragmatic treated in order to facilitate a general and hematological recovery.

The doses received by the normal structures during a treatment cycle of 4000 rad to the affected lymph-node areas have been studied by Lillicrap and Dickens at The Royal Marsden Hospital.[8] The average dose absorbed by the lungs is 350 rad. The heart receives a minimum dose of 400 rad and a maximum dose of 4000 rad.

The spinal cord absorbs different doses depending on the regions; thus the cervical receives a minimum dose of 4000 rad, the dorsal, 4000 rad, although some centers place a lead protection block in the posterior field after administrating 2000 rad in the medium mediastinic field, reducing the dose absorbed in these cases to 2600 rad.

A maximum dose of 4000 rad in absorbed by the lumbar spine cord.

The dose to the testicles in the inverted-Y field depends on the irradiation of the inguinal lymph node. With the purpose of reducing this dose, some authors use special lead protectors. Without the induinal fields, the dosage is generally below 1.5% of the lymph-node dose (60 rad per dose of 4000 rad). When the inguinal regions are irradiated, the dosage is increased to approximately 2.5% to the lymph-node dose (100 rad), applying a testicular protection in position. If this protection is not used, the doses are more than double of dose abovementioned with or without inguinal irradiation.

In young women at laparotomy, the ovaries can be placed behind the uterus and protected from direct irradiation by means of blocks of lead, thus preserving the menstrual function in some cases; although only a small number of women are capable of conceiving, as indicated by Baker, et al.[2] The doses measured by means of phantom or in vagina range from 520 rad when ovariopexy is performed, to 100% of the lymph-node dose when they are left in their normal position.

The tolerance of the mantle is astonishing, producing a depilation in the posterior cervical region, dryness, and pharynx oedema as well as esophagitis when the treatment is terminated, but these do not normally require an interruption of treatment. Also noted are a decrease in the number of leucocytes and platelets which do not interrupt therapy.

The tolerance of the inverted-Y is more problematic, although it also does not usually impede the termination of the treatment. Leuco- and thrombocytopenia may require interruption of treatment. Nausea and diarrhea may also contribute to interrupt the treatment, making it longer. It is probable that splenectomy will improve the tolerance of the radiochemotherapy.

Complications of treatment

A. Hematological complications

The anemia may be treated by means of blood transfusions, first excluding hemolysis or infiltration of the bone marrow. Leukopenia usually recovers when the treatment is interrupted or completed. The same remarks apply to thrombocytopenia. When this complication is due to hypersplenism or to an auto-immune cause, it may be treated with splenectomy. Platelet transfusions may be necessary for amounts below 20 000.

B. Jaundice

It can be produced as a consequence as a massive hepatic infiltration, hemolysis, transfusions, or drugs. Laparotomy has, in some cases, demonstrated the existence of enlarged lymph node of the porta hepatis nodes, producing an obstructive jaundice.

C. Lhermitte's syndrome

It seldom appears. This syndrome is characterized by a sharp pain in the lower part of the back, in particular, when the neck is flexed and disappears a few months after the treatment is applied. Jones has suggested that the cause may be a transient radiation-induced demyelination of the nerve fibers in the spinal cord.[5]

D. Hyperuricemia

It is produced by the rapid destruction of the tissues affected by the tumor. The renal function must be known before beginning the treatment and, in the course of the same, the amounts of uric acid must be regularly verified. It can be treated by administrating Allopurinol during the treatment.

E. Hypothyroidism

The proportion of presentation ranges from 20% for the series of Prager, Sembrot, and Souttard[9], 10% for Kaplan's[6] to 2% for Smithers and Peckham's.[11] These percentages seem to be in proportion with the administrated doses of 4600, 4400, and 3500 rad, respectively.

F. Pericarditis

This may appear as a consequence of the mediastinic irradiation by one single field, to apply a dose of 4000 rad to the midplane. Thus the cardiac

surface receives from 5 to 7000 rad; however, this complication seldom appears when opposed anterior and posterior fields are utilized. It is important recognize it on time because it may result in constriction which can be relieved by pericardiectomy.

G. Pneumonitis

A certain degree is inevitable and can be reduced by means of an adequate planification. The irritable transitory cough produced in the first weeks is spontaneously dissipated after the radiotherapy, and the patient is soon free from symptoms. An apical and paramediastinic fibrosis can be demonstrated in a thorax radiography, and the lung function tests can show a restrictive defects. Glucocorticoids are helpful in treating symptoms.

Brief review of our experience

All patients treated in our department had their diagnosis histologically confirmed and a complete clinical study.

From 1955 to December 1978 a total of 269 patients have been treated at the Radiotherapy Department of the Fundación Jiménez Díaz. 152 patients treated from April 1970 to December 1978 are the subject of the present work since their cases have been studied and treated in accordance with the above-mentioned guidelines.

The series includes more men than women (88 and 64). The age of greater incidence was the 20–30-year decade with 41 patients, closely followed by that of 30–40 years of age (40 patients) and lastly 40–50 years of age (28 patients).

Nodular sclerosis constituted the histological type with the most number of cases (60 and 39.48%), respectively followed by the mixed cellularity (51 patients and 33.56%) and with lymphocytic depletion (15 patients and 9.86%).

The presentation of the nodular sclerosis in women was most common, and cellularity is comparatively higher in female patients, whereas lymphocytic deplection has appeared more often among men (Table 1).

Laparotomy has been used in 100 patients, and we have thus demonstrated the great utility of this procedure in order to learn the degree of infradiaphragmatic extension.

TABLE 1

Sex and Histological Type

Histological type	Sex		Total
	Male	Female	
Lymphocytic predominance	14 (15.90%)	12 (18.75%)	26 (17.10%)
Nodular sclerosis	33 (37.58%)	27 (42.18%)	60 (39.48%)
Mixed cellularity	28 (31.82%)	23 (35.93%)	51 (33.56%)
Lymphocytic depletion	13 (14.78%)	2 (3.12%)	15 (9.86%)
Total	88	64	152

Combined chemotherapy has been widely used. We have followed the following strategy: In early stages with favorable histological types, radiotherapy has been the method chosen, using chemotherapy in the relapses and, in a few patients, as a complement to the therapy previously administered. On the other hand, in advanced stages with unfavorable histologies, combination chemotherapy with MOPP has played a prominent role. The number of cycles administrated has been between three and six.

The largest number of patients included stages III and IV, with 63 cases and 41.44% of the total amount. Patients with stages I and II were 63 and 58.56% (Table 2).

We should like to point out that these figures have improved in the last years, and the improvement may be attributable to a better knowledge of the therapeutic possibilities (1).

For radiotherapy we have used a Cobalt-60 unit with different DFS, depending on the technique applied.

The therapeutic modality most employed has been the total nodal irradiation on 96 occasions, and extend the field of treatment to include the spleen in another 10 patients.

We have performed the mantle alone on 13 occasions and this same technique including the para-aortic nodes in two other patients. Locally therapy in 28 patients was confined to relapses, post-chemotherapy, palliation. In three cases we have applied the inverted-Y (Table 3).

Survival in all cases presented is calculated by an actuarial method. We have not obtained relapse-free survival.

After 5 years, the actuarial survival of all our patients was 72.5%, with the curve remaining practically flat after the third year (Fig. 1).

In stages I and II, without distinction of histological types the actuarial survival at 5 years is 93.1% (Fig. 2). The figure declines to 59.6% in stages III and IV (Fig. 3).

We have carefully reviewed the patients with relapses in regions previously treated with radiotherapy. The total number of them has been 17: 13 cases were marginal relapses, that is, located in the margins of the treatment fields. They were all located either on the axillary or upper cervical regions, except for two cases in the mediastinum.

Dorso-lumbar compressions, post-irradiation, histologically demonstrated, have appeared in four patients. Two patients also had similar affectations in nontreated regions. The treatment of these relapses has been the association of local radiotherapy and chemotherapy.

In May 1973 we began to treat patients with bad prognosis by radiochemotherapy consisting of the administration of two cycles of MOPP, total nodal irradiation and, lastly, four cycles of MOPP.

Since then we have treated 15 men and 12 women; mixed cellularity was present in 15 cases followed by lymphocytic predominance in five cases, lymphocytic depletion in four and nodular sclerosis in four cases.

This therapeutic tactic was applied in a I-B stage, 7 II-A, 1 II-B, 7 III-A, 1 IV-A, and 3 IV-B.

TABLE 2

Histological Type and Stage of 152 Patients Treated with Radiotherapy

Histological type	Stage								Total
	I-A	I-B	II-A	II-B	III-A	III-B	IV-A	IV-B	
Lymphocytic predominance	2		4		9	7	1	3	26
Nodular sclerosis	6		16	9	9	10	2	8	60
Mixed cellularity	5	2	10	4	6	14		10	51
Lymphocytic depletion			5		2	4		4	15
Total	13	2	35	13	26	35	3	25	152

TABLE 3
Stage and Radiotherapeutic Modality

Radiotherapeutic modality	Stage								Total
	I-A	I-B	II-A	II-B	III-A	III-B	IV-A	IV-B	
Total nodal irradiation	7	2	30	8	20	22	2	5	96
Total nodal irradiation & spleen			3	1	4	2			10
Mantle	2		2	1	1	2		5	13
Inverted-y	1					1		1	3
Mantle + para-aortic	2								2
Local	1			3	1	8	1	14	28
Total	13	2	35	13	26	35	3	25	152

All patients received two MOPP cycles followed by total nodal irradiation in 24 and mantle in three. The remaining four MOPP were only applied in 11 patients. The main reason for lack of completion was the appearance pancytopenias that, together with the patient's complete remission, did not make its administration advisable. ABVD cycles were added in two relapse cases.

At the time of writing the present study, there are 19 patients alive and eight have died. The main causes of death have been one erythroleukemia, five due to a generalization of the disease, and, on two occasions, death from pancytopenia, sepsis, and shock.

This experience adds to the conclusions of Rosenberg, et al.,[10] regarding combined regimens. They do not advise the utilization of MOP(P) after irradiation of this disease, since a survival advantage cannot be demonstrated. The possibility of second primary reoplasms, particularly leukemia, adds to this cautionary note.[3]

Conclusions

The best results obtained in patients with Hodgkin's disease have been thoroughly analyzed by Jelliffe in his 1977 Knox lecture which is based on five premises which have changed the spectrum of this disease.[4]

The first one is that the majority of physicians agree that this disease can be cured.

The second one is the improvement in the histological interpretation of the lymphomas that has allowed a more logical treatment and a better

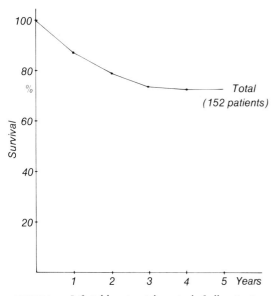

FIGURE 1.   Life table actuarial survival of all patients.

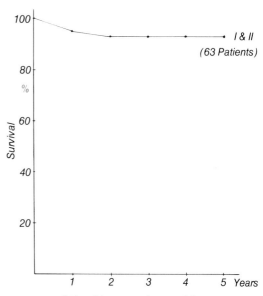

FIGURE 2.   Life-table actuarial survival for stages I–II.

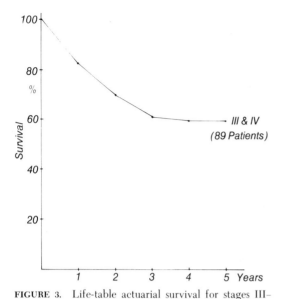

FIGURE 3. Life-table actuarial survival for stages III–IV.

comparison of the therapeutic results among the various centers.

Thirdly, there has been a clear advance in the evaluation of the extension of the disease, making possible more logical strategies. In 20 years we have evolved from a simple chest x-ray and blood tests to more accurate techniques of tumor visualization and routine staging.

Fourthly, the improvements in machines and radiotherapeutics techniques have allowed a more adequate treatment of many patients.

Lastly, there has been a great increase in the number of effective cytotoxic agents with a clear demonstration of efficacy of the MOPP regimen.

References

1. Albert Solis, J.: La radioterapia en la enfermedad de Hodgkin. *Bol Fund Jiménez Díaz 6: 575–582, 1974.*

2. Baker, J. W., Morgan, R. L., Peckham, M. J., and Smithers, D. W.: Preservation of ovarian functión in patients requiring radiotherapy for para-aortic and pelvic Hodgkin's disease. *Lancet 1307–1310, 1972.*

3. Coleman, C. N. Williams, C. J., Flint, A., Glatstein, E. J., Rosenberg, S. A., and Kaplan, H. S.: Hematologic malignancy in patients treated for Hodgkin's disease. *N Engl J Med 279: 1249–1252, 1977.*

4. Jelliffe, A. M.: Hodgkin's disease: The pendulum swings. Knox Lecture, Royal College of Radiologists, 1977. *Clin Radiol 30: 121–137, 1979.*

5. Jones, A. E.: Transient radiation mielopathy (with reference to Lhermitte's sign of electrical paraesthesia). *Br J Radiol 37:727–731, 1964.*

6. Kaplan, H. S.: Radiation therapy with curative intent in the malignant lymphomas. In *Recent Results in Cancer Research: Current Concepts in the Management of Lymphomas and Leukaemia,* J. E. Ultman, et al., Eds., 1971, Vol. 36, pp. 52–56.

7. Kaplan, H. S.: Evidence for a tumoricial dose level in the radiotherapy of Hodgkin's disease. *Cancer Res 22: 1221–1224, 1966.*

8. Lillicrap, S. C., and Dickens, C. W.: Radiation technique and dosimertry. *Hodgkin's Disease,* Sir David Smithers, Ed. Edinburgh and London, Churchill Livingstone, 1973, pp. 214–220.

9. Prager, D., Sembrot, J., and Southard, M.: Cobalt-60. Therapy of Hodgkin's disease and subsequent development of hipothyroidism. *Cancer 29: 458–465, 1972.*

10. Rosenberg, S. A., Kaplan, H. S., Glatstein, E. J., and Portlock, C. S.: Combined modality therapy of Hodgkin's disease. A report on the Stanford trials. *Cancer 42: 991–1000, 1978.*

11. Smithers, D. W., and Peckham, M. J.: Management of complications. In *Hodgkin's Disease,* Sir David Smithers, Ed. Edinburg and London, Churchill Livingstone, 1973, p. 234.

26

Non-Hodgkin's lymphomas: Introduction

J. A. Moreno-Nogueira

A. Casas

L. Iglesias Perez

F. Andrev-Kern

In recent years, knowledge of malignant lymphomas, particularly in the area of lymphoproliferative pathology, has reached a very high level thanks to recent discoveries about lymphocytes; previously, Erhlich had denied that they had the capacity of movement, and for a long time they were considered terminal cells.

Currently we are witnessing the "great lymphocytic revolution" which is transforming the concepts and classifications of this malignant lymphoproliferative pathology, and the great revolutionary is the lymphocyte.[27]

Before embarking on the study of the lymphoid cells, it is necessary to recall the history of the last 150 years of this lymphoproliferative pathology; this will bring us to the conclusion that our work has only just begun, as we can foresee a much more promising future.

It may be said that everything really began in 1832, when T. Hodgkin described the clinical pathological characteristics which he had observed in seven patients with tumors in the lymph nodes and spleen, which led to death. In 1846, Wiks revised the casuistry of Hodgkin and brought new cases and proposed the term Hodgkin's disease. In those years (1846 and 1856), Virchow described what he called leukemia of the spleen, later separating another variety related to the lymph nodes which corresponded to chronic lymphatic leukemia.[11]

In 1860, Connhein remarked that diseases existed with enlargement of the lymph nodes very similar to the leukemia described by Virchow, in which an increase of leukocytes in the peripheral blood was never shown, and which he called pseudoleukemia. It was Virchow himself who delimited the concept of lymphosarcoma for the primary tumor of the lymphoid parenchyma.[20]

In 1886, Trousseau established the concept of "adenia," and in 1893 Dreschfeld and Kundrat pointed out the macroscopic and microscopic differences between lymphosarcoma and Hodgkin's disease; but above all it was Kundrat who better recognized the peculiar quality of lymphosarcoma, where an aggressive growth existed with invasion of the capsule of the lymph nodes.

In 1892, Paltaut described a histological pattern which differed from the concept of pseudoleukemia of Connhein, and which corresponded to the clinical pattern described years before by Hodgkin. Later, Sternberg and then Reed completed the histology of this disease.[2]

Until 1925, Hodgkin's disease and lymphosarcoma were the two basic types of malignant lymphomas, and within the denomination of lymphosarcoma a range of cytological varieties. In that same year, Goormagtigh distinguished another type of neoplasia, also primitive of the lymph nodes, but which was considered to be derived from the reticular stromatic elements of the lymph node.[20] In 1929 and 1932, Roulet and Rössle proposed for this type of lymphatic tumor the name of retothelial sarcoma, later denominated reticulosarcoma, separating it from the wider concept of lymphosarcoma.

In 1925 in the United States, Brill, Baehr and

From the Department of Internal Medicine and Postgraduate Medical School and the Division of Clinical Oncology Ciudad Sanitaria, Sevilla, Spain.
Reprinted from Cancer Clinical Trials 2: 63–69, 1979.

Rosenthal and in 1927 Symmers described separately cases of generalized enlargement of the lymph nodes with splenomegaly which was interpreted as secondary to a hyperplasia, benign but massive or gigantic of the lymphoid follicles. Baehr, however, considered that it was a malignant process, proposing the term "gigantic follicular lymphoblastoma." Ten years later, Symmers also recognized that it was of the malignant kind. In 1940, Gall et al. studied the differential histological criteria between the benign follicular hyperplasia and this follicular lymphoid neoplasia, the key to which was in distinguishing the architecture of a reactive follicle from a neoplastic pseudofollicle.

It may be observed that during the 1940s, various neoplastic entities existed within the generic concept of malignant lymphomas: Hodgkin's disease, lymphosarcoma, retothetical sarcoma and the gigantic follicular lymphoma of Brill-Symmers. But all these entities once used proved to be confusing; thus, schemes of classification came into being such as the one proposed by Robb-Smith, which turned out to be very complex and only increased the existing confusion. This explains why in 1948 Willis said that "in no part of Pathology exists a chaos of names so lacking in clear concepts as in the subject of lymphoid tumors."[30] It seems that history is repeating itself, in part, at the present.

Gall and Mallory in 1942 proposed a new order of malignant lymphomas; this was widely accepted, being basic to posterior classifications. They used the term lymphomas of germinal cells, when they were constituted by highly undifferentiated cells, and that of clasmocytic, when they were constituted by well-differentiated cells, and which corresponded to the concept of reticulosarcoma.[9] The term follicular lymphoma was maintained, eliminating that of lymphosarcoma, and they speak only of lymphoblastic and lymphocytic forms.

In 1947, Jackson and Parker subclassified Hodgkin's disease, which was incorporated in the classification proposed in 1958 by Gall and Rappaport which turned out to be a variant of the former. The term nodular was introduced in the different forms of lymphomas, and the gigantic follicular lymphoma was eliminated as it was considered a nodular form. The term germinal cells was maintained, substituting clasmocytic for the term histiocytic. The type lymphocytic–histiocytic was included for those lymphomas composed of both cytological types without a clear predomi-

nance of either one. The lymphoblastic form was substituted for that of poorly differentiated lymphocytic lymphoma.[10]

In 1966, Rappaport foretold a modification of the former classification, introducing the modality of the undifferentiated lymphoma in the place of the lymphoma of germinal cells.[24] In general, he distinguished between nodular or follicular forms and diffuse forms. The studies of electronic microscopics of Lennert, published in 1966, give support to the origin of the nodular lymphomas from the germinal centers.[2] Also in that year, Lukes proposed a new classification of malignant lymphomas, emphasizing the typification of Hodgkin's disease, which slightly modified was accepted at the Rye Reunion (Washington) that same year, and still has not been rendered obsolete.[16]

Finally, the figure of Burkitt must be remembered. Working in Uganda, he observed the presence of a special kind of cancer with regional characteristics and which he described with O'Conor in 1961, being characterized histologically by Wright in 1963.[18]

It is the classification proposed by Rappaport which has been most widely accepted recently and which is based on the presence or absence of nodularity and in the degree of differentiation of the two cellular series, the lymphocytic and the histiomonocytic. This classification is still in force clinically, for the great deal of research that has been done, but which does not impede advancement in the new typifications of the malignant lymphomas with an immunological and morphofunctional base.

So far, this report has provided a historical and evolutionary summary of the lymphomas; but in the 1960s the "great lymphocytic revolution" was in gestation, when the lymphocyte was discovered anew thanks to the rebirth of immunology, when it was thought that antibodies could be formed and transformed into plasmatic cells. Since then it has been transformed into the central cell of the immune response, which has been of vital importance for the knowledge of this tumoral pathology. It is the cell charged with specific immunity in its different phases: antigenic recognition, primary response, immunological memory and secondary response. In order to fulfill these functions, the lymphocyte must undergo a series of transformations which for the most part are known, but not totally. Today we recognize the existence of two distinct populations of lymphocytes, the T-lymphocytes of the thymus and in charge of cellular immunity, and the B-lymphocytes processed in the equivalent of the "bursa" (bone marrow, fetal liver, etc.) in charge of immunity of the plasma, but in intimate relation to the T-lymphocytes. Both populations proceed from a common multipotential cell, or stem-cell, existing first in the yolk sac and in the fetal liver and later in the bone marrow. The monocytes appear to come from the same source.

A third population of lymphocytes is distinguished, which does not present the characteristics of T- or B-cells, named null-cells, and which could be cells of a period previous to the differentiation in one direction or the other.

The T-lymphocytes processed in the thymus are those which populate the T-dependent lymphoid tissue, such as the interfollicular zones of the lymph nodes, peri-arterial areas of the spleen and zones which surround the follicles of the intestinal lymphatic tissue.

The B-lymphocytes processed in the territories equivalent to the "bursa" populate the B-dependent peripheric zones such as the lymphoid follicles of the lymph nodes, the spleen and the medular region of the lymph nodes and follicles of the intestinal lymphoid tissue. The locality of the monocytes is less well known, but it is known that they are present in the lymphoid follicles, in lymphatic sinus and in the paracortical zone.

In order to bring about the immune response from the lymphoid cells, the presence of macrophages, whose forerunning cell seems to be the same as that of the lymphocytes, through the differentiation in monocytes is necessary. These macrophages are those which present in an adequate form the antigens to be recognized by the lymphocytes. Once the virgin lymphocyte has been placed in contact with the antigen, they undergo a process of blastic transformation, and the immunoblasts T and B appear with the capacity of proliferation and which generate a clone of specifically reactive cells, comprised by a determining antigen. The processes take place in the T- and B-dependent peripheric lymphoid areas. The B-immunoblasts, specifically compromised, give rise to plasmatic cells by maturing, memory cells, etc. The T-immunoblasts give rise to T-lymphocytes specifically compromised by the antigens, and different subpopulations are distinguished according to the function they exert (effectoral cells, memory, suppressors, amplifiers, helper, etc.) in close cooperation with the B-population.

One fact that must be emphasized is that the B-lymphocytes, once stimulated, undergo the blastic transformation at the follicular level, as may be seen in Figure 1 taken from Lukes and Collins, and the cellular division at the interfollicular level. Something similar must happen to the T-lymphocytes at the level of the paracortical zones. These facts have served as a basis to these authors for in-

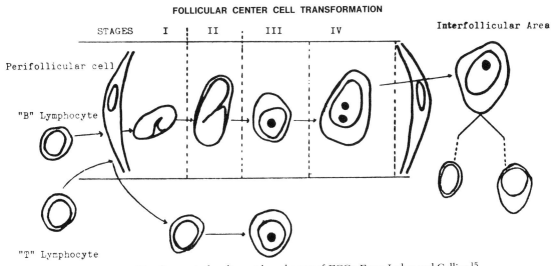

FIGURE 1. Development of malignant lymphomas of FCCs. From Lukes and Collins.[15]

terpreting the origin of the different non-Hodgkin's lymphomas as they represent blocks at different levels.[15]

From the above, the importance of recognition of the different lymphoid populations may be seen. As their application in the field of malignant lymphoproliferative pathology is fundamental, so we must admit that the lymphomas are nothing other than the malignant pathology of the immunological organ. The recognition of the different lymphoid populations is reached by the study of cellular markers. These markers may be antigenic, specific receptors of membrane and enzymatic markers. The presence of one of these markers at the level of the lymphoid cell may be limited to a determined phase in the course of cellular differentiation, disappearing or being inhibited in posterior phases. When applied to the neoplastic lymphoid cell the interpretation must be made with great care, as these cells may have lost some markers or acquired a new one. Another interesting fact is that the study of these markers can enable us to find out about the ontogenic evolution of the T- and B-cells. The ontogenia of the monocyte is not well known.

The study of the antigenic markers is carried out by means of antiserum against determined antigens of the different cellular lines. Thus, antithymocyte and anti-T-lymphocytes antiserums are obtained (Hu-TLA). The antigen "Ia" revealed with heteroantiserums of leukemic cells are not safe markers of the B-cells, as they have also been shown in cells of myeloblastic leukemia. The T-lymphocytes react with an antihuman brain antibody, something which does not happen with the B-lymphocytes. Altogether these markers are of little use, because of the difficulty in interpreting them and for the difficulty in obtaining specific antiserums in sufficient quantity. The specific markers of membrane are the most used to try to identify the different populations as represented in Table 1, principally the first five. The test of spontaneous rosettes with lambs' blood corpuscles presents the majority of the T-lymphocytes and is negative for B-lymphocytes and monocytes. The peripheral T-lymphocyte forms only E-rosettes at 4°C, while the thymocyte does also at 37°C, which is applicable to neoplastic cells.[7]

The immunoglobulins of the surface are one of the safest markers of B-lymphocytes. They may be detected by immunofluorescence, above all when

TABLE 1
Main Cellular Markers

	"B"	"T"	"M"
"E"-Rosettes	−	+	−
IgS	+	−	
Fc	+	−	+
"EA"-rosettes	+	−	+
C$_3$ (EAC-rosettes)	+	−	+
Hu-TLA	−	+	−
Hu-BLA	+	−	−
Hu-MA	−	−	+
EB virus	+	−	−
Measles virus	−	+	−
"E"-rosettes (mouse)	+	−	−
Acide phosphatase	+	+++	−
Response to mitogens			
Phitahemaglutinine		+	
Bacterians lipopolysaccharides	+		

monospecific antiserums are used. However, it must be mentioned that there are cells which are not B-lymphocytes that can present immunoglobulins on their surface and not necessarily produced by them. Monocytes and nonlymphoid cells can present Fc receptors, where immunoglobulins of type IgG serum may be joined, or immunocomplexes, or complement, or even direct antibodies against antigens of the lymphocyte membrane or the neoplastic cell. It is very important to identify the cell in question, and so it is advisable to use the fraction "Fab" marked with fluorescein, instead of a complete immunoglobulin, submitting the cells to an enzymatic digestion and posterior culture.[7]

The intracytoplasmatic immunoglobulins are considered authentic markers of the B-cells since only these cells produce them. They have been studied with the technique of the marked immunoperoxidases, but one must be careful with their interpretation as they can also be detected inside the monocytes. Applying this to Stenberg's cell, intracytoplasmatic immunoglobulins have been found which would give them a B-origin.[5,28]

The receptors "Fc" are markers of the B-lymphocytes, but they are also present in the monocytes and in some T-subpopulations with suppressive function. These cells are capable of forming EA-rosettes.

Receptors for the complement C$_3$ have been detected not only in the B-lymphocytes, but also in the monocytes and even in some small T-subpopulations, especially in thymocytes. In the presence of C_3 receptors, the formation of EAC-rosettes is based.

The E-rosettes mouse are characteristic of the B-cells, but in the most differentiated subpopulation. This test is positive in the majority of the chronic lymphatic leukemias, but negative in the B-lymphomas.

The viral markers may be of great value, such as the EB-virus for the B-lymphocytes and the measles virus for the T-lymphocytes.

The enzymatic markers are very useful. One of those most used is the determination of acid-phosphatase which is frankly positive in the T-lymphocytes and plasmatic cells and to a lesser degree in the B-lymphocytes. Of equal value is the determination of its isoenzymes.[7,26]

The deoxynucleotidyl-transferase is also an enzymatic marker principally of the prothymocytes and thymocytes, being negative in the peripheric T-lymphocytes.

Another enzymatic marker is betaglucuronidase which is valid for being positive in T-type chronic lymphatic leukemias and in the Sezary syndrome. Also valid are the sterases such as A-EST, B-AEST, NASDA, etc.[12,26]

In fact, with all these markers, differentiation of each of the lymphoid populations is attempted. With the same objective, the study of markers to lymphomas has been applied, as it has been in general to all the lymphoproliferative syndrome, to try to typify the neoplastic cell.

It is possible to confirm that the well-differentiated lymphocytic lymphomas, the histiocytic lymphomas, the Burkitt lymphomas, etc., are B-type monoclone proliferations in their majority and less frequently T-type.

The poorly differentiated lymphocytic lymphomas diffuse in the adult are essentially of B origin, which can be recognized by the presence of cleaved cells. In 10% they have T-characteristics.

The group of diffuse histiocytic lymphomas immunologically is an heterogeneous group; some present characteristics of B-cells and correspond to lymphomas of uncleaved cells according to the classification of Lukes and Collins. In a lesser proportion they are of T-type, and in a very small proportion of monocytic origin. In others, receptors are not demonstrated.[12]

The cellular origin of the Sezary syndrome is uncertain, but in general it is accepted to be of T-cells. Recently, Broder has pointed out that this syndrome is a lymphoma proceeding from the "helper" T-cells.[15] Immunological studies have also defined the lymphoblastic lymphoma as a subgroup of non-Hodgkin's lymphomas in the child, included previously in the poorly differentiated lymphocytic lymphomas, suspected by the clinical aspect of being of thymic origin. In the majority T-immunological markers have been shown, and great positivity of acid phosphatase, the same as in the leukemia phase, similar in every way to acute T-type lymphatic leukemia.

Immunoblastic sarcoma is of B origin in the majority of cases and more rarely of T-type. Burkitt's lymphoma corresponds to lymphoma of little uncleaved cells of the Lukes and Collins classification, and from the immunological point of view a diffuse proliferation of B-cells, the same as its leukemic transformation. In the endemic and nonendemic Burkitt lymphomas it occurs that the evolution may differ a great deal; in some, survival may be very prolonged with the possibility of cure after chemical therapy while in others nothing is of avail. These variations show us the limitations as far as prognostical value is concerned, which could presuppose the existence of superficial markers and the histology itself. Yet the diffuse lymphomas typified as B present a great survival, as is shown in the diffuse histiocytics in which long survivals in 25–30% of the cases after intensive chemotherapy are reached, which leads us to presuppose the existence of immunological subgroups in these types of lymphomas.[28]

Definitively, the study of all these antigenic markers, of surface or enzymatic types known to date, leads us towards an immunological classification of prognosis value, but in itself at present is not satisfactory for clinicians. This is why a combination is attempted with the morphological classification sufficiently reproducible, essential for clinical analysis, judgments of prognosis and even therapeutical indications.

We have come a long way since Hodgkin in 1832 described the illness which bears his name, but while this curriculum is generous and even fascinating, the character is ambiguous and fleeting, hiding much more than it reveals. Its name is well known, but we still do not know the most important aspect: its etiology.[25] Yet progress has been made here also. Possibly most arguments in favor of an etiological cause exist in the endemic lymphoma of Burkitt. In patients with this type of lymphoma, high levels of antibodies are regularly found against different antigens of the EB virus. Sequences of EB-DNA virus in tumoral biopsies are also regularly found. Authors like Noyonama and Olweny find viral genoma in Burkitt's African lymphomas. It seems possible that this virus is an oncovirus for man. Klein also considers that the endemic Burkitt lymphomas are a proliferation of a genome of the EB virus, but proof did not exist for the nonendemic lymphomas.[13] Still, tubular structures in the cytoplasm of the cells of these tumors have been described, which could reflect an increase in the production of antibodies as a response to a viral aggression.[22] What is certain is that the genome of the EB virus can be used as a differentiating marker of the Burkitt African lymphoma, with small margin for error.[17] It has been thought that malaria could play some part in the appearance of these types of lymphoma in Africa as the endemic regions coincide in both processes. O'Connor points out that lymphocytal proliferation in response to the antigenic stimulation of malaria would be the ideal environment for its transformation under the influx of the EB virus, but there are still many doubts to resolve with regard to this matter. Palmblad thinks that certain nutritive antigenic proteins could lead to a chronic stimulation of the lymphoid system, which in some way would induce the appearence of lymphomas. A diet rich in fats probably plays some role, as it has been seen that lipids interfere in the function of the lymphocytes and the phagocytosis of the granulocytes which would act as a facilitating mechanism.[19]

The greater frequency of lymphomas in autoimmune diseases (Sjögren syndrome, thyroiditis of Haschimoto, L.E.D., etc.) is something which is demonstrated. In the case of L.E.D., where an imbalance of the T- and B-populations exists with proliferation of the B-lymphocytes which would give rise to the production of autoantibodies responsible for the disease, this could lead in certain cases to the development of malignant lymphomas. Possibly the immunosuppressive treatments which these patients undergo also play an important role, without ruling out of course the possible role of an oncovirus. The same hypothesis could be applied to the greater incidence of lymphomas in patients treated with immunosuppressives for another kind of pathology.[3,4,21,22]

The family studies have also brought towards something concerning the etiology of lymphomas. In Duncan's syndrome, a complaint linked to the X chromosome and which comes with a certain degree of immunodeficiency to infections which could bring about alterations in the function of T- and B-lymphocytes, comes with a greater incidence of lymphomas. Families carrying an immunity deficit genetically regulated have also been described in which there has also been detected a greater incidence of malignant lymphoproliferative processes. It is interesting to note that in some members of these families, an increase in the titre of antibodies against the EB virus has been shown.[8] The immunodeficiency as favorable to the appearance of a lymphoproliferative pathology has also been studied in experimental animals, which is one more fact in favor of the role of the immunity deficit in the etiology of the lymphomas.[6] Also pointing in this direction is the appearance of lymphomas in patients already diagnosed and treated for the chronic lymphoproliferative syndrome of the macroglobulinemia type, chronic lymphatic leukemia, etc.

Finally, the role of the hydantoins in the etiological field of the lymphomas is notable, having been published in epileptic patients treated with these drugs over a prolonged period a greater incidence of lymphomas (Hodgkin's and non-Hodgkin's), myelomas, macroglobulinemias, etc. The mechanism by which they act would be an immunosuppressive effect as much in the cellular immunity as plasmatic.[29] However, the existence of latent lymphoproliferative pathology cannot be ruled out, and which the treatment with hydantoins merely manifest.[14]

From the study of all these possible etiological factors, we gather that there may possibly be a sum of etiological factors in which immunity complaints and the action of an oncovirus play a principal part in the genesis of this interesting pathology.

Many others aspects will be displayed in this Symposium on non-Hodgkin's lymphomas, such as the analysis of the ranges of extension in this type of pathology after the experience of the Hodgkin's lymphomas, the study of prognosis factors where in the near future the determination of the immunological markers will play a leading part, the possibilities of the new classifications, and finally the most important aspect for the clinician, the treatment, as it is time to ask ourselves whether the non-Hodgkin's lymphomas are curable.

References

1. Batlie Fonrodona, J., Vincente Garcia, V., Alberca Silva, I., Corral Alonso, M., Vidal Catala, V., and Lopez Borrasca, A.: Hidantoinas y neoplasias linfoides. *Sangre* 22: 486–491, 1977.

2. Berard, C. W.: Histopatologia de los linfomas. In *Hematologia, Tomo II*, W. J. Williams, E. Bentler, A. J. Erslev, and R. W. Rundles, Eds. Salvat, Barcelona, 1975, pp. 919–931.

3. Betourne, C., Cassan, P., Franc, B., Bacri, J. L., and Levy, R.: Lymphopathie maligne chez un malade ayant un lupus érythémateux aigu disséminé. *Nouv Presse Med 31: 2753–2756, 1977.*

4. Blanc, A. P., Gastaut, J. A., Dalivoust, Ph., and Carcassonne, Y.: Hemopathies malignes survenant au cours d'un traitement immunosuppresseur. *Nouv Presse Med 28: 2503–2509, 1977.*

5. Diebold, J., Reynes, M., Paczynski, and Galtier, M.: Origine lymphocytaire B de la cellule de Reed-Sternberg. Arguments fournis par l'immunocytochimie ultrastructurale. *Nouv Presse Med 41: 3835–3837, 1977.*

6. East, J.: Immunopathology and neoplasms in New Zealand black (NZB) and SJL-J mice. *Progr Exp Tumor Res 13: 84, 1970.*

7. Esponis, D., Diaz Mediavilla, J., Villegas, A., and Del Rio Vazquez, M.: Clasificación funcional de los linfomas no hodgkinianos. *Sangre 22: 677–696, 1977.*

8. Fraumeni, J. F., Jr., Werlelecki, W., Blattner, W. A., and Jensen, R. D.: Manifestaciones de un trastorno linfoprolilerativo familiar. *Am J Med 2: 108–113, 1975.*

9. Gall, E. A., and Mallory, T. B.: Malignant lymphoma. A clinicopathologic survey of 618 cases. *Am J Pathol 18: 381, 1942.*

10. Gall, E. A., and Rappaport, H.: Seminar on diseases of lymph nodes an spleen. In *Proceedings of 23rd Seminar,* J. R. McDonald, Ed. *Am Soc Clin Pathol,* 1958.

11. Hodgkin, T.: On some of the morbid appearance of the absorbent glands and spleen. *Trans Med Chir Soc Lond 17: 68, 1832.* Reported in *Hematology, Vol. II,* W. J. Williams, E. Bentler, A. J. Erslev, and R. Rundles, Eds. Salvat, Barcelona, 1975.

12. Jaffe, E. S., Braylan, R. C., Nanba, K., Frank, M. M., and Berard, C. W.: Functional markers: A new perspective on malignant lymphomas. *Cancer Treat Rep 61: 953–962, 1977.*

13. Klein, G.: The Epstein-Barr virus and neoplasia. *N Engl J Med 293: 1353, 1975.*

14. Li, F. P., Willard, D. R., Goodman, R., and Vawter, G.: Malignant lymphoma after Diphenylhydantoin (Dilantin) therapy. *Cancer 36, 1359–1362, 1975.*

15. Lukes, R. J., and Collins, R. D.: Lukes-Collins classification and its significance. *Cancer Treat Rep 61: 971–979, 1977.*

16. Lukes, R. J., Craver, L. F., Hall, T. C., Rappaport, H., and Rubin, P.: Report of the nomenclature committee. *Cancer Res 26: 1311, 1966.*

17. Olweny, Ch. L. M., Atine, I., Kaddu-mukasa, A., Owor, R., Andersson-Anvret, M., Klein, G., Henle, W., and De-The, G.: Epstein-Barr virus genome studies in Burkitt's and non-Burkitt's lymphomas in Uganda. *J Natl Cancer Inst 58: 1191 1196, 1977.*

18. O'Connor, G. T.: Malignant lymphoma in African children. II. A pathological entity. *Cancer 14: 270, 1961.*

19. Palmblad, J.: Lymphomas and dietary fat. *Lancet 1: 1977.*

20. Pedro-Pons, A.: *Patologia y Clinicas Médicas, Tomo V.* Salvat, Barcelona, 1963, p. 499.

21. Penn, I.: Second malignant neoplasms associated with immunosuppressive medications. *Cancer 37: 1024–1032, 1976.*

22. Popoff, N. A., and Malinin, T. I.: Cytoplasmic tubular arrays in cells of American Burkitt's type lymphoma. *Cancer 37: 275–284, 1976.*

23. Purtilo, D. T., Yang, J. P., Allegra, S., DeFlorio, D., Hutt, L. M., Soltani, M., and Vawter, G.: Hematopathologia y patogenia del sindrome linfoproliferativo recesivo ligado al cromosoma X. *Am J Med 5: 169–176, 1977.*

24. Rozman, C.: Neuvas tendencias en el estudio y clasificación de los linfomas malignos. *Med Clin 64: 257–261, 1975.*

25. Rozman, C., Estape Rodriguez, J., San Miguel, J. G., Hernandez Nieto, L., Rivas Mundo, M., Romagosa, V., Sans Sabrafen, J., and Woessner, S.: *Aspectos Actuales de la Enfermedad de Hodgkin.* Salvat, Barcelona, 1974.

26. Rozman, C., Woessner, S., and Lafuente, R.: Aspectos citologicos, citoquimicos y ultraestructurales de los sindromes linfoproliferativos cronicos de expresión leucemica. *Sangre 22: 697–715, 1977.*

27. Sanchez Fayos, J., and Outeirino, J.: Problemas conceptuales conflictivos en torno a la leucemia linfatica cronica. *Sangre 22: 792–809, 1977.*

28. Seligmann, M., Brouet, J-C., and Preud'homme, J-L.: Immunologic classification of non-Hodgkin's lymphomas: Current status. *Cancer Treat Rep 61: 1179–1183, 1977.*

29. Sorrell, T. C., Forbes, I. J., Burnes, F. B., and Rischbleth, R. H. C.: Depression of immunological function in patients treated with phenytoin sodium (sodium diphenylhydantoin). *Lancet 2: 1233, 1971.*

30. Willis, R. A.: *Pathology of Tumors.* Mosby, St. Louis, 1948, Chap. 49, p. 760.

Pathology and classification

27

Carmen Rivas, M.D.

Horacio Oliva, M.D., Ph.D.

Lymphoid tumors were first recognized at the end of the last century[14] and at the beginning of the present century. The concept of their pathological significance, evolution, and treatment has changed in recent years.[9,19,27]

Hodgkin's disease was reclassified in 1966 by Lukes[16] concomitantly with a change in its evolution. A survival of at least 70%, 5 years after treatment, became the rule and Hodgkin's disease became regarded as a curable entity.

Non-Hodgkin's lymphomas were described as lymphosarcomas[14,19] (Lymphoid proliferations), reticulosarcomas (histiocytic proliferations,[9,27] and giant follicular lymphoblastoma (nodular proliferation of follicular center cells).[3,28,32] Rappaport introduced a new classification.[20,21] He stated that the proliferating cells are lymphoid or histiocytic and grow in a nodular or diffuse pattern, indicating only the beginning or the evolution of the tumor. Thus he changed the concept of lymphoid tumors, denying the existence of true neoplasm of follicular centers. Prognosis was better in nodular than diffuse forms.

In recent years, at the same time as the new classification of Hodgkin's disease was being made, new techniques in the study of lymphoid tissue were being applied in pathology laboratories (histochemistry[31] and electron microscopy[2,11,13,17,33]). Immunological concepts led to better understanding of lymphoid cells and were applied to the study of neoplasms.[5,12,18,22,24] Therefore, with this, other classifications have appeared, but have not been generally accepted.[1,4,7,8,10,11,15,16,26,34] Great variability in the terminology has led to a lack of agreement up to now, and therefore the Rappaport classification has been retained.[18] We shall therefore examine the application of immunological techniques and particularly their implications within this last classification.

Histochemistry: T lymphocytes showed focal cytoplasmic positivity with acid phosphatase and beta glucuronidase. B lymphocytes are negative in these two techniques. Hstiocytes showed diffuse and intense cytoplasmic positivity with the same techniques (acid phosphatase and nonspecific sterase).

Electron microscopy: T lymphocytes in tumors manifest a cerebriform nucleus, scant cytoplasm with few organelles, abundant polyribosomes, and scarce lysosomes grouped together. B lymphoid cells show unequal development of ergastoplasm in a medium sized cytoplasm. Histiocytes show big cytoplasm with active phagocytosis. These T and B characteristics can be compared with *immunological reactions* in cellular suspensions (E rosettes and immunoglobulins fixation) or in histological sections with immunofluorescence and immunoperoxidase.[5,12,31]

Conceptually it is most important to decide if the knowledge of these different lymphoid neoplasms will provide different prognosis and therapeutic attitudes. Until now the majority of clinicopathologic published series in lymphoid neoplasms has been made using Rappaport's classification. This year, therefore, the Kiel classification has been introduced,[4,15,26] coupling these cellular lymphoid differentiation characteristics and clinical features: low and high degree of malignancy. T neoplasias are known in adult as Mycosis fungoides or Sézary syndrome and in children as mediastinal convoluted lymphoma.[31]

The majority of lymphoid tumors are B neoplasias[30]; the possibility of a primary histiocytic tumor is discussed, because the majority of so-called "histiocytary tumors" are composed of cells with immunoblastic pattern and evident formation of ergastoplasm and immunoglobulins.

In these B lymphomas we can observe cellular

Department of Pathology, Fundacion, Juménez Díaz, Universidad Audonoma, Madrid, Spain.

transformation similar to the physiological lymphoid modifications. Also there are:

1) Cells similar to mature lymphocytes
2) Cells with plasmacytic or plasmocytoid differentiation
3) Cells with a similarity to follicular center cell: centroblast (large noncleaved blasts) and centrocytes (small cleaved blasts)
4) Cells with a picture of immunoblasts (previously commented on) called histiocytic neoplasias
5) Nondifferentiated neoplasms

The distinction among these different cells requires routine histochemistry and possibly electron microscopy and immunofluorescence or immunochemistry. Approximately 10% of lymphoid tumors are not classifiable by these techniques and are divided according to their degree of malignancy. The clinico-morphological characteristics are therefore as follows:

A) Low degree of malignancy:
   1) Slow growing neoplasm
   2) High frequency
   3) More often in adults (20–70) years
   4) High level of dissemination
   5) Bone marrow affected
   6) Better evolution
   7) Low response to therapeutical agents

B) High degree of malignancy:
   1) Accelerated clinical course
   2) Less frequency
   3) Occurrence in extreme ages of life; above all in children
   4) Possibility of diagnosis in the early stages of affectation
   5) Bone marrow affected by leukemic peripherial picture
   6) Bad evolution
   7) Rapid response to therapeutical agents with unusual recurrences

Comparison of the Kiel and Lukes-Collins classifications with Rappaport's is shown in Table 1. Each entity will now be reviewed separately.

I. Low degree of malignancy lymphocytic type

CLL (chronic lymphocytic leukemia) (Fig. 1)

This is the true neoplasm of mature lymphocytes. The cells cannot evolve into plasmocytes because of an enzymatic lack. The three cells responsible for this tumor are lymphocytes, prolymphocytes, and paraimmunoblasts. The growing pattern is diffuse or pseudonodular. No plasmocytic differentiation is found. There are no special histochemical cellular

TABLE 1

Kiel	Lukes-Collins	Rappaport
Low-grade malignancy	I. Undefined (not B or T)	Nodular Diffuse
CLL	II. B-Cell (lymphocytic) Types	Lymphocytic well differentiated
Lymphoplasmocytoid	1. Small lymphocytic type (CLL)	Lymphocytic poorly differentiated
Germinal center	2. Plasmocytoid lymphocytic	Mixed
Centrocytic	3. Follicular center	Histiocytic
centroblastic-	cleaved	Undifferentiated
centrocytic	small noncleaved	
High-grade malignancy	large cleaved	
Centroblastic	noncleaved.	
	4. Immunoblastic	
Convoluted		
Lymphoblastic		
Burkitts	III. T-cell	
Immunoblastic	Mycosis fungoides	
	Convoluted	
	IV. Histiocytic	
	V. Unclassified	

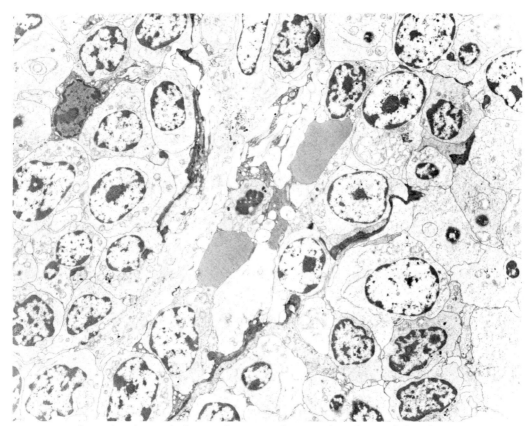

FIGURE 1. Chronic lymphocytic leukemia. Ultrastructural pattern of neoplastic cells lymphocytes and paraimmunoblasts. EM 9254 × 2000.

properties. Electron microscopy shows lymphoid cellular pattern, round nucleus with large amounts of marginal chromatin and well-developed nucleoli, scant cytoplasm with scarce organelles, and polarization of the mitochondria. This morphology changes in prolymphocytes (more cytoplasm) and paraimmunoblasts) bigger nucleus and nucleoli), less chromatin and a larger cytoplasm with many ribosomes.[15,16,21]

Mycosis fungoides (MF) and Sézary syndrome

This is a T neoplasm of adults which affects skin primarily and can extend to lymph nodes and other hematopoietic organs. The finding of tumoral cells in peripheral blood indicates Sézary syndrome without apparent involvement of bone marrow. The morphological lymphoid characteristics are cerebriform nucleus with scant cytoplasm. The lymphoid proliferation is accompanied by a small amount of dendritic cells as is usual in T neoplasias.

The lymph node affectation in MF differs depending on the stage of the skin tumor. Thus, paravenular localization of cerebriform cells or diffuse tumors with T immunoblasts can be seen. The tumoral cell shows with acid phosphatase and beta-glucuronidase in small punctuated positive amounts.

In electron microscopy the nucleus show concentrated chromatin and multiple convolutions. The cytoplasm has few organelles, scanty lysosomes, and also some glycogen.

Lymphoplasmacytic lymphomas (Fig. 2)

These are constituted by a proliferation of B lymphocytes which are able to transform themselves into plasmacytoid or plasmacytic cells. Histologically they are divided into three groups:

1) Lymphoplasmocytoid: lymphocytes and plasmocytoid cells
2) Lymphoplasmacytic: lymphocytes and plasmocytes

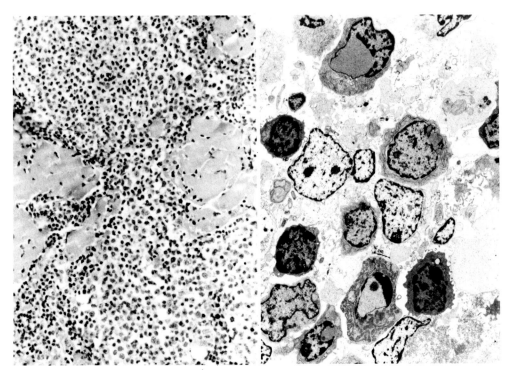

FIGURE 2. Optic and ultrastructural pictures in a lymphoplasmacytic lymphoma. Tumoral cells with high content in ergastoplasm and proteic intranuclear amounts. Interstitial proteinaceous material (IgM positivity with immunofluorescence). 78B801. EM 9727 reduced from × 3000.

3) Polymorphous: lymphocytes, immunoblasts, follicular center blasts, and lymphoplasmocytoid cells

These tumors frequently show mastocytosis, epithelioid cells, amyloid interstitial amounts, and intracellular or intranuclear PAS positive immunoglobulins depots. The latter can be identified by immunofluorescence techniques. These tumors can appear in lymph nodes, spleen, skin, or eyes. They also constitute one of the most important varieties of primary visceral tumors, above all in the digestive tract. Perhaps the majority of so-called pseudolymphomas correspond to these neoplasias. They can change into neoplasias with a high grade of malignancy: immunoblastic lymphoma.

Bone marrow involvement is common, but there are seldom leukemic manifestations. Perhaps the CLL described with a monoclonal gammapathy corresponds to lymphoplasmocytoid variety. These neoplasias can be clinically diagnosed because the appearance of a monoclonal gammopathy occurs in the blood of 30% of patients.

The histochemical findings help the diagnosis demonstrating the lymphoplasmacytic feature. The immunofluorescent and immunochemical data show positive cellular depots. The electron microscope demonstrates the abundance in ergastoplasmic reticulum, with proteinaceous substance in the interior which corresponds to optical depositions. In some cases the immunoglobulins appear also in the interstitial space.[15,16]

Follicular center tumors (Figs. 3 and 4)

These are neoplasms formed by proliferations of follicular center cells. When the tumor is constituted by the two cells of this region, the tumor is nodular. If the proliferation is made by only one type of cell, the tumor is diffuse.

The nodular pattern in follicular center tumor implies a better prognosis than the other diffuse varieties and occurs in young and old people (30–60). The lymphoid cytology in follicular tumors correspond to centrocytes (small cleaved cells) and centroblasts (large noncleaved cells). There is preservation of dendritic follicular center cell with "histiocytic" pattern without phagocytosis, with a positive coloration by lysosomal techniques, and

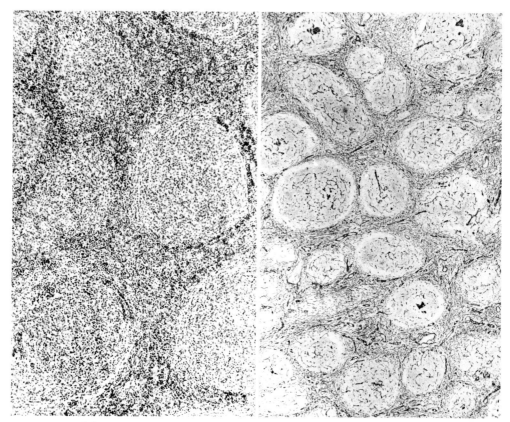

FIGURE 3.   Nodular pattern in a centroblastic-centrocytic lymphoma (HE and argentic coloration). 78B911.

desmosomes visible by electron microscope. With this last technique the morphology of centrocytism is like a lymphoid blast 10–12 μm in diameter, medium size cytoplasm with ribosomes, mitochondria, and cleaved nucleus with dense chromatin.

The centroblasts are larger than centrocytes based in greater nucleus with nonmarginal chromatin, with several constant peripherial hypertrophic nucleoli. The cytoplasm shows more ribosomes and polirobosomes.

The described cells constitute the nodular proliferation. Between the nodules there are normal T cells or hypertrophic or invaded T areas.

Centrocytic lymphoma

This is a diffuse proliferation of centrocytes without nodular pattern. Dendritic cells can be conserved (17%). This tumor occurs in older adults, and the prognosis is worse than the nodular variety.

II. High degree of malignancy

Centroblastic lymphoma

This is the second diffuse follicular neoplasm, the least frequent of non-Hodgkin's lymphomas. The cellularity is made by centroblasts. The prognosis is the worst of these follicular tumors. It can appear *de novo* or in a nodular pattern indicating the further evolution of this malignant tumor (Fig. 5).

Lymphoblastic lymphomas

This type of lymphomas is formed by proliferation of lymphoid nondifferentiated cell: They occur in extreme ages in life, above all in children. The cells show a lymphoid habit with blastic nucleolus and cytoplasm rich in ribosomes and polyribosomes, with scant mitochondria and occasional ergastoplasmic reticulum. The special

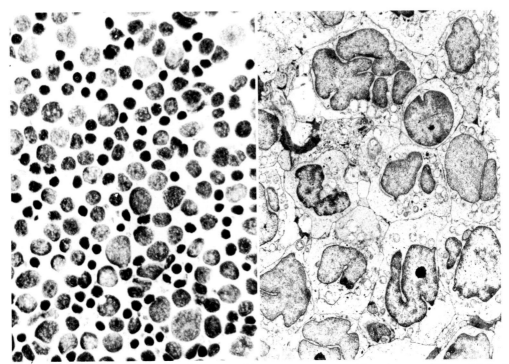

FIGURE 4. Imprints of a follicular lymphoma centroblastic-centrocytic type. They show two different kinds of cells. The bigger round cells are centroblast (large noncleaved) and the middle size, centrocytes. Ultrastructural findings which show predominantly cleaved cells with multiple nuclear invaginations, scant organelles, sometimes polarization of mitochondria, and absence of rough reticulum. Giemsa stain. 78B452.EM 1217 reduced from × 3000.

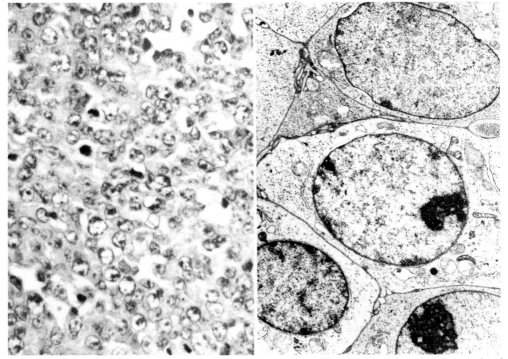

FIGURE 5. Diffuse centrofollicular tumor, large cleaved type, optic and estructural view. Centroblasts and with oval nucleus with margination of hypertrophic nucleoli. Few organelles, abundant, ribosomes, and diffuse localization of mitochondria. HE 76B5010. EM 6427 reduced from × 6000.

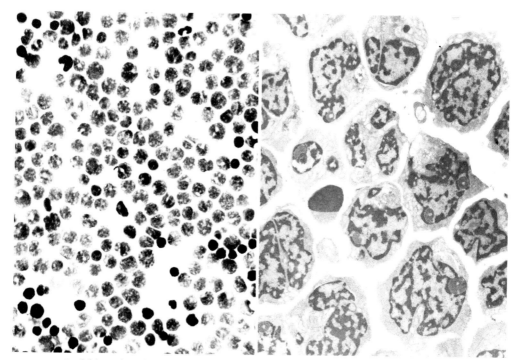

FIGURE 6.   Linfoblastic lymphoma convoluted type. Optic blood smear which presents characteristic cells with cerebriform nucleus and scant cytoplasm. Ultraestructural view with similar blasts in which nucleus there are abundant and irregular chromatine and constant invagination. Cytoplasms with abundant ribosomes and mitochondria and focal lysosomes. Giemsa 78B710. EM 1923 reduced from × 4000.

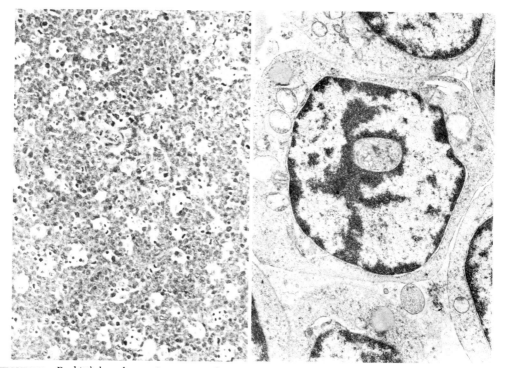

FIGURE 7.   Burkitt's lymphoma. Optic starry sky pattern. Neoplastic blasts with oval and smooth nucleus and medium-size cytoplasm with abundant ribosomes, diffuse mitochondria, and constant lipidic vacuoles. HE 78B423. EM 1229 reduced from × 10 000.

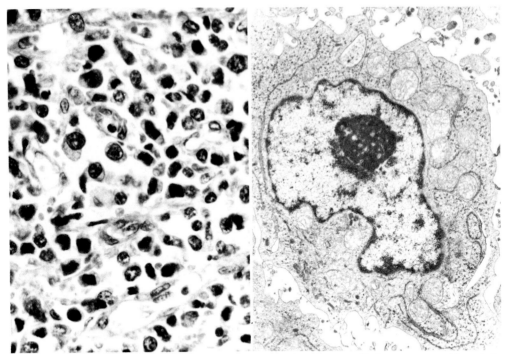

FIGURE 8.   Immunoblastic lymphoma. Diffuse optic view with characteristic cells showing immunoblastic habit, ultrastructural characteristics, oval nucleus and large cytoplasm with abundant ergastoplasm. Ribosomes and Golgi hypertrophic. HE 78B3740. EM reduced from × 10 000.

histochemistry and immunologic studies demonstrate the nonspecific cytoplasm of these cells.

Two entities are included in this group: convoluted lymphoma and Burkitt's lymphoma.

Convoluted lymphoma (Fig. 6) is a tumor arising in the thymus and coexisting in a high degree with acute leukemia and infiltration of nervous system. The cells which constitute this neoplasia show scant cytoplasms and large nucleus with cerebriform contour because of frequent invaginations. The chromatin is dense and the nucleolus with moderate hyperplasia. The ribosomes are abundant, only a few mitochondria exist, and the scarce lysosomes are located together and are responsible for the punctiform positivity of acid phosphatase and beta glucuronidase.

The tumoral cells grow without coalescence, their size is variable, and the nuclear convolution is not constant. These cells form E rosettes and have no immunoglobulins or complement, then they are derived from T lymphocytes. The prognosis for patients with this entity is poor.[21,23,29]

Burkitt's lymphoma[6,25,35]. This was described in African children by Dennis Burkitt in 1958. The first manifestation was a swelling of facial bones

followed by cranial, orbital, and buccal growth. In the rest of the body abdominal and thoracic affectation was common and also bone marrow, liver, spleen, and kidney metastasis. Peripheral adenopathies and leukemic picture were not frequent. In our experience affectation begins in the abdomen most frequently.

The tumor was identified as a lymphoma with special characteristics. The histological grow is diffuse with a "starry-sky" pattern because, among the tumoral cells, there are several histiocytes. The blast of Burkitt's lymphoma shows medium sizes, the nucleus is large without invagination, the chromatin is diffuse, and the nucleolus hyperplastic and marginated. The cytoplasm has numerous poliribosomes and fat vacuoles Oil-Red-O positive (Fig. 7). The tumor in the infiltration of the organs adopt a pseudocordonal pattern.

This entity can occur outside Africa. Its etiology has been related to a viral origin and particularly to the Epstein Barr virus.

Immunoblastic lymphoma

This high degree of malignant tumor is formed by tumoral immunoblast. The neoplastic cells can

TABLE 2

Total number of cases	303				
Lymphocytic lymphomas					
CLL	1				
MF	5				
MF + Sèzary	2 5.6%				
HCL	6				
T-zone lymphoma	1				
Lymphoplasmacytic lymphomas					
(Immunocytomas)	74 (27.61%)				
Nodal	40				
Extranodal	34				
Plasmocytoma	1 (0.38%)				
Centrocytic lymphoma	23 (8.58%)				
Centroblastic-centrocytic	51 (20.15%)				
Borderline (cb-cc, immunocyt.)	3				
Centroblastic lymphoma	6 (2.23%)				
Lymphoblastic	51 (19.02%)				
Lymphomas					
Burkitts	16				
Convoluted	14				
Unclassified	21				
Immunoblastic	21 (7.85%)				
Lymphoma					
Unclassifiable (anaplastic)	23 (8.58%)				
Rejected 35					
Diagnostic error	23				
Insufficient material	2				
Bad technique	10				

Sex	Men	Women	Ratio
Total	35	39	1/1.14
Nodal			
Lpl	11	9	1.2/1
Poli	8	12	1/1.5
Extranodal			
Lpl	6	6	1/1
Poli	7	15	1/2.1

Immunocytomas

Ages

Total		
Limits	16–75	
Average	55	
Nodal		
Limits	26–75	Lpl. 26–66
Average	56	Poli. 40–75
Extranodal		
Limits	16–70	Lpl. 16–70
Average	48.8	Poli. 16–62

Evolution
Of 40 cases (54%)

Average survival	4–6 years
Lpl	6 years
Poli	3 years

Immunoelectrophoresis
Of 27 cases (36.5%)
Monoclonal paraproteinemia: 7 cases (26%)
IgA-alpha: 1 case
IgM-lambda: 3 cases
IgM-kappa: 3 cases (urine with Bence Jones-kappa)

Lymphoplamocytoid Lymphomas (Immunocytomas)

General statistic

Total number	74 (27.6%)
Nodal	40 (54%)
Extranodal	34 (46%)
Stomach	9
Small bowel	16
Skin	4
Spleen	2
Lung	1
Nervous system	2

Histological types
Nodal

Lymphoplasmacytoid	20 (50%)
Polymorphous	20 (50%)
Extranodal	
Lymphoplasmacytoid	13 (38.2%)
Polymorphous	15 (44.2%)
Possible	6 (17.6%)

Follicular Lymphomas (Centroblastic-Centrocytic)

Total number	51 (20%)
Sex	
Men	29
	Ratio 1.3/1
Women	22

Ages

Total	
Limits	19–80
Average	45.3
Men	
Limits	19–80
Average	45.3
Women	
Limits	30–72
Average	49.12

Evolution
Of 26 patients   (51%)
Average survival:
6 years

TABLE 2 (cont.)

Centrocytic Lymphoma

Total number	23 (8.58%)
Sex	
Men	16
	Ratio 2.2/1
Women	7
Ages	
Total	
Limits	46–89
Average	65
Men	
Limits	50–76
Average	64
Women	
Limits	46–89
Average	65
Localization	
Lymph nodes	18
Small bowel	1
Nasal cavity	2
Skin and orbit	3
Evolution	
Of 11 patients (47.8%)	
Average survival: 2.3 years	

Centroblastic Lymphoma

Total number	6 (3.2%)
Sex	
Men	3
	Ratio 1/1
Women	3
Ages	
Total	
Limits	32–76
Average	55.8
Men	
Limits	32–66
Average	46.3
Women	
Limits	58–76
Average	65.3
Evolution	
Of 4 patients (66.6%)	
Average survival: 1.75 years	

Lymphoblastic Lymphomas

Total number	51 (19.02%)
Historical types	
Burkitt	16 (31.37%)
Convoluted	14 (27.45%)
Unclassifiable	21 (41.18%)

Sex:	
Male	37
	Ratio 2.6/1
Female	14
Ages	
Limits	1–61
Average	18

Convoluted Type

Total number	14 (27.4%)
Sex	
Male	12
	Ratio 6/1
Female	2
Ages	
Limits	4–50
Average	19.7
Evolution	
Only three adults were in remission.	
The rest died in less than 1 year.	

Burkitt Type

Total number	16 (31.3%)
Sex	
Male	6
	Ratio 1/1
Female	6
Ages	
Children	
Limits	5–9
Average	7
Adults	
Limits	5–61
Average	30
Evolution	
Only two adults living after 1 year.	
The rest died. Average: 1–30 days.	

Lymphoblastic Type

Unclassifiable	
Total number	21 (41.17%)
Sex	
Male	19
	Ratio 9.5/1
Female	2
Ages	
Limits	1–51
Average	15.6

TABLE 2 (cont.)

Immunoblastic Lymphomas

Total number	21 (7.85%)
Sex	
Male	13
	Ratio 1.8/1
Female	8
Ages	
Limits	22–80
Average	54
Evolution	
Of 17 cases (80.9%)	
Average survival: 2.4 years	

appear to be normal immunoblasts with atypias and several mitotic figures. The nucleolus is big with coarse chromatin and hypertrophic nucleolus. The cytoplasm is big, with ribosomes, mitochondrias, and rough reticulum more or less developed. In the interior, proteinaceous substance can exist. The monoclonal positivity of the cytoplasm with immunological studies identifies this substance with immunoglobulins which can appear also in the serum of the patient (15%) (Fig. 8).

There are two varieties of immunoblastic lymphoma, with or without plasmocytic proliferation. The acid phosphatase and nonspecific sterase are negative; for this reason, the nature is not histiocytic, as was previously believed.[23,15]

Our material using the Kiel classification in a group of 303 patients, diagnosed since 1973 are shown in Table 2.

References

1. Berard, C. W.: Reticuloendothelial system: An overview of neoplasia. In *The Reticuloendothelial System*. The International Academy of Pathology, Waverly Press, New York, 1975, p. 30.

2. Bernhard, W., and Leplus, R.: *Fine Structure of the Normal and Malignant Human Lymph Node*. Macmillan, New York, Gautiers-Villars, Paris, 1964.

3. Brill, N. E., Baehr, G., and Rosenthal, N.: Generalized giant lymph follicle hyperplasia of lymph nodes and spleen. A hitherto undescribed type. *JAMA 84: 668–671, 1925*.

4. Brittinger, G.: Prospektive multizentrische Studie der Kieler Lymphomgruppe tiber klinische Bedeuntung der Kiel-Klassifikation der malignen Non-Hodgkin-Lymphome. *Blut. 36:111–116, 1978*.

5. Bryland, R., Jaffe, E. S., Berard, C. W.: Malignant lymphomas: Current classification and new observations. In *Hematologic and Lymphoid Pathology De-*

cennial (1966–1975), Sheldon Sommers, Ed., Appleton-Century-Crofts, New York, 1975, p. 333.

6. Burkitt, D.: A sarcoma involving the jaws in African children. *Br J Surg 46:218–223, 1958*.

7. Carr, I., Hancock, B. W., Henry, L., and Ward, M.: *Lymphoreticular Disease*. Blackwell Scientific Publications. Oxford, Edimbourg, Melbourne, 1977.

8. Dorfman, R. F.: The non-Hodgkin's Lymphomas. In *The Reticuloendothelial System*. The International Academy of Pathology, Waverly Press, New York, 1975, pp. 262–282.

9. Gall, E. A., and Mallory, T. B.: Malignant lymphoma. A clinicopathologic survey of 618 cases. *Am J Pathol 18:381–429, 1942*.

10. Gerard-Marchant, R., Hamlin, I., Lennert, K., Rilke, F., Stansfeld, A. G., Van Unnik, J. A. M.: Classification of non-Hodgkin's lymphomas. *Lancet 17:405–408, 1974*.

11. Henry, K., Bennet, M. H., and Farrer-Brown, G.: Morphological classification of non-Hodgkin lymphomas. In *Recent Results in Cancer Research. Lymphoid Noplasias I*. Springer-Verlag, Berlin, Heidelberg, New York, 1978.

12. Jaffe, E. S., Bryland, R. C., Frank, M. M., Green, I., and Berard, C. W.: Heterogeneity of immunological markers and surface morphology in childhood lymphoblastic lymphoma. *Blood 48:213–222, 1976*.

13. Kaiserling, E.: Non-Hodgkin lymphome. Gustav-Fisher-Verlag, Stuttgart, New York.

14. Kundrat, H.: Ueber Lympho-Sarcomatosis. *Wien Klin Wochenschr 6:211, 1893*.

15. Lennert, K.: *Malignant Lymphomas. Other than Hodgkin's Disease*. Springer-Verlag, Berlin, Heidelberg, New York, 1978.

16. Lukes, R. J., and Collins, R. D.: New approaches to the classification of the lymphomata. *Br J Cancer (Suppl II) 31:1–28, 1975*.

17. Mori, Y., and Lennert, K.: *Electron Microscopic Atlas of Lymph Node Cytology and Pathology*. Springer-Verlag, Berlin, Heidelberg, New York, 1969.

18. Natwani, B., Kim, H., Rappaport, H., Solomon, J., and Fox, M.: Non-Hodgkin's lymphomas. A clinicopathologic study comparing two classifications. *Cancer 41:303–325, 1978*.

19. Oberling, C.: Les réticulosarcomes et les réticuloendotheliosarcomes de la moelle osseùse. *Bull Assoc Fr Cancer 17:259–296, 1928*.

20. Rappaport, H.: Tumors of the hematopoietic system. In *Atlas of Tumor Pathology*, AFIP, Washington, D.C., 1966, Sec. 3, Fasc. 8.

21. Rappaport, H., Winter, W., and Hicks, E. B.: Follicular lymphoma. A re-evaluation of its position in the scheme of malignant lymphoma, based on a survey of 235 cases. *Cancer 9:792–821, 1956*.

22. Rivas, C.: Los linfomas. Variedades Histologicas. *Bol Fund Jim Díaz 6:531–535, 1974*.

23. Rivas, C., and Oliva, H.: El diagnóstico óptico de reticulosarcoma revisado y corregido por la microscopía electrónica. *Bol Fund Jim Díaz 7:37–48, 1975*.

24. Rivas, C., Oliva, H., G. de la Concha, E., Vicente, J.,

and Albert, J.: *Linfomas no Hodgkin*. Salvat, Barcelona, 1979.

25. Rivas, C., Vicente, J., Murias, A., and Oliva, H., Linfoma de Burkitt. *Rev Clin Esp 6:412–420, 1979*.

26. Rilke, F., Pilotti, S., Carbone, A., and Lombardi, L.: Morphology of lymphatic cells and of their derived tumors. *J Clin Pathol 31:1009–1056, 1978*.

27. Rössle, R.: Das retotelsarkom der Lymphdrüssen. Seine formen und Verwandts-chaften. *Beitr Pathol Anat 103:385–415, 1930*.

28. Rosenthal, N., Dreskin, O. H., Vural, I. L., and Zak, F. G.: The significance of hematogenes in blood, bone marrow and lymph node aspiration in giant follicular lymphoblastoma. *Acta Haematol (Basel) 8:368–337, 1952*.

29. Smith, J. L., Barker, C. R., Clein, G. P., and Collins, R. D.: Characterization of malignant mediastinal lymphoid neoplasm (Sternberg sarcoma) as thymic in origin. *Lancet 1:74–77, 1973*.

30. Stein, H., Lennert, K., and Parwaresch, M. R.: Malignant lymphomas of B-cell type. *Lancet 2:855–857, 1972*.

31. Stein, H., Petersen, N., Gaedicke, G., Lennert, K., and Landbeck, G.: Lymphoblastic lymphoma of convoluted or acid phosphatase type. A tumor of T precursor cells. *Int J Cancer 17:292–295, 1976*.

32. Symmers, W. S. C.: Follicular lymphadenopathy with splenomegaly. A newly recognized disease of the lymphatic system. *Arch Pathol 3:816–820, 1927*.

33. Tanaka, Y. and Goodmann, J. R.: *Electron Microscopy of Humanoid Cells*. Harper and Row, New York, London, 1972.

34. Taylor, C. R.: *Hodgkin's Disease and the Lymphomas*, D. F. Horrobin, Ed. Churchill-Livingstone, Edinburg, Montreal, 1977, p. 2.

35. Wight, D. H.: Burkitt's lymphoma. A review of the pathology, immunology and possible etiologic factors. In *Hematologic and Lymphoid Pathology Decennial*, Sheldon Sommers, Ed. Appleton-Century-Crofts, New York, 1966–1975, pp. 433–463.

28

Staging and prognostic factors in non-Hodgkin's lymphomas

J. J. Lopez Lopez

A MULTIFACTORIAL RETROSPECTIVE STUDY on a series of 149 non-Hodgkin's Lymphoma (NHL) patients is presented. Staging procedures were sequentially performed in order to avoid unnecessary invasive explorations. Diagnostic techniques were stopped as soon as a disseminated disease was determined. Prognostic factors with a positive correlation with survival were: stage at diagnosis, presence of general symptoms, site of origin, and some biological parameters such as hemoglobin and albumin level. A brief discussion is presented comparing our protocol with some of the most relevant papers in literature.

Introduction

Classification of non-Hodgkin's Lymphoma (NHL) is still a challenging problem. Under the same terminology of NHL we are including a variety of histological entities with different prognosis and different clinical courses.

Pathologists are proposing new classifications still difficult to correlate with clinical prognosis and survival because of a lack of experience.[1–3] Rappaport's[4] original work is still being used as our routine methods.[5]

The staging procedures used in Hodgkin's disease have been used as a model for NHL, but the diversity of sites of origin and the great frequency of advanced disease make the model only of limited value.

Ann Arbor's clinical classification[6] introduced the *extranodal* category, allowing for a greater flexibility of the stage grouping. Even though correlation with survival has not been proved as effective as in Hodgkin's disease,[7] we still use it since no better choice is available.

With these limitations in mind, there is still a basic need for staging, in order to select the therapy in NHL. Advanced stages (III, IV) are eligible for systemic treatment such as chemotherapy or total body irradiation, whereas localized disease is, in some cases, treated and even cured with local radiation therapy. Obtaining accurate information of the extent of the disease at diagnosis has thus a first implication in selecting one or another form of therapy for the patient.

Prognostic factors are useful in both planning the treatment for an individual patient and analysing clinical trials. The results of a multifactorial analysis of the main prognostic factors on a personnal series of 149 cases of NHL treated for the period 1972–1977 are presented with comments on literature findings.

Hospital Santa Cruz y San Pablo, Unidad Medicina Oncológica, Barcelona, Spain.

Table 1 summarizes the main steps in our diagnostic protocol for NHL. As a general rule, exploration is stopped as soon as an advanced stage is diagnosed, and so our techniques are sequentially ordered from the less to the more aggresive ones.

Non-Hodgkin's lymphomas originate in extranodal sites with proportions ranging from 11% to 50%.[5,8,9] In our experience primary extranodal lymphomas were 46%.

Systemic symptoms (stage B) are present at diagnosis with a lower frequency than in Hodgkin's disease,[10] and this lowers its prognostic implications.[5] Generalized forms are frequent. Stages III and IV at diagnosis are not only more common than in Hodgkin's disease, but the spreading pattern is also different. Infradiaphragmatic disease, for instance, occurs in Hodgkin's disease following a logic pattern of lymphatic drainage through lumboaortic or retroperitoneal fields with little impact on mesenteric nodes, whereas in non-Hodgkin's lymphoma we frequently find a total abdominal invasion.

TABLE 1

Staging in Non-Hodgkin's Lymphoma

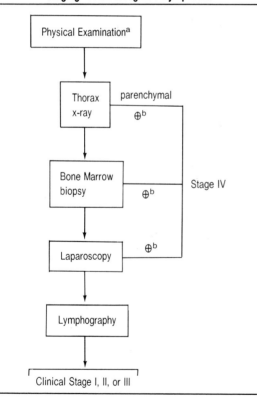

a Extranodal origin require special diagnostic strategies, G.I. ray, endoscopy.
b ⊕ Infiltration by lymphoma.

I wish to emphasize the importance of the routine exploration of Waldeyer's ring. In Freeman's experience,[11] 28% of extranodal NHL originated in this area, while Rosenberg[12] reported 8.7% of all NHL. In our experience 57% of the extranodal cases were first localized in this region, which represents 26% of all cases. The reasons for such differences are unclear.

Some authors have advocated multiple blind tonsil biopsies when a NHL is diagnosed though a cervical node biopsy without any other clinical evidence of a primary.[13]

A frequent association with NHL of Waldeyer's ring origin is the gastrointestinal tract,[14,15] and we routinely advise an x-ray exploration with special attention to the gastric region. In our study 10 cases (6.7%) were positive.

Primary NHL of the gastrointestinal tract have been described in 5–10%.[11,12] In our experience, 18% of the cases were of gastrointestinal tract origin. This represents 38% of all the extranodal primaries with stomach and terminal ileum being the most frequent locations, followed by jejunum, cecum, and duodenum.[16] Diagnostic procedures are the standard ones for intra-abdominal tumors including x-ray study, endoscopy, and open biopsies.

Thorax x-ray in NHL reveals invasion of mediastinal lymph nodes in a lower percentage than in Hodgkin's disease. Some series described mediastinal mass in 18, and 25% of the cases.[10,17] Pulmonary parenchymal lesions were seen in 5% and 10%. This finding, although rare, allows ready identification of stage IV. Diagnosis of infra-diaphragmatic disease has been a difficult matter in all lymphomas. Lymphography, which proved to be useful in Hodgkin's disease, has also shown accuracy in NHL.

Goffinet found 12% of false negatives and 13% of false positives in a series of patients who underwent both lymphography and laparotomy.[10] Organ involvement such as spleen, liver, and bone marrow was significantly correlated with a positive lymphography.

Histology has been reported to be relative to lymphography results.[17] Nodular lymphoma presented a positive lymphography in 90% of the cases, whereas diffuse forms were positive in 66%.

Intravenous pyelogram might detect retroperitoneal invasion with ureteral obstruction or impairment of excretory renal function.

Cavography yielded 7% false-positive and 53% false-negative rates. The procedure might be useful whenever lymphography is not feasible.

Liver involvement is present in 58% of nodular NHL and 27% of the diffuse types.[19] Laparoscopy with liver biopsy in both hepatic lobes is a technique with a high yield and low risk. We routinely use it in all stage III cases.

Bone marrow invasion occurs frequently. Positive biopsies have been reported in Reference 16 to 39% of all NHL.[20,17] The biopsy techniques are mandatory since they yield the highest percentage of positives.

Staging laparotomy has evolved following the model developed in Hodgkin's disease. It has permitted a better understanding of the natural history and patterns of presentation and spread of there neoplasms. Nodular lymphomas with negative linphography were positive in mesenteric nodes and spleen in 50% of the cases in Goffinet's series,[10] whereas diffuse forms showed visceral involvement in only 4% and mesenteric nodes in 9% of the cases.

Nodular lymphomas are diagnosed in localized forms—stage I and II—in less than 10% of the cases in several series.[10,19,21] Moreover, nonsurgical exploratory techniques yield the highest percentages of positivity in nodular lymphomas.[19] One must consider also that the use of laparotomy has some risks, particularly since the age of these patients is usually higher than in Hodgkin's disease. In most cases easy classification as stage III or IV through nonsurgical techniques can be made. Therefore, staging laparotomy cannot be recommended as a routine procedure in NHL. We shall illustrate staging and prognostic factors by reviewing our personal experience with 149 patients.

Patients Studied

These were treated by the Servicio de Oncologia

TABLE 3

Non-Hodgkin's Lymphoma. Histopatologic Subgroups

	Nodular	Diffuse
Lymphocytic, well differentiated	3	25
Lymphocytic, poorly differentiated	19	40
Histiocytic	2	31
Undifferentiated	—	3
Nonclassified	8	7
Total	34	111

of the Hospital de San Pablo in Barcelona between January 1972 and December 1977. We used Rappaport's histological classification and Ann Arbor's clinical stages. Our staging protocol was the model described previously. All patients with stages III and IV received CVP chemotherapy,[22] and stages I and II were treated either with surgery or radiotherapy. Stage distribution histology architectural pattern and sites of origin are shown in Tables 2–4.

The parameters studied at diagnosis were: age, sex, histology and architectural pattern, stage, general symptoms, Hemoglobin level, WBC, differential count, platelets, ESR, total protein and fractions, BUN, creatinine SGOT, SGPT, alkaline phosphorese, α-GTP, cholesterol level were determined in 60 patients. Computer techniques have been employed to developed the survival curves utilizing the statistical methods of Berkson and Gage.[23]

Results

Out of the 30 parameteres only seven were significantly correlated to survival. These were histology, architectural pattern, general symptoms, stage, hemoglobin and total protein and albumin levels.

Figure 1 relates the survival of patients according to histology. The well-differentiated lymphocytic

TABLE 2

Non-Hodgkin's Lymphoma

Stage	Nodular	Diffuse	Unknown
I	5	21	2
II	7	30	—
III	15	21	1
IV	7	39	1
Total	34	111	4

TABLE 4

Non-Hodgkin's Lymphoma. Site of Origin

	Cases	%
Nodal	79	53
Extranodal	70	47
Waldeyer	40	27
Gastrointestinal tract	27	18
Skin	3	2

Lymphoma (WDL) did significantly better, whereas no difference was found between poorly differentiated lymphocytic (PDL) and the histiocytic (H).

Figure 2 reflects the most favorable prognosis of nodular lymphomas when compared to diffuse

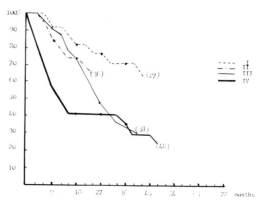

FIGURE 4. Survival on non-Hodgkin's lymphoma. Stages.

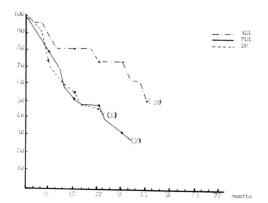

FIGURE 1. Survival of non-Hodgkin's lymphoma. Histopatologic subgroups.

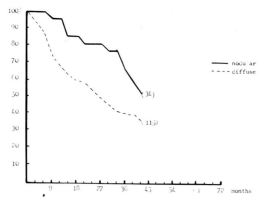

FIGURE 2. Survival on non-Hodgkin's lymphoma. Histologic type.

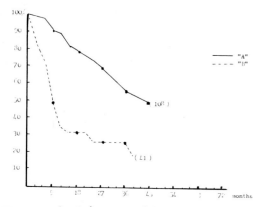

FIGURE 3. Survival on non-Hodgkin's lymphoma. General clinical symptoms.

forms. In our series, the proportion of nodular types is lower than generally reported in the U.S., accounting for a worse total survival rate.

Figure 3 shows the effects of general clinical symptoms. The difference is highly significant ($p < 001$) especially for the first 15-month period. Weight loss over 10% was the most significant symptom in our series.

Figure 4 relates survival with stage survival after 30-months clearly differentiates stages I and II versus III and IV even if, for the first period, stage III does not significantly differ from others.

Four hemoglobin levels do separate groups with varying outlook. Statistical significance was reached only when comparing patients with Hb levels lower than 11.8 g% with levels above 13 g%. A difference was observed among the four levels, but was not significant.

Similarly a significant difference in survival is found when total albumin is greater or less than 35 g% or 65 g% for total protein albumin. Both pa-

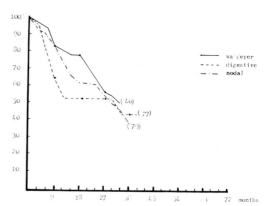

FIGURE 5. Survival on non-Hodgkin's lymphoma. Site of origin of the process.

rameters were significant when below 35 g% for the former and 65 g% for the latter. No differences were found according to origin, as shown in Figure 5. The multiple correlation test selected four clinical parameters—stages, architecture, general symptoms, and site of origin—and three biological tests—cholesterol, albumin, and ESR—demonstrating interactions highly significantly associated with survival (R: 0.624, p <0.001).

Our results confirm the well-known importance of stage and architecture in predicting survival. Research on tumor markers and biochemical parameters could be integrated with these variables and help pathology reports in determining the appropriate clinical evaluation and treatment.

References

1. Lukes, R. J., and Collins, R. D.: Immunological cloracterization of human malignant lymphomas. *Cancer* 34: 1488–1503, 1974.

2. Bennett, M. H., Farrer-Brown, G., and Henry, K.: Classification of Non-Hodgkin's lymphoma. *Lancet* 2: 406–408, 1974.

3. Ronald, F., and Dorfman, K.: Pathology of the non Hodgkin's lymphomas: New classifications. *Cancer Treat Rep* 61: 945–951, 1977.

4. Rappaport, H.: Tumors of the hematopoietic system. In *Atlas of Tumor Pathology*. Armed Forces Institute of Pathology, Washington, D.C., 1966, Sec. 3, fasc. 8, p. 270.

5. Jones, S. E., Fuks, Z., Bull, M., Kadin, M., Dorfman, K., Rosenberg, S. A., and Kim, M.: Non-Hodgkin's lymphomas IV. Clinicopathologic correlation in 405 cases. *Cancer* 31: 806–823, 1973.

6. Carbone, P. P., Kaplan, H. S., Musshoff, K., Smithers, D. W., and Tubiana, M.: Report of the comunittee on Hodgkin's disease classification. *Cancer Res 31:* 1860–1861, 1971.

7. Rosenberg, S. A.: Validity of the Ann Arbor Staging Classification for the Non-Hodgkin's lymphomas. *Cancer Treat Rep* 61: 1023–1027, 1977.

8. Peters, M. V., Hasselback, R., and Brown, T. C.: The natural history of the lymphomas related to the clinical classification. In *Proceedings of the International Conference on Leukemia-Lymphoma*, C. J. Zaratonetis, Ed. Lea & Febiger, Philadelphia, 1968, pp. 357–371.

9. Gall, E. A., and Mallory, T. B.: Malignant Lymphoma. A clinico-pathologic survey of 618 cases. *Am J Pathol* 18: 381–429, 1942.

10. Goffinet, D. R., Warnke, R., Dunnick, N. R., Castellino, R., Glasteni, E., Nelsen, T. S., Dorfman, R. F., Rosenberg, S. A., and Kaplan, H. S.: Clinical and surgical laparotomy evaluation of patients with non Hodgkin's lymphomas. *Cancer Treat Rep* 61: 981–992, 1977.

11. Freeman, C., Berg, J. W., Cutler, S. J.: Occurrence and prognosis of extranodal lymphomas. *Cancer 29:* 252–260, 1972.

12. Rosenberg, S. A., Diamond, H. D., Jaslowitz, B., et al.: Lymphosarcoma: A review of 1269 cases. *Medicine* 40: 31–84, 1961.

13. Banfi, A., Bonadonna, G., Rieci, S. B., Milani, F., Molinosi, E., Monfardini, S., and Zneali, R.: Malignant lymphomas of Waldeyer's ring natural history and survival after radiotherapy. *Br. Med J* 3:140–143, 1972.

14. Banfi, A., Bonadonna, G., Carnevali, G., et al.: Lymphoreticular sarcoma with primary involvement of Waldeger's ring: Clinical evaluation of 225 cases. *Cancer* 26: 351–351, 1970.

15. Bruguse, J., Schliengs, M., Gerard-Marchant, R., Tubiana, M., Pouillart, P., and Cachin, Y.: Lymphosarcomas et reticulosarcomas des voies aerodigestives supèrieures. Histoire naturelle et resultats de la radiotherapie. *Bull Cancer* 61: 79–91, 1974.

16. Berg, J. W.: Primary Lymphomas of the human gastrointestinal tract. *Nat. Cancer Inst Monogr* 32: 211–220, 1969.

17. Chabner, B. A., Johnson, R. E., De Vita, V. T., Canellos, G. P., Hubbard, S. P., Johnson, S. K., and Young, R. C.: Sequential staging in non-Hodgkin's lymphoma. *Cancer Treat Rep* 61: 993–997, 1977.

18. Moran, E. M., Ultmann, J. E., Ferguson, D. J., et al.: Staging laparotomy in non Hodgkin's lymphomas. *Br J Cancer (Suppl II)* 31: 228–236, 1975.

19. Chabner, B. A., Johnson, R. E., Young, R. C., Cannellos, G. P., Hubbard, S. P., Johnson, S. K., and De Vita, V. T., Jr.: Sequential nonsurgical and surgical staging of non-Hodgkin's lymphoma. *Ann Intern Med* 85: 149–154, 1976.

20. Jones, S. E., Rosenberg, S. A., and Kaplan, H. S.: Non-Hodgkin's lymphomas I. Bone marrow involvement. *Cancer* 20: 954–960, 1972.

21. Rosenberg, S. A., Dorfman, R. F., and Kaplan, H. S.: The value of sequential bone marrow biopsy and laparotomy in a series of 127 consecutive untreated patients with non-Hodgkin's lymphoma. *Br. J Cancer (Suppl II)* 31: 221–227, 1975.

22. Bagley, C., De Vita, V. T., Berard, C. W., et al.: Advanced lymphosarcoma: Intensive cyclical combination chemotherapy with cyclophosphamide, vincristine and prednisone. *Ann. Intern Med* 76: 227–234, 1972.

23. Berkson, J., and Gage, R. P.: Calculation of survival rates for cancer. *Mayo Clin Proc* 25: 270–286, 1950.

29

The non-Hodgkin's lymphomas

Two main clinicopathological subtypes: NLPD and DH

Manuel Ribas-Mundo, M.D.[†]

Saul A. Rosenberg, M.D.

IN THE GROUP OF NON-HODGKIN'S LYMPHOMAS, in spite of the multiple classifications existing, there are two main histological subtypes with a clear-cut clinicopathological personality: nodular lymphocytic poorly differentiated (NLPD) and diffuse histiocytic (DH). NLPD affects older patients and presents at the time of diagnosis as a widespread disseminated disease. The majority of patients have bone marrow involvement, thus making unnecessary a staging laparotomy in most of the cases. DH affects a younger population, is localized in about half the patients, and shows a low percentage of bone marrow involvement at the time of diagnosis. Following these two major subtypes, the other minor subtypes may be related to one or the other: nodular mixed histiocytic–lymphocytic (NM) is more related to NLPD and DLPD and nodular histiocytic (NH) to DH.

Introduction

One of the most urgent problems of the moment is to find a suitable classification of the non-Hodgkin's lymphomas acceptable for both pathologists and clinicians. Although the classification by Rappaport et al.[16] was adopted by the majority of investigators, it became apparent that the new immunological concepts and the functional differentiation of the lymphatic system in the B- and T-lymphocyte series might play an important role in the classification of the non-Hodgkin's lymphomas. Lukes and Collins[14] presented this new approach which was followed in Europe with a different classification by Lennert et al.[13] from Kiel. During the last few years, many other classifications have been published,[1,6,9] creating at least among clinicians a sense of confusion which was openly commented on with a marvelous sense of British humor by Kay.[12]

The purpose of this communication is to emphasize from a clinical point of view that in spite of the multiple classifications of the non-Hodgkin's lymphomas, two main subtypes emerge that each present a clear-cut clinicopathological entity. These observations were obtained from the analysis of 200 consecutive previously untreated patients with the diagnosis of non-Hodgkin's lymphoma studied under strict protocol conditions at the time of diagnosis.[19]

Materials and methods

A consecutive series of 200 previously untreated patients was studied as part of a prospective ther-

From the Division of Medical Oncology, Department of Medicine, Stanford University School of Medicine, Stanford, California.

[†] Present address for Prof. M. Ribas-Mundo: Chief of the Department of Medicine, Autonomous University of Barcelona, Barcelona, Spain.

Reprinted from Cancer Clinical Trials 2: 171–174, 1979.

apeutic trial which was initiated in July 1971. The selection of patients, criteria for eligibility for protocol study, preoperative studies and laparotomy techniques have been described elsewhere.[7,10,18]

In summary, the following criteria were used: 1) diagnostic biopsy was reviewed by the Stanford Division of Surgical Pathology, confirmed as a malignant lymphoma other than Hodgkin's disease and classified according to the Rappaport classification[16]; 2) patient was previously untreated; 3) patient lived within 300 miles of the Stanford Medical Center; 4) age was between 10 and 70 years inclusive; 5) patient and referring physician agreed to entry into protocol after being carefully informed about the investigative nature of the diagnostic and therapeutic programs; 6) patient did not have the clinicopathological diagnosis of chronic lymphocytic leukemia based on previously defined criteria[11]; 7) there existed no previous or concurrent medical condition which would seriously compromise the patient's ability to withstand the diagnostic and therapeutic program planned.

The preoperative evaluation included bilateral pedal lymphography and needle biopsy of the bone marrow, in addition to other and routine studies described elsewhere.[17,18]

Results

In our series of 200 patients, the nodular pattern was observed in 114 patients and the diffuse pattern in 86 patients. In each pattern we find a main cytological subtype: nodular lymphocytic poorly differentiated (NLPD) with 72 cases and diffuse histiocytic (DH) with 56 cases. Both subtypes together account for 64% of all cases. If we add the third subtype nodular mixed histiocytic–lymphocytic (NM) with 30 patients, these three subtypes represent 80% of the patients. Only 13 patients were classified in the diffuse lymphocytic poorly differentiated (DLPD) subtype and 12 patients in the nodular histiocytic (NH) subtype. The rest of the patients were considered: nine as diffuse mixed histiocytic–lymphocytic (DM), six as diffuse lymphocytic well differentiated (DLWD), and two as diffuse undifferentiated (DU).

In the NLPD group 85% of the cases were older than 40 years, as were 83% of the patients in the NM group. By contrast, 35% of the patients in the

DH group were younger than 40 years, 30% in the DLPD group, and 33% in the NH group.

After complete diagnostic study, 98 of 200 patients (49%) changed stage, but the data were very different in the two main subtypes. In NLPD, 55 of 72 patients (76%) changed stage, all of them to a higher pathological stage. In the DH, only 12 of 56 patients (21%) changed stage and only seven (13%) to a higher pathological stage. In NM, 15 of 30 patients (50%) changed stage, 14 (46%) to a higher pathological stage. Only three of 13 patients (23%) in the DLPD group and two of 12 (16%) in the NH group changed to a higher pathological stage.

Thus, at the time of diagnosis, 67 patients (93%) of the NLPD subtype were classified in pathological stages III and IV as were 26 patients (87%) of the NM subtype. On the contrary, 29 patients (52%) of the DH subtype were classified at the time of diagnosis in pathological stages I and II; the same was observed in seven patients (54%) of the DLPD subtype and in four (33%) of the NH subtype.

One of the most remarkable results of this study was the frequency of bone marrow involvement at the time of diagnosis in the different subtypes. In the NLPD group, 55 of 72 patients (76%) presented bone marrow involvement, while in the DH group only seven of 56 (13%) could be detected by bone marrow biopsy. In the other minor subtypes, the results were: 11 of 30 patients (36%) in the NM group, two of 13 patients (15%) in the DLPD group, and two of 12 patients (17%) in the NH group.

In the NLPD subtype, 67 of 72 patients (93%) presented with peripheral lymph node involvement, while in 25 of 56 patients (45%) of the DH subtype no apparent peripheral adenopathy was felt. In the NM subtype, 26 of 30 patients (86%) showed peripheral lymph node involvement.

Discussion

The data presented show clearly that in the non-Hodgkin's lymphoma there are two main subtypes, one in each histological pattern, with a clear-cut difference in their clinicopathological characteristics at the time of diagnosis.

NLPD affects mainly an older population, has a high frequency of bone marrow involvement as a manifestation of a widespread dissemination of the disease at the time of diagnosis, making a staging laparotomy unnecessary in the majority of cases. On the contrary, DH, the most frequent subtype of the diffuse patterns, affects a younger population, and in half of the patients the disease is still localized at the time of diagnosis.

The other minor subtypes follow in their clinical presentation one of the two major prototypes. NM presents many clinical aspects very similar to NLPD, the only important difference being the lower percentage of bone marrow involvement at the time of diagnosis. On the contrary, DLPD and NH present many clinical aspects, including bone marrow involvement, very similar to the DH subtype.

The distribution of cases in our series is not comparable with other published series[3,5,20] that show a great predominance of the diffuse patterns over the nodular patterns. However, in two other series published by Chabner et al.[4] and by Nathwani et al.,[15] we find a very similar distribution of cases with two major subtypes: NLPD and DH. In the latter publication, of 202 patients in the series, 111 patients had a nodular pattern and 91 a diffuse pattern. Of the 111 nodular lymphomas, 98 (88%) were classified as NLPD, six as NM and seven as NH. Of the 91 diffuse lymphomas, 54 (59%) were classified as DH and 18 as lymphoblastic, which in the classical Rappaport's classification would be considered in the DLPD, DM or DH subtypes. Their translation to the Lukes and Collins classification also indicates the predominance of two types: of 98 NLPD cases, 96 were considered small cleaved and of 54 DH cases, 42 were considered large noncleaved.

It is actually clear that the "histiocytic" cells in the Rappaport classification are not really histiocytes, but "large lymphoid (pironinophilic) cells" as indicated in Dorfman's classification,[6] and accepted by most of the pathologists.

In a recent paper, Bitram et al.[2] analyzed 100 patients with poorly differentiated lymphocytic and mixed cell types. Of them, 74 belong to NLPD, 12 to NM, 12 to DLPD and two to DM. They found important similarities between NLPD and NM patients and between DLPD and DM patients. These latter diffuse subtypes had the best responses to combination chemotherapy and possibly "cures" in contrast with the results obtained in the nodular patterns NLPD and NM. These results are comparable to the results reported by Fisher et al.[8] in the DH patients.

ACKNOWLEDGMENT

The authors wish to thank Dr. Ronald Dorfman and Dr. Hun Kim for the pathological diagnoses of the patients studied and for their valuable comments on most of the pathological slides reviewed with them. They are also grateful to the physicians and nurses of the Oncology and Radiotherapy Divisions of the Stanford Medical Center who made possible the collection of the data and cared for the paitents included in this series.

This study was supported in part by Grants CA-05838 and CA-08122 from the National Cancer Institute, N.I.H. Dr. Ribas-Mundo was supported by a Grant from the Commission of Cultural Exchange between Spain and the United States.

References

1. Bennet, M. H., Farrer-Brown, G., Henry, K., and Jelliffe, A. M.: Classification of non-Hodgkin's lymphomas. *Lancet 2: 405–406, 1974.*

2. Bitram, J. D., Golomb, H. M., Ultmann, J. E., Sweet, D. L., Lester, E. P., Stein, R. S., Miller, J. B., Moran, E. M., Kinnealey, A. E., Vardiman, J. E., Kinzie, J., and Roth, N. O.: Non-Hodgkin's lymphoma, poorly differentiated lymphocytic and mixed cell types. *Cancer 42: 88–95, 1978.*

3. Castellani, R., Bonadonna, G., Spinelli, P., Bajetta, E., Galante, E., and Rilke, F.: Sequential pathologic staging of untreated non-Hodgkin's lymphomas by laparoscopy and laparotomy combined with marrow biopsy. *Cancer 40: 2322–2328, 1977.*

4. Chabner, B. A., Johnson, R. E., Young, R. C., Canellos, G. P., Hubbard, S. P., Johnson, S. K., and DeVita, V. T., Jr.: Sequential nonsurgical and surgical staging of non-Hodgkin's lymphoma. *Ann Intern Med 85: 149–154, 1976.*

5. Dick, F., Bloomfield, C. D., and Brunning, R. D.: Incidence, cytology and histopathology of non-Hodgkin's lymphomas in the bone marrow. *Cancer 33: 1382–1398, 1974.*

6. Dorfman, R. F.: Classification of non-Hodgkin's lymphomas. *Lancet 1: 1295–1296, 1974.*

7. Enright, L. P., Trueblood, H. W., and Nelsen, T. S.: The surgical diagnosis of abdominal Hodgkin's disease. *Surg Gynecol Obstet 130: 583–589, 1970.*

8. Fisher, R. I., DeVita, V. T., Jr., Johnson, B. L., Simon, R., and Young, R. C.: Prognostic factors for advanced diffuse histiocytic lymphoma following treatment with combination chemotherapy. *Am J Med 63: 177–182, 1977.*

9. Gerard-Marchant, R., Hamlin, I., Lennert, K., Rilke, F., Stansfeld, A. G., and Van Unnik, J. A. M.: Classification of non-Hodgkin's lymphomas. *Lancet 2: 406–408, 1974.*

10. Goffinet, D. R., Castellino, R. A., Kim, H., Dorfman, R. F., Fuks, Z., Rosenberg, S. A., Nelsen, T., and Kaplan, H. S.: Staging laparotomies in unselected previously untreated patients with non-Hodgkin's lymphomas. *Cancer NY 32: 672–681, 1973.*

11. Jones, S. E., Fuks, Z., Kadin, M. D., Dorfman, R. F., Kaplan, H. S., Rosenberg, S. A., and Kim, H.: Non-Hodgkin's lymphomas. IV. Clinicopathologic correlation in 405 cases. *Cancer NY 31: 806–823, 1973.*

12. Kay, H. E. M.: Classification of non-Hodgkin's lymphomas. *Lancet 2: 586, 1974.*

13. Lennert, K., Mohri, N., Stein, H., and Kaiserling, E.: The histopathology of malignant lymphoma. *Br J Haematol 31(Suppl): 193–203, 1975.*

14. Lukes, R. J., and Collins, R. D.: New approaches to the classification of the lymphomata. *Br J Haematol 31(Suppl): 1–28, 1975.*

15. Nathwani, B. N., Kim, H., Rappaport, H., Solomon, J., and Fox, M.: Non-Hodgkin's lymphomas. A clinicopathologic study comparing two classifications. *Cancer 41: 303–325, 1978.*

16. Rappaport, H., Winter, W. J., and Hicks, E. B.: Follicular lymphoma: A re-evaluation of its position in the scheme of malignant lymphomas. Based on a survey of 253 cases. *Cancer NY 9: 792–821, 1956.*

17. Rosenberg, S. A., Dorfman, R. F., and Kaplan, H. S.: A summary of the results of the review of 405 patients with non-Hodgkin's lymphoma at Stanford University. *Br J Cancer 31(Suppl II): 168–173, 1975.*

18. Rosenberg, S. A., Boiron, M., DeVita, V. T., Jr., Johnson, R. E., Lee, B. J., Ultmann, J. E., and Viamonte, M.: Report of the Committee on Hodgkin's disease staging procedures. *Cancer Res 31: 1862–1865, 1971.*

19. Rosenberg, S. A., Ribas-Mundo, M., Goffinet, D. R., and Kaplan, H. S.: Staging in adult non-Hodgkin's lymphomas. In *Lymphoid Neoplasias II: Clinical and Therapeutic Aspects,* G. Mathé, Ed. (*Recent Results in Cancer Research, Vol. 65*) (in press).

20. Stein, R. S., Ultmann, J. E., Byrne, G. E., Moran, E. M., Golomb, H. M., and Oetzel, N.: Bone marrow involvement in non-Hodgkin's lymphoma. *Cancer 37: 629–636, 1976.*

30

Radiotherapy of non-Hodgkin's lymphomas

J. Otero Luna, M.D.

Patients with non-Hodgkin's lymphomas present a broad spectrum of pathologies and clinical evolutions; this fact forcibly leads to a wide variety of therapeutic approaches and alternatives. These vary from minimal and well-tolerated treatments, such as local irradiation or single agent chemotherapy, to aggressive treatments such as total abdominal irradiation or complex multiple agent regimens.

Any line drawn between indications for irradiation and chemotherapy would be artificial, but this presentation will focus on radiotherapy.

The first use of radiotherapy in lymphoproliferous disease dates back to March 1902 when Dr. William A. Pusey from Chicago treated a 44-year-old patient who presented voluminous adenopathies in the neck, axilla, and groin. Radiotherapy was administered in daily divided doses. The adenopathies decreased notably within the first few days. This observation triggered the use of irradiation in other lymphoproliferous processes. The effect of irradiation on lymphatic masses is often produced quickly, and it was observed how large conglomerates of adenopathies disappeared within a few days under the action of moderate doses of radiotherapy. This spectacular effect inspired the widely published metaphor that adenopathies "melted" like dew under the sun, and it served to promote the indication of radiotherapy in the treatment of lymphomas. Unfortunately, divided doses of a few hundred rads were administered. The limited amount of penetration of radiotherapy used up to 1950 also conditioned a heterogenous distribution of radiation within the interior of the lymphomatous mass. Although the effect was spectacular in its immediate manifestations, considerable disappointment followed when the majority of adenopathies inexorably grew back again in a few weeks to months.

The introduction in daily clinical practice of linear accelerators and units of tele-cobalt-therapy as well as other methods of high-energy radiation has liberated radiotherapeutists from the limitations of the old 200-kV alternators. Before such means could be employed, a small group of radiotherapists, headed by René Gilbert of Geneva and followed by Richard and Peters of Toronto, started applying radiotherapy in more systematic fashion to Hodgkin's disease. A reasonable number of definitive controls of disease were noted. Systematization of this treatment was carried out by Henry Kaplan at Stanford,[1] who promoted what he called the "cardinal features" of radiotherapy in Hodgkin's disease. These criteria were fundamentally three points: 1) A tumoricidic dose of approximately 4000 rad had to be administered within 4 weeks. 2) The treatment should be applied to a wide field in such a way that irradiation should encompass the volume in which the affected lymphatic chains are included, while at the same time the vital structures such as the heart, the liver, and the kidney are excluded. 3) The use of the megavoltage energy was essential.

Advances in radiotherapy of non-Hodgkin's lymphomas have come as a result of those obtained in the use of radiotherapy in Hodgkin's disease. The cardinal features stated by Kaplan for Hodgkin's disease are also valid in the field of non-Hodgkin's lymphomas. While the first and third features, the dose and the energy, are distinctly applicable to either one or both groups of diseases, the second feature, that is, the volume to be irradiated, is very different. This is due to certain peculiarities of localization and extension of non-Hodgkin's lymphomas which differ from the classical patterns of extension and localization characteristic of Hodgkin's disease.

Clinica Puerta de Hierro, Madrid, Spain.

Radiotherapy techniques

The modalities of radiotherapy which are used more in the treatment of non-Hodgkin's lymphomas can be classified as the following:

1) Locoregional
2) Nodal supradiaphragmatic (modified mantle)
3) Nodal infradiaphragmatic (modified inverted Y)
4) Modified total nodal
5) Total abdominal
6) Total body
7) Neuromeningeal, prophylactic, or therapeutic
8) Palliative

1) Locoregional. This type or irradiation technique is applicable to the very early stages of favorable pathology. It consists of irradiating a volume which should include the primary localization and the first site of lymphatic drainage. One of the types most frequently used in this technique is that which is called the "Waldeyer" type. The volume treated includes all the lymphatic tissue of the Waldeyer ring, pre- and post-auricular lymphatic areas, superior parapharyngeal lymphatic chains, and those on both sides of the neck as far as the clavicle. Conformed fields are used, that is to say, of irregular shape adopted to the geometry of the lesion and of the anatomical region. This technique is indicated particularly in extended lymphomas, frequent in the head and neck area. Lymphomas of the cavum and oropharynx stand out the most because of their frequency.

2) Nodal supradiaphragmatic (modified mantle). Since Kaplan's classical technique some modifications have been introduced by the different disseminating patterns of non-Hodgkin's lymphomas with respect by Hodgkin's disease. The latter adopts a clear "centripetal" pattern which facilitates the irradiation of volumes (the majority of such lie on the middle line). Non-Hodgkin's lymphomas have a "centrifugal" distribution. Thus, it is frequent to see patients with preauricular or epitrochlear adenopathies. The classical mantle does not cover these localizations, and it must be modified by performing an irradiation of the Waldeyer type in the superior volume, a normal mantle or without mediastinum, and the addition of isolated epitrochlear fields.

3) Nodal infradiaphragmatic. This technique includes lumboaortic, iliac, bilateral inguinal and femoral, lymphatic chains with partial exclusion of the rectum and the bladder. The spleen and splenic hilum are included in specific cases.

4) Total modified nodal. This consists in successive irradiation, with a resting interval, of all supra- or infradiaphragmatic lymphatic areas with the modifications defined by the different non-Hodgkin's lymphomas.

In general it can be said that techniques 2, 3, and 4, which were widely used some time ago, are used to a lesser degree than wider irradiations (see the next point) which adapt themselves more adequately to the extent and sometimes spreading of these lymphomas.

5) Total abdominal. Patients affected by non-Hodgkin's lymphoma have at least mesenteric involvement in more than 50% of the cases. As the lymphatic mesentery is not covered by the usual technique used in Hodgkin's (inverted Y), Goffinet, et al.[2] emphasize the inadequacy of this technique in the treatment of abdominal localizations of non-Hodgkin's lymphomas. In these patients irradiation should cover the total abdominal cavity. For many years now, we have known techniques which are adequate for this purpose, such as that described by Patterson as "abdominal bath."[3] This technique has been simplified by the availability of high energy. There is no technical problem in administering a 2000–3000-rad dose to all of the abdomen within 3–4 weeks, but this dose is only adequate in the treatment of very vulnerable tumors such as the seminoma. Lymphomas require doses superior to 3000 rad. However, when this dose is exceeded, lesions with repercussions and clinical sequela in the intestine and liver are produced. The critical abdominal organ is the kidney, which has a tolerance limit of 1500–2000 rad in 3–4 weeks.

In order to obviate these inconveniences, various techniques have been devised, one of which, the "mobile band,"[4] may be used in certain cases, although for abdominal irradiation of non-Hodgkin's lymphomas the more adequate is the one proposed by Goffinet, et al.,[5] which consists of initiating the irradiation throughout the anterior and posterior fields, opposite and parallel, which cover all the abdominal content, excluding the right hepatic lobule. During a second phase, horizontal beams are projected through one and then another side of the patient. The fields are arranged so that they just touch the anterior pole of the kidneys, while fully affecting the lymboaortic chains and the mesenteric nodes. During the third phase, restricted fields are used, such as a wide inverted Y, in order to raise the dose from 4000 to 4500 rad within 6–7 weeks.

6) *Total body* irradiation consists in the administration of ionized radiation to the whole body in the most homogeneous way possible. Its trial and clinical use in a number of pathological processes is almost as old as radiotherapy itself. This technique of irradiation has again been introduced with appreciable results by del Regato,[6] especially on patients with chronic lymphatic leukosis. This reintroduction was after a long period of disuse, due to its poor therapeutic results, conditioned by inadequate indications and by inefficiently penetrating energy. Following the development of chemotherapy this form of treatment again fell into disuse until Johnson[7] recently demonstrated its effectiveness in non-Hodgkin's lymphomas.

The mechanism of action of total body irradiation is not clearly known. It is an obvious paradox that moderate doses of 100 or more rads can provide complete and prolonged remissions in patients with large tumoral localizations, whose local treatment, according to the classical point of view, would require thousands of rads. We can speculate on the harm that sublethal doses could provoke by interfering mitochondriac enzymatic processes or other processes, but any interpretation of this surprising therapeutic effect should obviously be related to its "systematic" character.

Special facilities for total body irradiation are needed. It is essential to have high energy available (telecobalt or linear accelerator) and space for treatment wide enough so that the size of the field can cover the whole body of the patient. In our hospital, the patient is treated in a sitting position; the cobalt unit is arranged for a horizontal beam and the patient is situated at a distance of 3–4 m from the source. The patient is treated through lateral fields, from right to left. Dosimetric tests must be conducted during the irradiation. The total dose ranges between 100 and 150 rad, and the daily dosage between 5 and 10 rad, administered 3–5 days/week. The tendency is to administer two cycles, with an interval of 2 or more months, or to follow a maintenance therapy of moderate doses of total irradiations repeated once or twice a year.

7) *Neuromeningeal, prophylactic, or therapeutic.* The development of an effective chemotherapy has changed the evolution in certain types of leukemia, postponing meningeal involvement, which is almost always fatal. Recently, DeVita, et al.[8] and Schein, et al.[9] have reported their experience with a series of patients with non-Hodgkin's lymphomas with unfavorable pathology where chemotherapy has provided complete remission in one-third of the cases. The same group of authors[10] have also reported that, in the "histiocytic diffuse" as well as in the "undifferentiated" forms, 29% developed neurologic complications; the risk is greater in patients with bone marrow involvement so that meningeal invasion is expected in two-thirds of these patients. This circumstance is only applicable to diffuse lymphomas since in the group of nodular lymphomas, with a high degree of marrow involvement, meningeal invasion is extremely rare.

The prophylactic or therapeutic pattern of neuromeningeal complications is carried out by combining irradiation and intrathecal chemotherapy. Irradiation is limited to the cranial volume and to the first two cervical segments. The irradiation technique consists of disposing two lateral fields, parallel and opposite, conformed in such a way that the eyeballs, thyroid gland, and all extracranial marginal structures are protected. The dose, estimated in the medial plane, is 2400 rad, comparable to the one which is effective in acute lymphoblastic leukosis as prophylactic treatment. In the case of known focal involvement with tumoral expression, the dose must be raised to 3000–4000 rad.

8) *Palliative.* Radiotherapy has a precise indication in many evolutive circumstances with lymphomas, not with a radical intention but with a palliative one. A bone pain, a nerve compression, a conflictive situation of space in the thorax or knee may be reduced or even remitted with local irradiation performed in just one or a few treatment sessions.

Therapeutic alternatives

The wide diversity of clinical and pathological forms makes therapeutic systematization different. As a minimum, we are obliged to distinguish three large groups:

—lymphomas
—extra lymphatic lymphomas
—lymphomas in children

Lymphomas

Stages I and II—favorable pathology. In these cases, which in practice are rare, the treatment indicated is locoregional irradiation. The response rate is very positive and a good part of the failures are due to a badly plotted radiotherapeutic technique, deficient in its dosage or poorly performed.

Stages I and II—unfavorable pathology. Radiotherapy may be locoregional or total nodal. We are more inclined toward a locoregional radiotherapy with a more or less aggressive and prolonged chemotherapy according to the pathologic form.

Stages III and IV—favorable pathology. Body radiotherapy followed by total nodal radiotherapy is usually considered for young patients in good general condition or for older patients in poor general condition on prolonged single-agent chemotherapy.

Stages III and IV—unfavorable pathology. Radiotherapy as total body irradiation provides a valid alternative to programs of aggressive chemotherapy. In any case, its indication must be considered from the beginning as well as in cases already treated, even though the response rate is lower. Previous total irradiation does not appear to compromise the effectiveness of chemotherapy.

Two basic characteristics may be derived from a total consideration of the therapeutic problem of non-Hodgkin's lymphomas:

—Most of the failures after radiotherapy occur in marginal nodes which were not irradiated, or in extralymphatic localizations.

—Most of the failures after chemotherapy occur in the known involved areas where the tumoral mass is more voluminous.

It is obvious that both therapies should complement each other in the majority of these patients. The main value of chemotherapy is the eradication of the microscopic foci of the disease. The crucial problem, as Glatstein, et al.[11] indicate, lies in how to integrate both therapies in order to get the most benefit. How much radiotherapy and how much chemotherapy is the first main question in the development of therapeutic research in the field of non-Hodgkin's lymphomas.

Non-Hodgkin's lymphomas in children

The individualized consideration of infantile lymphomas is motivated, at least, for two reasons: its specific pathologic characteristics and the high frequency of leukemic evolution. Almost all infantile lymphomas are diffuse lymphomas, which would condition dissemination patterns that are not approachable by radiotherapy.

Indications for radiotherapy still seem to be valid in all cases of localized lymphomas and extralymphatic lymphomas, and especially in those cases of badly differentiated nodular lymphomas and diffuse histiocytic lymphoma. Even in these cases the simultaneous or sequential addition of chemotherapy should be considered. The chemotherapy will be, in general, of the same kind as that applied in acute leukemia.[12] In some localizations such as the mediastinum, the role of irradiation appears very doubtful, except to help overcome a critical situation. Its administration in high doses offers a high risk of complications for the organs contained in the mediastinum especially when total doses are also administered with adriamycin and other chemotherapeutic agents.

With respect to the indication of neuromeningeal prophylaxis with cranial irradiation and intrathecal metrothexate, it should also be considered in all lymphomas with high evolutive potential toward leukemia. It does not appear to be indicated in certain extended lymphomas (intestine, Waldeyer ring, primitive osseous) nor in Burkitt's lymphoma.

Radiotherapy in infantile lymphomas has a precise indication with a radical intention, in all localized forms, as has been mentioned before. These indications coincide with these localizations that tend to evolve toward leukemia with less frequency.

In general, it can be said that those which do not require prophylactic neuromeningeal irradiation are those which have a higher indication of radiotherapy.

Extranodal non-Hodgkin's lymphomas

Extranodal lymphomas present evolutive characteristics that with certain considerations and reservations resemble the evolution of an epithelial or glandular tumor of the same localization. Many times the extranodal lymphoma follows the oncologic model of a tumor-lymphatic-metastasis.

In extranodal lymphomas, besides the clinical stage and the pathological varieties, a third factor, the primary site, is going to condition the therapeutic indication.

In our casuistics, extralymphatic lymphomas are over one-third of the totality, 37% to be exact. Out of a total of 187 non-Hodgkin's lymphomas treated from 1964 to 1976, 69 cases initially appeared as extralymphatic forms, and among them 52 were in adults and 17 were in children.

It is not possible to generalize with respect to the indications of radiotherapy, since the techniques of irradiation are as many as the possible locations. In order of frequency in our series, head and neck lymphomas come first. In these cases the technique indicated is locoregional irradiation, Waldeyer type. Digestive localizations are next, in which the indication is constituted by total abdominal irradiation, according to the above-mentioned technique.[5] Bone lymphomas are a precise indication for radiotherapy, by irradiating the whole bone at relatively high doses.[13] Lymphomas of the CNS require total cranial irradiation with overdosification over the primary site.[14] The rare primary cutaneous lymphomas are a controversial matter between irradiation with electron beam and topic or systematic chemotherapy.[15,16]

Extranodal non-Hodgkin's lymphomas form the group of patients in which radiotherapy has its most adequate indication. In its early stage they are susceptible to local or locoregional irradiation procedures, when accessible, which are well-tolerated and with a minimum of sequels. In our series, the survival (actuarial) of these patients is greater than the general survival and that of the infantile lymphomas. Survival after 10 years was 25% in the total series of 187 patients including those with relapses. Lymphomas have a lower survival rate, only 17.7% of a total of 90 patients. In children, survival was 22.5% of a total of 45 patients. In the extranodal-lymphoma group, whose treatment has been predominantly radiotherapeutic, survival 10 years later was 47.8% of a total of 52 adults and 17 children.

References

1. Kaplan, H. S.: *Hodgkin's Disease*. Harvard University Press, Cambridge, Mass., 1972.

2. Goffinet, D. R., Castellino, S. A., Kim, H., et al.: Staging laparotomies in unselected previously interested patients with non-Hodgkin's lymphomas. *Cancer 37: 2797, 1976.*

3. Paterson, R.: *The Treatment of Malignant Disease by Radiotherapy*, 2nd ed. Arnold, London, 1963, p. 441.

4. Delclos, L., Baun, E. J., Herrera, R. J., et al.: Whole abdominal irradiation by Cobalt-60 moving strip technique. *Radiology 81: 632, 1963.*

5. Goffinet, D. R., Glatstein, E., Furs, et al.: Abdominal irradiation in non Hodgkin's lymphomas. *Cancer 37: 2797, 1976.*

6. delRegato, J. A.: Total body irradiation in the treatment of chronic lymphogenus Leukemia: Janeway Lecture, 1973. *Am J Roentgenol 120: 504, 1974.*

7. Johnson, R. E.: Evaluation of fractionated total body irradiation in patients with leukemia and diseminated lymphomas. *Radiology 86: 1085, 1966.*

8. DeVita, V. T., Canellos, G. P., Chabner, B. A., et al.: Advanced diffuse histiocitic lymphoma, a potentially curable disease. *Lancet 1: 248, 1975.*

9. Schein, Ph.S., Chabner, B. A., Canellos, G. P., et al.: Non Hodgkin's lymphoma: patterns of relapse from complete remission after combination chemotherapy. *Cancer 35: 354, 1975.*

10. Bunn, P. A., Schein, P. S., Banks, P. M., et al.: Central nervous system complacations in patients with diffuse histiocytic and undifferentrated lymphoma: Leukemia revisited. *Blood 47: 3, 1976.*

11. Glatstein, E., Donaldson, S. S., Rosenberg, S. A., and Kaplan, H. S.: Combined modality therapy in malignant lymphomas. *Cancer Treat Rep 61: 1199, 1977.*

12. Aur, R. J. A., Hustu, H. O., Pinkel, D., et al.: Therapy of localized and regional lymphosarcoma of childhood. *Cancer 27: 1328, 1971.*

13. Boston, H. CH., Dahlin, D. C., and Ivins, J. C.: Malignant lymphoma (so-called reticullum-cell sarcoma) of bone. *Cancer 34: 1131, 1974.*

14. Littman, P., and Wang, C.: Reticulum cell sarcoma of the brain. A review of the literature and study of 19 cases. *Cancer 35: 1412, 1975.*

15. Tetenes, Ph. J., and Goodwin, P. N.: A comparative study of superficial whole-body radiotherapeutic techniques using a 4-MeV electron beam. *Radiology 122: 219, 1977.*

16. van Scott, E. J., Grein, D. A., Kalmanson, J. D., et al.: Frequent low dose of intravenous mechlorethamine for late-stage mycosis fungoides lymphoma. *Cancer: 1613, 1975.*

31

Chemotherapy in non-Hodgkin's lymphoma

Experience of the Argentine Group for the Treatment of Acute Leukemia (GATLA)*

Santiago Pavlovsky, M.D.

Since the discovery of nitrogen mustard in the 1940s, many drugs have been incorporated in our therapeutic arsenal. Non-Hodgkin's lymphomas along with Hodgkin's disease and acute leukemias are included among the most chemosensitive neoplastic processes. Many antineoplastic drugs have shown some cytolytic action and efficacy in their treatment (Table 1). The initial studies were performed using most of these drugs as single agent. There were often 40–50% objective responses. Nevertheless, the percentages of complete remissions were low and not above 20–30%, and these were often of short duration, lasting only a few weeks. The average of survival, therefore, was not longer than 2 years. With the arrival of drug combinations at the end of the 60s, there also came a significant increase in the percentages of complete remission and in their length of duration.

In 1968 Gatla started the first study with combined chemotherapy in non-Hodgkin's lymphoma following the COPP scheme (Table 2). Out of 52 patients, 10 were excluded because they abandoned the treatment before having completed six cycles. In this protocol, as in the following ones, the only patients considered as nonevaluable were those who refused to continue with combination chemotherapy, or who did not return for consultation before having completed six cycles. Those patients who

showed an obvious advance of their disease and/or who died of their disease before having completed six cycles, were evaluated as no response or as deceased.

Out of 42 patients, 33 (79%) obtained complete remission (Table 3). The average of complete remission was 18 months, although 43% of those patients were disease-free up to 60 months later. The average survival of the 42 patients was 49 months, and 44% were still alive 60 months later.

After a 60-month period, 67% of the patients of stages I–II, 45% in stage III, 32% in stage IV, 73% of asymptomatic patients, and 28% "B" symptomatic patients are still in complete remission.

If we compare the survival rate in accordance with the therapeutic response, a marked difference is observed ($p < 0.005$) among patients with complete remission versus partial or no remission. After a 60-month period, 53% of the patients with complete remission are still alive, whereas none of those with partial or null remission are alive.

With the purpose of searching for new combinations which could be equally effective but less toxic, more economic, and easier to administer, protocol 11–lymphoma-72 was designed which compared CVPP versus CCVPP (Table 2).

Out of 191 patients included in the study from November 1972 to November 1975, 166 were evaluated; 83 were treated with CVPP and 83 with CCVPP. The percentage of complete remissions was slightly higher in the CCVPP group (55%) than in the CVPP group (49%), although the difference was not significant (Table 3). However, we must point out the greater number of deaths in the

Instituto de Investigaciones Hematológicas, Pacheco de Melo 3081, Buenos Aires, Argentina.

TABLE 1

Effective Drugs in the Treatment of Lymphomas

Drug	Way of Administration	Dose	Toxicity Which Limits Its Use	Other Toxic Effects
Nitrogen mustard	IV	0.4 mg/kg every 3–4 weeks	leukopenia thrombocytopenia	nausea, vomiting, bone marrow depression
Cyclophosphamide	Oral	1–4 mg/kg day	leukopenia	nausea, vomiting, hemorhagic cystitis;
	IV	15 mg/kg/ week		alopecia, bone marrow depression
Vinblastine	IV	0.1–0.3 mg/kg/ week	leukopenia thrombocytopenia	bone marrow depression, polyneuritis
Vincristine	IV	0.025–0.05 mg/kg/ week	intestinal paralysis polyneuritis	alopecia
Procarbazine	Oral	3–5 mg/kg/day	leukopenia thrombocytopenia	bone marrow depression, nausea, and vomiting; hepatic failure
Prednisone	Oral	1 mg/kg/day	osteoporosis diabetes GI bleeding	Cushing syndrome, immunosuppression
Adriamycin	IV	30–50 mg/m^2/week	cardiac	alopecia, oral ulcerations
Nitrosoureas	Oral and IV	100 mg/m^2 every 6–8 weeks	myelodepression	nausea and vomiting
DTIC	IV	100 mg/m^2/day $\times$ 5	myelodepression	nausea and vomiting; phlebitis
Bleomycin	IV	100 mg/m^2/week	lung fibrosis	vomiting, temperature

TABLE 2

Treatment Schemes

COPP
  Cyclophosphamide 600 mg/m^2 IV days 1 and 8
  Vincristine 1.5 mg/m^2 IV days 1 and 8
  Procarbazine 100 mg/m^2 oral days 1–10
  Prednisone 40 mg/m^2 oral days 1–14 of the first and fourth
    cycle
CVPP
  Cyclophosphamide 600 mg/m^2 IV day 1
  Vinblastine 6 mg/m^2 IV day 1
  Procarbazine 100 mg/m^2 oral days 1–14
  Prednisone 40 mg/m^2 oral days 1–14
CCVPP
  CVPP plus CCNU 75 mg/day 1, cycles 1, 3, and 5
COPP-CCNU
  COPP plus CCNU 40 mg/m^2 day 14, cycles 1, 3, and 5
DOP-E
  Cyclophosphamide 400 mg/m^2 IV days 1, 14, 28, 48, 68,
    98, and 128
  Vincristine 1.5 mg/m^2 IV same days
  Daunomycin 40 mg/m^2 IV days 7, 21, 38, 58, 83, and 113
  Prednisone 40 mg/m^2 oral $\times$ 10 days and 10 days rest

CCVPP group occurred before having completed the six cycles. Both combinations were significantly inferior to COPP ($p < 0.05$), and for this reason this protocol was concluded. The duration of complete remission and of survival in scheme CCVPP was paradoxically inferior to scheme CVPP, although this was not a significant difference (Fig. 1).

Due to the lower percentage of complete remissions obtained with the CVPP-CCVPP combination, another protocol was started comparing COPP with the inclusion of CCNU with another combination. (DOP-E) which resembled regimens employed in acute leukemia. (Table 2). These regimens were initiated to attempt to avoid lymph-node relapses during the period of rest. A total of 123 patients were included from December 1975 to October 1977, of which 90 were evaluable. A greater response in the percentages of complete remission was observed in scheme CCOPP (66%) than in DOP-E (46%) (Table 3). The duration of complete remission was greater with CCOPP, although the results are too preliminary to draw up a conclusion. Survival was similar in both groups.

TABLE 3
Results of Treatment with Combination Chemotherapy

Scheme	COPP	CVPP	CCVPP	CCOPP	DOP-E
No. of patients	42	83	83	47	43
No. CR	33	41	46	31	20
% CR	79	49	55	66	46
Median CR (months)	18	>36	22	>18	>18
Median survival (months)	49	41	28	>18	>18
% Survival 4 years	51	37	37	—	—

Prognostic factors in non-Hodgkin's lymphoma

To evaluate the factors which could influence the response to drug combinations, as well as the duration of complete remissions and survival, 166 patients with non-Hodgkin's lymphoma treated with protocol 11-lymphoma-72 from October 1972 to November 1975 have been analyzed. (Table 4).

Complete remission: If we compare the percentage of therapeutic response according to prognostic factors, significant differences can be observed in the following parameters: stage II versus stage IV, $p < 0.05$, stage III versus stage IV, $p < 0.05$, "A" versus "B" symptoms, $p < 0.001$, well-differentiated (WD) versus histiocytic (H), $p < 0.01$, and poorly differentiated (PD) versus H, $p < 0.05$. We conclude that the adverse prognostic factors are stage IV, presence of symptoms, histiocytic type. A decrease in the response is also observed in older patients, diffuse structure, and previous chemotherapeutic treatment, although they do not reach significant values.

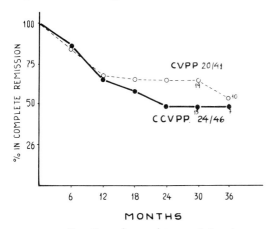

FIGURE 1. Duration of complete remission in non-Hodgkin's lymphoma.

Duration of complete remission: According to the histologic type, differences are observed between WD versus H, $p < 0.025$.

If we take into account the previous treatment, a significant difference is observed between radiotherapy versus chemotherapy with or without previous radio therapy ($p < 0.005$) and between nonprevious treatment versus chemotherapy ($p < 0.01$). Differences were not observed between "without treatment" and "only radiotherapy." It was observed that 82%, 92%, 63% of patients included in each group of "non-treatment, chemotherapy, radiotherapy," respectively, were stages III and IV; 19%, 8%, 9% were histiocytic type and 66%, 61%, 45% were symptomatic.

The inclusion of a greater percentage of patients with a worse prognosis in the non-prior-treatment group was the cause of the lower duration of complete remission as compared with "only radiotherapy." In fact, the presence of previous chemotherapy alone was an adverse prognostic factor.

Prognostic factors and survival: Age was useful as a prognostic factor. There are differences among the 15–30-year-old groups versus 31–45-year-old, $p < 0.0025$, and the 15–30-year-old versus less than 45-year-old ($p < 0.005$), and 31–45-year-old versus less than 60-year-old ($p < 0.05$).

Stage: Differences were observed only between stages III and IV ($p < 0.05$).

Symptomatology: There were significant differences between "A" versus "B" ($p < 0.005$); at 36 months 75% versus 45% were alive, respectively.

Histologic type: Differences between WD and PD versus H ($p < 0.025$) were observed; at 36 months 68% WD, 59% PD, 51% mixed (M), and 29% H were still alive (Fig. 2).

Structure: A better survival was observed among the nodular forms than among the diffuse forms ($p < 0.05$); at 36 months 73% and 51% were still alive,

TABLE 4

Percentage of Complete Remission. Duration of Complete Remission and Survival in Non-Hodgkin's Lymphoma According to Different Prognostic Factors (Prot. 11-Lymph.-72)

Parameter	CR/Total	%	Media		% after 36 months	
			CR	Survival	CR	Survival
Age						
15–30 years	8/11	73	>36	>36	62	100
31–45 years	16/27	59	11	>36	44	73
46–60 years	38/73	52	34	29	49	46
>60 years	25/55	45		22	19	44
Sex						
Male	51/98	52	19	>36	36	52
Female	36/68	53	>36	>36	63	56
Stage						
II	17/23	74	34	29	47	46
III	48/85	56	24	>36	45	68
IV	22/58	38	36	16	50	35
Symptoms						
A	37/52	71	36	>36	50	75
B	50/114	44	24	24	45	44
Histological Type						
WD	27/41	66	>36	>36	63	68
PD	37/64	58	29	>36	44	59
H	14/39	36	11	11	14	29
M	9/22	41	>36	>36	67	51
Structure						
Nodular	21/35	60	>36	>36	54	73
Diffuse	38/74	51	36	>36	50	51
?	28/57	49	20	24	43	45
Previous Treatment						
No.	63/116	54	36	23	50	48
Rd.	11/22	50	>36	>36	66	51
Q ± Rd.	13/28	46	8	>36	17	77

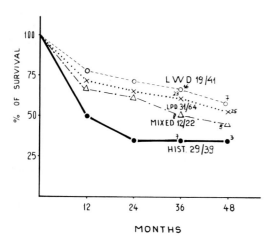

FIGURE 2. Survival of non-Hodgkin's lymphoma according to histology.

respectively. Structure data were not given in an important number of cases, having to call the attention of pathologists to this fact, due to its prognostic importance.

In conclusion, adverse values for the prediction of survival are: age above 45 years, stage IV, the presence of "B" symptoms, histiocytic type, and diffuse forms. Sex has no prognostic value.

There is no doubt that a better knowledge of the prognostic factors will aid in the stratification of the patients in order to allow the performance of randomized studies, as well as the choice of therapy according to the patient's risk.

Pediatric non-Hodgkin's lymphoma

Contrary to what has been observed in other neoplastic processes of the hematopoietic system,

TABLE 5

Pediatric Non-Hodgkin's Lymphoma (Prot. 6-Lymp.-73)

Induction		Maintenance
Daily prednisone VCR[a] VCR VCR VCR	CO60 CNS	COPP × 6 cycles—COPP only 1 cycle every 2 months A
CO60	IT MTX[b] × 5	6MP[c] + MTX + CPM[d]—every 3 months VCR 1 dose B PRED[e] × 7 days

[a] VCR: 1.5 mg/m^2 IV weekly.
[b] MTX: IT 12 mg/m^2 × 5 doses. Oral 15 mg/m^2 × week.
[c] 6MP: 2.5 mg/kg/day oral.
[d] CPM: 300 mg/m^2/week oral.
[e] PRED: 40 mg/m^2/day oral.

advances in pediatric non-Hodgkin's lymphomas have been few. One of the reasons for this is that the diffuse lymphoblastic lymphoma which is the predominant type is prone to early dissemination in the cerebrospinal fluid and in the bone marrow.

Recently, with the new immunological advances in the classification of lymphomas, it has been observed that the majority of poorly differentiated diffuse lymphomas of the adult are type "B," while among children they are type "T" (thymic derived).

A therapeutic protocol was initiated with the purpose of improving the complete remission percentages and of increasing survival in patients under 15 years of age with non-Hodgkin's lymphomas. It combined different therapeutic methods: surgery, chemotherapy, radiotherapy, and CNS prevention. Two methods for maintenance were also evaluated: COPP type "A" lymphoma and leukemia type "B" with 6-mercaptopurine, methotrexate and cyclophosphamide (Table 5). The protocol was initiated in June 1973 and ended in December 1975. In November 1977, it was evaluated. Out of 61 patients, 49 were considered evaluable, and 12 were not evaluable due to an initial infiltration of the bone marrow.

Thirty-two (65%) of the 49 patients obtained complete remission (Table 6). The percentage of complete remission was lower in stage IV than in the others ($p < 0.05$). The average duration of complete remission was 10 months with no differences between the maintenance scheme or stage. A significant difference was observed ($p < 0.001$) when comparing the average survival according to therapeutic response among patients who obtained complete remission versus partial or no remission, 12 and 7 months. The average of survival according to clinical staging was; stage I and II, 12 months; III and IV, 8 months; with 32% and 20%; respectively, still alive 36 months later ($p < 0.02$). It is concluded that 27% of the total number of patients and 40% of those with complete remission were still alive 36 months later, with no deaths having occurred in any of the children after 24 months.

There is no doubt that more aggressive schemes including other drugs are needed to raise the percentage of complete remissions and of survival in this disease, and other unfavorable non-Hodgkin's lymphomas.

TABLE 6

Results of Induction Treatment According to Clinical Stage

Stage	CR. No.	CR. %	PR	Null	Died	Total
I	4	100	—	—	—	4
II	12	80	1	2	—	15
III	9	82	1	1	—	11
IV	7	37	4	4	4	19
Total	32	65	6	7	44	49

References

1. Cebrian Bonesana, A., Schvartzman, E., Roca García, C., Pependieck, C., Sackmann Muriel, F., Ojeda, F., Kuicala, R., Pavlovsky, S., Lein, J. M., and Penchansky, L.: Non-Hodgkin's lymphoma in childhood. An analysis of 122 cases from Argentina. *Cancer 41: 2372–2378, 1978.*

2. Morgenfeld, M. C., Pavlovsky, A., Suarez, A., Somoza, N., Pavlovsky, S., Palau, M., and Barroz, C. A.: Combined cyclophosphamide, vincristine, procarbazine and prednisone (CVPP) therapy for malignant lymphoma.

Evaluation of 190 patients. *Cancer 36: 1241–1249,* *1975.*

3. Murphy, S. B.: Management of childhood non-Hodg-kin's lymphoma. *Cancer Treat Rep 61: 1161–1173,* *1977.*

4. Somoza, N., Morgenfeld, M. C., Magnasco, J., Pavlovsky, S., Cavagnaro, F. J., Saslavsky, J., de Maria, H., Macchi, A., and Suarez, A.: Estudio comparativo de dos combi-naciones de drogas en linfoma no Hodgkin. *Sangre 23:* *418–425, 1978.*

32

Issues in therapy of non-Hodgkin's lymphomas

Franco M. Muggia, M.D.[†]

Hernán Cortes-Funes, M.D.[‡]

O ver the past two decades the outlook of patients with Hodgkin's disease has been drastically altered, initially by improvement in radiotherapy and later by the development of effective combination (MOPP) chemotherapy. In the treatment of other lymphomas, similar degrees of success have not been achieved. Moreover, the complexity of histopathologic conditions has slowed delineation of optimal treatment methods for each disease category. The purpose of this paper is to define the status of current treatments and to focus on current therapeutic issues.

A major recurrent theme is the variable success of combination chemotherapy according to histology. Whereas in aggressive ("unfavorable") lymphomas combination regimens have drastically altered the course of disease, in the indolent ("favorable") lymphomas new drug combinations have not convincingly proven superior to single alkylating agent therapy or other conservative approaches of the past. However, obvious gaps persist in our knowledge. Future clinical trials may be expected to provide information on treatment according to stage and histology, on the integration of chemotherapy with radiotherapy, and on the development of new drug regimens.

Introduction

The terminology "non-Hodgkin's lymphoma" (NHL) has been applied to malignant lymphomas

exclusive of Hodgkin's disease. While expedient, this definition belies the vast complexity of conditions encompassed under it, and it will be outlined below. This paper will comment on therapeutic issues dealing with some of these malignant lymphomas and indicate areas of potential progress. Variable success has been achieved in the treatment of patients with these diseases which generally have lagged behind the remarkable strides made in Hodgkin's disease during the past two decades.

Classification

Histopathology

Increasingly since the 1960s, the Rappaport classification has been widely applied to NHL,[6,37] replacing the terminology of "lymphosarcoma, reticulum cell sarcoma, and giant follicular lymphoma," which was previously in vogue. This new classification proved generally reproducible and clinically useful in characterizing types of *diffuse* and *nodular* lymphomas with variable prognosis, from the very unfavorable diffuse histiocytic to the most favorable nodular lymphocytic lymphomas. Figure 1 indicates the basic features of this classification. The nodular histology is mainly constituted by types 2, 3, and 4.

More recently, new classifications have been introduced which utilize ultrastructural and/or immunological concepts.[12,25,36] For example, morphologic features have replaced the histiocytic terminology because the lymphocytic origin of these cells has been identified. The practical superiority of these new systems over the Rappaport classification remains to be demonstrated. A study was initiated by the National Cancer Institute in 1977 to help resolve these questions. The analysis

[†] Cancer Therapy Evaluation Program, Division of Cancer Treatment, Bethesda, Maryland 20205. Present address: NYU Cancer Center, New York, NY 10016.

[‡] Sección Quimioterapia Oncológica, Hospital 1° de Octubre, Madrid.

NODULAR   DIFFUSE

1. Lymphocytic, well-differentiated

2. Lymphocytic, poorly differentiated

3. Mixed cell
   (lymphocytic and histiocytic)

4. Histiocytic

5. Undifferentiated
   (Burkitt's and non-Burkitt's)

FIGURE 1.   Rappaport classification (1966).

of clinicopathologic correlations in malignant lymphomas at four major centers is awaited before alternate proposals to the Rappaport classification can be readily endorsed by clinicians.

Staging

The Ann Arbor classification applicable to Hodgkin's disease has been widely utilized in the non-Hodgkin's lymphomas as well. Its relevance for therapeutic decisions in many instances, however, remains conjectural. A major drawback in the practical application of such staging is the great propensity of NHL to present in stage IV. Furthermore, extranodal involvement occurs to a much greater extent than in Hodgkin's disease, and different sites may have specific prognostic implications. Also, the proper use of staging procedures, such as laparoscopy and laparotomy, is likely to be quite different for histiocytic as opposed to lymphocytic tumors. For instance, liver involvement is considerably less prevalent in diffuse histiocytic lymphoma than in the diffuse poorly differentiated lymphocytic lymphoma. In arriving at appropriate staging sequences, therefore, both the histologic type and the therapeutic decisions required relative to stage must be considered.[8,18] The value of systematic restaging has also been stressed.[19]

Treatment Modalities

Optimal therapy is difficult to define in view of complexities of histology and staging. Some basic concepts will be outlined herein, with future research areas to be discussed subsequently.

Radiotherapy

As with other radiosensitive tumors, radiotherapy has been utilized in the localized stages of disease. High doses of radiation (greater than 3500 rad in conventional fractionation schemes) are considered necessary to control the majority of these tumors.[14,16] Long-term control is generally obtained in Stages I and II, particularly with nodular histologies.[5,15,17,22,31,33,34,42]

The total body irradiation (TBI) approach used by Johnson and other authors[9,21,41] has achieved survival results comparable to chemotherapy in stages III and IV non-Hodgkin's lymphomas in some studies. However, such treatment has been disappointing in terms of curative potential.

Chemotherapy

Since the introduction of cyclophosphamide and other alkylating agents, the sensitivity of these tumors to chemotherapy has been generally recognized. Such single agent therapy is, in fact, curative in Burkitt's lymphoma.[45] The combination of CVP, reported by Bagley, et al.[2] and later by Luce, et al.,[24] indicated improvement in results relative to those achieved with single agent chemotherapy. C-MOPP was introduced by DeVita and co-workers initially as an alternative to MOPP in Hodgkin's disease, and subsequently applied widely to treat patients with aggressive non-Hodgkin's lymphoma.[1] Other combinations, such as CHOP, BACOP, and M-BACOD[7,10,38,39] (Table 1), were developed after the initial success of CVP and upon recognition of variability of responsiveness to chemotherapy among histological types of NHL. In addition, the availability of newer active drugs, such as bleomycin and adriamycin, permitted the development of drug combinations such as ABP[3] exhibiting no cross-resistance to CVP. Various histologies are associated with different response rates to these drugs, but, in almost every instance, complete remission rates in excess of 50% have been obtained. However, the duration of these complete responses varies greatly from one histologic type to another. Combined approaches of radiotherapy and chemotherapy have not been widely explored until recently.

TABLE 1

Combination Chemotherapy in Non-Hodgkin's Lymphomas

Combination—Day Cycle (Institution—Ref.)	Drug[a]	Dose	Route	Schedule
CVP—21 days (NCI—2)	CTX	400 mg/m^2	IV	days 1–5
	VCR	1–4 mg/m^2	IV	day 1
	PRD	100 mg/m^2	PO	days 1–5
C-MOPP—28 days (NCI—1)	CTX	650 mg/m^2	IV	days 1 and 8
	VCR	1.4 mg/m^2	IV	days 1 and 8
	PCZ	100 mg/m^2	PO	days 1–14
	PRD	40 mg/m^2	PO	days 1–14
ABP—21 days (NCI, Milano—3)	ADM	75 mg/m^2	IV	day 1
	BLM	15 mg/m^2	IV	days 1 and 8
	PRD	100 mg/m^2	PO	days 1–5
CHOP—21 days (M. D. Anderson/ SWOG—10)	CTX	750 mg/m^2	IV	day 1
	ADM	50 mg/m^2	IV	day 1
	VCR	1.4 mg/m^2	IV	day 1
	PRD	100 mg/m^2	PO	days 1–5
BACOP—28 days (NCI—39)	BLM	5 mg/m^2	IV	days 15–22
	ADM	25 mg/m^2	IV	days 1 and 8
	CTX	650 mg/m^2	IV	days 1 and 8
	VCR	1.4 mg/m^2	IV	days 1 and 8
M-BACOD—21 days (Sidney Farber, Peter Bent Brigham Hospital, Harvard Medical School—38)	MTX-CF	1 mg/m^2–10 mg × 12	IV	day 14
	BLM	4 mg/m^2	IV	day 1
	ADM	45 mg/m^2	IV	day 1
	CTX	600 mg/m^2	IV	day 1
	VCR	1 mg/m^2	IV	day 1
	DM	6 mg/m^2	PO	days 1–5

[a] Abbreviations: CTX = cyclophosphamide; VCR = vincristine; PRD = prednisone; PCZ = procarbazine; ADM = adriamycin; BLM = bleomycin; MTX-CF = methotrexate-citrovorum factor rescue; DM = dexamethasone.

Future Directions

Localized tumors arising at extranodal sites have been managed optimally in the past with radical radiotherapy. In addition, in the gastrointestinal tract and occasionally in other areas, surgical resection is a common occurrence.[30] The contributions of chemotherapy in situations of high risk to relapse are now being systematically explored. A study from Dr. Bonadonna's group in Milano indicates benefit from the addition of CVP in stages I and II.[23] A recent study also raises the question of chemotherapy *alone* being potentially very effective in histiocytic lymphoma, but this must be regarded as an investigational approach.[27] Studies such as the Southwest Oncology Group trial in Figure 2, should also lead the way in testing combined modalities in localized forms of this disease. In the intraabdominal, nongastric diffuse lymphomas, the study evaluates a single arm of RT + CHOP, in view of their generally poor outlook when radiotherapy alone is used.

Aggressive approaches have fallen short of expectations in the group currently classified under nodular or favorable lymphomas. In the Stanford experience with these types, conservative policies employing single alkylating agents and prednisone have fared as well as the more radical treatment including combination chemotherapy and/or total lymphoid irradiation (TLI) previously mentioned.[2,3,7,9,21,23,24,35,41,44,45] Results of the Eastern Cooperative Oncology Group also favor the least toxic arm (cyclophosphamide and prednisone) over C-MOPP and CVP.[13] The relatively long survival

RANDOMIZED PATIENTS

Laparotomy Required

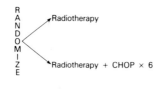

All Histologic Types, above diaphragm

Nodular Types, below diaphragm

Inguinal Nodes Only

No Laparotomy Required

Diffuse Types, above diaphragm

NON-RANDOMIZED PATIENTS

Laparotomy Required

Diffuse Types, below diaphragm ──────────────▶ CHOP × 6 + Radiotherapy

FIGURE 2.   Southwest Oncology Group 7411: Phase III study in non-Hodgkin's lymphomas (Stages I, I_E, II, II_E).

obtained by conservative means has also been recently emphasized.[4] Since the vast majority of these patients die of their disease, one should, nevertheless, not be complacent about these results. Additional trials of various therapeutic strategies are warranted.

Another active area of clinical research is induction chemotherapy in disseminated diffuse histiocytic and poorly differentiated lymphocytic lymphomas. Several new chemotherapeutic concepts, although not necessarily new chemotherapies, appear worth testing. Dr. Bonadonna's group has recently reported prolonged duration of response with their ABP/CVP alternating combination.[28] Studies building on these leads should be carried out, primarily to test concepts and not necessarily minor modifications of induction schemes.

One concept worth testing is the Norton-Simon hypothesis of *late intensification* as opposed to the more protracted maintenance schedules.[32] In addition, the concept of *non-cross-resistant combinations* must be further extended and explored; this concept includes the use of cycle-specific agents or drug combinations, some of which have been included successfully in some series.[40] Another concept that should be introduced is that of *flexible time courses* for these induction chemotherapies. Prevention of CNS recurrences by means of high-dose methotrexate and other drugs is now being evaluated.[43] More trials evaluating immunotherapy in a controlled fashion may be desirable. Finally, the relationship of timing and extent of local radiotherapy needs to be clarified.

In summary, these brief remarks present an overview of some areas where progress has recently been made and others where additional work is required. Much remains to be done in the development of optimal strategies. Hopefully, some of those areas where large questions exist are being addressed by cooperative group trials.[29]

References

1. Anderson, T., Bender, R. A., Fisher, R., DeVita, V. T., Jr., Chabner, B. A., Berard, C. W., Norton, L., and Young, R. C.: Combination chemotherapy in non-Hodgkin's lymphoma: Results of long-term follow-up. *Cancer Treat Rep 61: 1057–1066, 1977.*

2. Bagley, C., DeVita, V. T., Jr., Berard, C. W., and Canellos, G. P.: Advanced lymphosarcoma: Intensive cyclical chemotherapy with cyclophosphamide, vincristine and prednisone. *Ann Intern Med 76: 227–234, 1972.*

3. Bonadonna, G., Monfardini, S., and Villa, E.: New cross-resistant combinations in stage IV, non-Hodgkin's lymphomas. *Cancer Treat Rep 61: 1117–1123, 1977.*

4. Bonadonna, G., Narduzzi, C., and Monfardini, S.: Chemotherapy of non-Hodgkin's lymphomas with favorable histologies. In *Antibiotics and Chemotherapy,* H. Schonfeld, R. Brockman, and F. E. Hahn (Eds.). S. Karger, Basel, 1978, pp. 112–124.

5. Brugere, J., Schlienger, M., Gerard-Marchant, R., et al.: Non-Hodgkin's malignant lymphomata of upper digestive and respiratory tract: Natural history and results of radiotherapy. *Br J Cancer 31 (Suppl II): 435–440, 1975.*

6. Byrne, G. E., Jr.: Rappaport classification of non-Hodgkin's lymphoma: Histologic features and clinical significance. *Cancer Treat Rep 61: 935–944, 1977.*

7. Canellos, G. P., Lister, T. A., and Skarin, A. T.: Chemotherapy of the non-Hodgkin's lymphomas. *Cancer 42: 932–940, 1978.*

8. Chabner, B. A., Johnson, R. E., Young, R. C., Canellos, G. P., Hubbard, S. P., Johnson, S. K., and DeVita, V. T., Jr.: Sequential non-surgical staging of non-Hodgkin's lymphomas. *Ann Intern Med 85: 149–154, 1976.*

9. Chaffey, J. T., Hellman, S., Rosenthal, D. S., and Moloney, W. E.: Total body irradiation in the treatment

of lymphocytic lymphoma. *Cancer Treat Rep 61: 1149–1152, 1977.*

10. Coltman, C. A., Jr., Luce, J. K., McKelvey, E. M., Jones, S. E., and Moon, T. E.: Chemotherapy of non-Hodgkin's lymphoma: 10 years experience in the Southwest Oncology Group. *Cancer Treat Rep 61: 1067–1078, 1977.*

11. DeVita, V. T., Jr., Canellos, G. P., Chabner, B. A., et al.: Advanced histiocytic lymphoma, a potentially curable disease. Results with combination chemotherapy. *Lancet 1: 248, 1975.*

12. Dorfman, R. F.: Pathology of the non-Hodgkin's lymphomas: New classifications. *Cancer Treat Rep 61: 945–951, 1977.*

13. Ezdinli, E., Costello, W. G., and Silverstein, M. N.: Chemotherapy of prognostically favorable non-Hodgkin's lymphoma (Abstract). *Blood 52(5): 249, 1978.*

14. Fuks, Z., and Kaplan, H. S.: Recurrence rates following radiation therapy of nodular and diffuse malignant lymphomas. *Radiology 108: 675–684, 1973.*

15. Fuller, L. M., Bankes, F. L., Butler, J. J., et al.: The natural history of non-Hodgkin's lymphomata stage I and II. *Br J Cancer 31 (Suppl II): 270–285, 1975.*

16. Glatstein, E. Donaldson, S. S., Rosenberg, S., and Kaplan, H. S.: Combined modality therapy in malignant lymphomas. *Cancer Treat Rep 61: 1199–1207, 1977.*

17. Goffinet, D. R., Glatstein, E., Fuks, Z, et al.: Abdominal irradiation of non-Hodgkin's lymphomas. *Cancer 37: 2797–2805, 1976.*

18. Goffinet, D. R., Warnke, R., Dunnick, N. R., Castellino, R., Glatstein, E., Nelson, T. S., Dorfman, R. F., Rosenberg, S. A., and Kaplan, H. S.: Clinical and surgical (laparotomy) evaluation of patients with non-Hodgkin's lymphomas. *Cancer Treat Rep 61: 981–992, 1977.*

19. Herman, T. S., and Jones, S. E.: Systematic re-staging in the management of non-Hodgkin's lymphomas. *Cancer Treat Rep 61: 1009–1015, 1977.*

20. Johnson, G. J., Costello, W. G., Oken, N. M., Sponzo, R. W., Bennett, J. M., Silverstein, M. N., Glick, J. H., and Carbone, P. P.: Cyclophosphamide (C), vincristine (V) and prednisone (P) plus adriamycin (A), bleomycin (B) or BCNU: A prospective clinical trial in unfavorable diffuse non-Hodgkin's lymphomas (NHL). *Blood 52: 255, 1978.*

21. Johnson, R. E.: Management of generalized malignant lymphomas with "systemic" radiotherapy. *Br J Cancer 31 (Suppl): 450–455, 1975.*

22. Jones, S. E., Butler, J. J., Byrne, G. E., Jr., et al.: Non-Hodgkin's lymphoma. V. Results of radiotherapy. *Cancer 32: 682–690, 1976.*

23. Lattuada, A., Bonadonna, G., Milani, F., Banfi, A., Valagussa, P., DeLena, M., and Monfardini, S.: Adjuvant chemotherapy with CVP after radiotherapy (RT) in Stage I–II non-Hodgkin's lymphomas. In *Adjuvant Therapy of Cancer,* S. E. Salmon and S. E. Jones (Eds.). Elsevier/North Holland Biomedical Press, Amsterdam, 1977, pp. 537–544.

24. Luce, J. K., Gamble, J. F., Wilson, H. E., et al.: Combined cyclophosphamide, vincristine and prednisone therapy of malignant lymphoma. *Cancer 28: 306–317, 1977.*

25. Lukes, R. J., and Collins, R. D.: Immunological characterization of human malignant lymphomas. *Cancer 34: 1488–1503, 1974.*

26. McKelvey, E. M., and Moon, T. E.: Curability of non-Hodgkin's lymphomas. *Cancer Treat Rep 61: 1185–1190, 1977.*

27. Miller, T. P., and Jones, S. E.: Chemotherapy of localized histiocytic lymphoma. *Lancet 1: 358–360, 1979.*

28. Monfardini, S., Tancini, G., DeLena, M., Villa, E., Valagussa, P., and Bonadonna, G.: Cyclophosphamide, vincristine, and prednisone (CVP) versus adriamycin, bleomycin, and prednisone (ABP) in stage IV non-Hodgkin's lymphomas. *Med Pediatr Oncol 3: 67–74, 1977.*

29. Muggia, F. M., Davis, H. L., and Rozencweig, M.: Current cooperative clinical trials in non-Hodgkin's lymphomas. *Cancer Treat Rep 61: 1191–1197, 1977.*

30. Muggia, F. M., and Ultmann, J. E.: Exploratory laparotomy in reticulum cell sarcoma, a retrospective analysis. *Cancer 30: 454–458, 1972.*

31. Musshoff, K., and Schmidt-Vollmer, H.: Prognostic significance of primary site after radiotherapy in non-Hodgkin's lymphomata. *Br J Cancer 31 (Suppl II): 425–434, 1975.*

32. Norton, L., and Simon, R.: Tumor size, sensitivity to therapy and design of treatment schedules. *Cancer Treat Rep 61: 1307–1317, 1977.*

33. Peckham, M. J., Guay, J. P., Hamlin, I. M. E., et al.: Survival in localized nodal and extranodal non-Hodgkin's lymphomata. *Br J Cancer 31 (Suppl II): 413–424, 1975.*

34. Peters, M. V., Bush, R. S., Brown, T. C., et al.: The place of radiotherapy in the control of non-Hodgkin's lymphomata. *Br J Cancer 31 (Suppl II): 386–401, 1975.*

35. Portlock, C. S. and Rosenberg, S. A.: Chemotherapy of the non-Hodgkin's lymphomas: The Stanford experience. *Cancer Treat Rep 61: 1049–1055, 1977.*

36. Proceedings of the conference on non-Hodgkin's lymphomas. Discussion II: Roundtable discussion of histopathologic classification. *Cancer Treat Rep 61: 1037–1048, 1977.*

37. Rappaport, H.: Tumors of the hematopoietic system. In *Atlas of Tumor Pathology.* Washington, D.C., U.S. Armed Forces Institute of Pathology, 1966, Sec. 3, fasc. 8, p. 270.

38. Sarkin, A., Canellos, G., Rosenthal, D., Moloney, W., and Frei, E. III.: Therapy of unfavorable histology non-Hodgkin's lymphoma (NHL) with high dose methotrexate and citrovorum factor rescue (MTX/CF), bleomycin (B), adriamycin (A), cyclophosphamide (C), Oncovin[R] (O), and Decadron (D). *Proc Am Soc Clin Oncol and Am Assoc Cancer Res 19: 400, 1978.*

39. Schein, P. S., Chabner, B. A., Canellos, G. B., Young, R. C., Berard, C. W., and DeVita, V. T., Jr.: Potential for prolonged disease-free survival following combination chemotherapy and non-Hodgkin's lymphomas. *Blood 43: 181–190, 1974.*

40. Sweet, D. L., and Ultmann, J. E.: Chemotherapy of non-Hodgkin's therapy. The diffuse types. In *Antibodies and Chemotherapy*, H. Schonfeld, R. Brockman, and F. E. Hahn (Eds.). S. Karger, Basel, 1978, pp. 125–133.

41. Thar, T. L., Million, R. R., and Noyes, W. D.: Total body irradiation in non-Hodgkin's lymphoma. *Int J Radiat Oncol Biol Phys 5: 171–176, 1979.*

42. Tubiana, M., Pouillart, P., Hayat, M., et al.: Results of radiotherapy in stages I and II of non-Hodgkin's lymphoma. *Br J Cancer 31 (Suppl II): 402–412, 1975.*

43. Young, R., Howser, D., Anderson, T., Fisher, R., Jaffee, E., and DeVita, V. T., Jr.: CNS complications of non-Hodgkin's lymphoma. The potential role for prophylactic therapy. *Am J Med 66: 435–443, 1979.*

44. Young, R. C., Johnson, R. E., Canellos, G. P., Chabner, B. A., Brereton, H. D., Berard, C. W., and DeVita, V. T., Jr.: Advanced lymphocytic lymphoma: Randomized comparisons of chemotherapy alone or in combination. *Cancer Treat Rep 61: 1153–1159, 1977.*

45. Ziegler, J. L., Morrow, R. H., Fass, L., Kyalwazi, S., and Carbone, P. P.: Treatment of Burkitt's tumor with cyclophosphamide. *Cancer 26: 474–484, 1970.*

33

The role of clinical oncology in the general hospital

K. D. Bagshawe, M.D., F.R.C.P.

Perhaps the theme of my paper should have been traps and pitfalls for the oncologist, for there are many of these. On a subject like this I find the path between the transparent and the obvious on the one hand and the totally obscure on the other, is perilously narrow. One can attempt to be realistic and describe the scene as one sees it. Yet it is so varied from country to country and hospital to hospital that in reality, quite inadequate generalizations tend to be made. One can attempt to set the world aright and be Utopian. But one man's Utopia is another man's Hell. Nevertheless, the founding of oncology is not trivial, and I think we all recognize that our capacity to help the patient with cancer can be profoundly influenced by the organization within which we work.

Special cancer centers vs. general hospital oncology

There are, of course, those problems which are common to cancer wherever it is treated. There are also problems which are particular to the specialty cancer center and those which are particular to general hospitals where cancer forms a small but significant part of the total care provided. It can be argued that the nature of cancer is so complex that all cancer care should be undertaken in specialist hospitals. But this is unrealistic, and at present only a few major cities around the world have such institutions. The bulk of work is done in the general hospital. In the United Kingdom, 8% of all hospital admissions involve the diagnosis or treatment of cancer. Whether we should move towards a situation where there are more special cancer centers is

a question which it might well be untimely to ask and which is hardly relevant to the main theme of the present report. The issue will be settled in the long run by the form in which effective therapy for a wider range of tumors eventually evolves. The influence of geographic factors, transport, and density of population will always remain crucial. For the foreseeable future, cancer will continue to be diagnosed and treated largely in general hospitals.

Objectives of an oncology service

Perhaps it is appropriate to comment on the purpose of institutions and organizations and doctors in relation to the cancer patient. It is summarized, or one might say oversimplified, by suggesting that their purpose is to bring the totality of knowledge and skills and facilities to bear on the patient as an individual.

But of course, cancer is not a static problem. The cancer patient is not a static problem. We have to consider the evolution of the disease as it passes through its subclinical phase where ultimately screening for malignant disease may become important; the problems of diagnosis; the problems of staging the disease; the problems of therapy in all its different forms; those of follow-up; and finally, where cure is not achieved, those of terminal care. The knowledge, skills and facilities required at different phases of the disease form distinct and diverse subcultures within a vast body of collective information. The task of bringing this vast array of knowledge and experience to the benefit of any community often rests with a very small group of people.

Perhaps one of the most fundamental issues for the general hospital is whether it has or is to have a Department of Oncology. Many hospitals have of course made the commitment and many are already well established with radiotherapy facili-

Department of Medical Oncology, Charing Cross Hospital, London, England.
Reprinted from Cancer Clinical Trials 2: 77–81, 1979.

ties. However, the development of chemotherapy has put into the hands of virtually all clinicians the means to be involved in the treatment of cancer. The view might be taken in some institutions that treatment with chemotherapeutic agents should best be left to the existing specialties. The contrary view, which I share, is that the complexity of cancer chemotherapy and the demands it makes are now such that it requires full-time commitment. If this latter view prevails, it follows that every general hospital where cancer therapy is undertaken should have on its staff at least one full-time oncologist. For the rest of this report, I shall assume that we are discussing the problem of oncology in those general hospitals that are prepared to make the commitment of having an oncology service of this nature. The position of the oncologist in relation to the patient and the other specialties can of course be presented in this way, with the oncologist acting as the means of focusing the other specialist services as well as providing his own expertise.

Even with an established Oncology Department, it must still be recognized that the oncologist does not have a universal function in relation to cancer. The primary diagnosis of cancer is almost exclusively a function of the general hospital and for the most part does not involve clinical oncologists. We would do well to recognize that the problem of establishing the diagnosis in the first place may be formidable. The diagnosis of symptomatic cancer, involving as it does many new techniques, can certainly not be embraced even within the most ambitious Department of Clinical Oncology. However, the thesis of early diagnosis appears so fundamental in the articles of faith of the oncologist that it is not an area which can be permanently ignored. In the U.K., the role of the general hospital has been changing in recent years. They are now called "District Hospitals" with District Administration and Nursing Services for the hospital and community, organized through a common administration. Despite our fears that the Health Service will eventually consist exclusively of administrators, this District orientation is useful because it emphasizes the importance of health within the community; in the long run, this should help to accommodate screening facilities and early diagnostic clinics, and thereby help to overcome the social and psychological factors which have so far proved difficult barriers in this area. The extension, then, of the general hospital's influence into community health care is something which should be encouraged in the context of early diagnosis.

Education

Questions of diagnosis lead us to the role of the clinical oncologist in education. The more one looks at the processes involved here, the more one is likely to be overwhelmed by their magnitude. Medicine as a whole becomes ever more complex and new techniques and knowledge appear faster than the capacity to assimilate them. At any time and in any place, complete knowledge and a full range of skills and all possible facilities are unlikely to coexist. Between the concept of all available knowledge and the patient lie various barriers or restrictions. These include the available facilities, the ability to access other sources of knowledge, and the time taken to access these sources.

These limitations can be overcome for the benefit of the individual patient, but the price that is paid is ultimately a question of the time the oncologist can afford. It is ultimately a question of economics and resources. If the restrictions on knowledge, skill and facilities are local in nature, the oncologist can call on the larger geographic region, or the national facilities, or on international facilities. How best to achieve this, in practice, is a question which probably has a different solution in different countries and probably in each hospital.

Not all knowledge can be conveyed readily, and sometimes it is in the patients' interest to go to another hospital. A major factor in the broad educational field of oncology is the readiness of doctors to refer patients to other doctors within their own local area or outside it. This remains a major determinant of the standard of care provided. It can be suggested that the biggest obstacle to the proper care of many patients with cancer lies in the way we work as doctors. It is common in some countries for doctors to regard any referral outside a particular hierarchy as a confession of ignorance, even as defeat. It matters little whether the restraint operates through considerations of income or personal pride because the effect is the same. We find it easier to blame lack of facilities than the faults which lie within our own professional methods.

One aspect of education in oncology that profoundly affects the capabilities of oncology services within the general hospital is the progressive increase in complexity. It is, of course, part of the overall increase in complexity of medicine in general. Indeed, one does not have to go back very far in the history of mankind to reach a point when remedies were claimed to have almost universal curative properties. In oncology we see a remarkable interaction between the process of morphological subclassification of disease and the identification of further subgroups in relation to the observed response to therapy. It can be assumed that this process of progressively increasing complexity will continue until the nature of disease at the molecular level is defined.

This complexity introduces educational problems over a vast range of disciplines. They range from the self-education of the oncologist to the education of medical students, junior doctors, senior doctors, nurses, pharmacists, and even politicians. It is not an area that the oncologist can afford to ignore. The problems are highly varied in nature. One of the best recognized problems, although seemingly trivial, is that of mis-prescribing which can occur as a result of errors by the doctor, the pharmacy, or the nurse administering the drug. To avoid such errors it is necessary to limit the rate of change of staff and to work as far as possible with a specialized team.

The process of training physicians and radiotherapists in oncology is not one which can be discussed here in any depth. It would, however, be an omission not to refer to the need to train nurses specifically in oncology, particularly with respect to knowledge of drugs and their administration.

The role of the oncologist in the education of the other medical disciplines both diagnostic and therapeutic is perhaps principally that of coordinator. The process of information exchange should be bidirectional. The oncologist has much to offer and equally much to learn.

Chemotherapy and radiotherapy

In some countries, such as the United Kingdom, where radiotherapy was a well-established discipline before chemotherapy, a part of the practice of chemotherapy has been accommodated within preexisting Departments of Radiotherapy. Nevertheless, medical oncology has now been recognized as a subspecialty of internal medicine. In the U.S., where radiotherapy was a notably understaffed discipline, the development of chemo-

therapy rapidly led to the recognition of Medical Oncology as a separate and very rapidly expanding area. It remains controversial whether one person can usefully practice in both areas. Many eminent radiotherapists as well as chemotherapists believe that no individual can successfully span both fields. However, it is important that each should have training in the other's area. Clearly, in the specialist cancer hospital one can afford to have higher degrees of specialization, and some general hospitals with large Oncology Departments will also retain some degree of specialization within this field.

The question of the division of oncological services within the general hospital has to be considered. Most patients enter such hospitals through Departments of Surgery, Medicine and Gynecology, and many of the practitioners of these disciplines claim, and rightly so, to be oncologists. The main distinction between their commitment to oncology and that of radiotherapists and medical oncologists lies in the fact that the latter two groups make a full-time commitment, whereas that of the others varies widely. Only an oncologist could have described an oncologist as a non-organ-specific full-time cancer worker. Some surgeons would say that they are fully, or nearly fully, engaged with cancer and that therefore they are oncologists. No one would wish to dispute this, but in the sense of trying to establish the nucleus of an oncology division or department in a general hospital there is much to be said for the two full-time disciplines of oncology merging their facilities and resources. In the United Kingdom at the present time, radiotherapy and medical oncology have separate training patterns, and although this diversity is valuable much will be gained from some sort of marriage or at least the evolution of teams with common purpose. Ideally, then, one would see the nucleus of the general hospital oncology team, including doctors trained primarily in radiotherapy and doctors trained primarily in internal medicine and chemotherapy.

Oncology in relation to other departments

Given that such duo-disciplinary Oncology Departments continue to evolve, then we should consider their relations with other colleagues involved in cancer care. The interface problems with diagnostic radiology and nuclear medicine appear to be small. Similar considerations apply to chemical pathology services, although here Oncology Departments may take the initiative in developing and providing certain types of tests such as those for tumor markers. There are advantages in the study of such substances when these are carried out within Oncology Departments. In the U.K., a system of specialized laboratories working on a national or supraregional scale has been established to provide services for tumor-associated products.

One area that has to be considered carefully is the relationship of the Hematology Department to oncology. No standard formula can be defined because of the widely varied interests of hematologists. The problems occur first at the service level for routine hematological investigations and, second, in the management of the leukemias and lymphomas. Oncology, particularly chemotherapy, places heavy demands on routine hematology services. The malfunction of blood-counting equipment results in long delays in oncology outpatient departments, and it is clear that modern oncology services cannot be created without parallel expansion in hematological facilities. The hematologist can expect the support of the oncologist.

Some oncologists, of course, started their careers as hematologists but largely gave up their laboratory functions. Other hematologists want to remain strictly confined to the laboratory, whereas some want to have beds, clinics and to be responsible for the care of leukemic patients and in some cases the lymphomas and other tumors also. The solution in any hospital tends to be determined by historical factors and there is no universal formula.

For the hematologist as for the surgeon, a deep penetration into the field of cancer chemotherapy can be effected only with a loss of competence in the primary discipline. Surgery remains one of the cornerstones in both the diagnosis and the treatment of cancer. In general hospitals, surgeons have a major responsibility for seeing that the pattern of treatment, as it emerges, calls for new disciplines. Equally, the newer disciplines recognize and depend on the large contribution of the surgeon.

The relatively complex problems of staging are of course best dealt with by multidisciplinary clinics in which the surgeons, radiologists and oncologists combine. Unfortunately, these are extremely time-consuming, and in practice more economic methods of communication often have to be employed.

The Oncology Department

The extent to which an Oncology Department can take on various aspects of cancer care in a general hospital depends on many factors and in particular the interests and wishes of other colleagues. At the therapeutic level we are confronted with ever growing work loads in the clinics. Patients may be under treatment for 1–3 years, and regular follow-up thereafter is necessary. The frequency of visits is high, and each visit is likely to involve one or more practical procedures. The demand on resources increases. The need for specially trained nursing staff and for venesectionists who can not only take blood but also give intravenous drugs and set up infusions is apparent if one is to make best use of medically trained staff. Graphic recording of data is often valuable but, again, is time-consuming and expensive. The need for an area reserved for the administration of drugs by infusion close to the outpatient clinic is obviously vital but is in practice difficult to achieve where there is severe competition for resources and facilities.

This progressive buildup of outpatients continues despite the failure of therapy to eradicate disease, and it is only choriocarcinoma where the laboratory monitoring is more sensitive and can entirely replace O.P. visits. This buildup is likely to prove to be one of the most acute problem areas as more tumors remit to therapy and the durations of remission lengthen.

Insofar as oncology has been accommodated at all in the general hospital scene, this has usually been on an *ad hoc* basis. At the other extreme, it may be the largest department in the hospital. The physical space requirements for a modern Oncology Department are considerable. In addition to the ward for inpatients, it is appropriate to have intensive care and isolation facilities, treatment rooms, day ward, an outpatient clinic, cell separator space and ready access to laboratory, radiotherapy, physiotherapy, etc.

Even the largest departments of this sort are, however, fully stretched to provide first-class care for the entire spectrum of cancer requirements. One issue is the extent of participation in multicenter trials. Some take the view that all patients should be in such trials; others find them a burden that distracts from patient care. Many find their capacity to participate in trials limited by clinical services, but the central issue is the extent to which treatment protocols should contribute to knowledge as well as demand on it. It can be argued that all patients should be treated on a defined protocol at least in the initial phase of therapy. To the lay person, the concept that treatment depends on which doctor one sees, even within a particular institution or department, is bewildering.

Multicenter trials have the important function, however, of diffusing knowledge and raising standards—at least provided they are well conducted. It is, I think, important to recognize this and to provide the clinician with the clerical support he requires to be able to enter patients into such trials.

There is, however, the question whether general hospitals can make a contribution to oncology beyond participation in such trials and beyond referring special classes of patients to specialist cancer centers. For instance, there is the possibility that many of the larger general hospitals might themselves become specialist centers for, say, one type of cancer. In this way, specific facilities can be concentrated on a regional basis. It provides local prestige and makes the referral of the patients to other hospitals, which would specialize in the same way, more acceptable. It is not a universal formula, but one that I believe would be used successfully in many places.

Index *

---

* Numbers in *italics* indicate charts or diagrams